Heart Failure in
Clinical Practice

HEART FAILURE IN CLINICAL PRACTICE

Edited by

John J V McMurray BSc MD MB ChB MRCP
Consultant Cardiologist
Western Infirmary, Glasgow
Senior Lecturer
MRC Clinical Research Initiative in Heart Failure
University of Glasgow, UK

John G F Cleland MD FRCP FESC FACC
Senior British Heart Foundation Fellow
MRC Clinical Research Initiative in Heart Failure
University of Glasgow
Glasgow, UK

With a foreword by

Stephen G Ball MA PhD FRCP
British Heart Foundation
Professor of Cardiology
Institute for Cardiovascular Research
University of Leeds
Leeds, UK

Mosby

St. Louis Baltimore Boston Carlsbad Chicago Naples New York Philadelphia Portland
London Madrid Mexico City Singapore Sydney Tokyo Toronto Wiesbaden

MARTIN DUNITZ

First published in the United Kingdom in 1996
by Martin Dunitz Ltd, The Livery House, 7–9 Pratt Street, London NW1 0AE

Mosby
Dedicated to Publishing Excellence

A Times Mirror Company

Distributed in the U.S.A. and Canada by

Mosby–Year Book	Times Mirror Professional Publishing Ltd.
11830 Westline Industrial Drive	130 Flaska Drive
St. Louis, Missouri 63146	Markham, Ontario L6G 1B8

A CIP catalogue record for this book is available from the British Library

ISBN 1-85317-225-1

Composition by Keyword Typesetting Services Ltd
Printed and bound in Great Britain

CONTENTS

List of contributors

Inder S Anand MD DPhil(Oxon) FRCP,
Professor of Medicine, Department of Cardiovascular Medicine, University of Minnesota Medical School, Veterans Affairs Medical Center, Minneapolis MN 55417, USA.

David B Barnett MD FRCP,
Professor of Clinical Pharmacology, Department of Medicine and Therapeutics, University of Leicester, Robert Kilpatrick Clinical Sciences Building, Leicester Royal Infirmary, Leicester LE2 7LX, UK.

Nicholas A Boon MD FRCP,
Consultant Cardiologist, Department of Cardiology, the Royal Infirmary of Edinburgh, Edinburgh EH3 9YW, UK.

T P Chua MB BS MRCP,
Department of Cardiac Medicine, Research Fellow, Department of Cardiac Medicine, National Heart & Lung Institute, London SW3 6LY, UK.

Andrew M Coats DM FRCP FRACP FESC,
Senior Lecturer and Honorary Consultant Cardiologist, National Heart & Lung Institute, London SW3 6LY, UK.

Stuart M Cobbe MD FRCP FESC,
Walton Professor of Medical Cardiology, Department of Medical Cardiology, Royal Infirmary, Glasgow G31 2ER, UK.

Alan J Cowley DM FRCP,
Senior Lecturer in Medicine, University Hospital, University of Nottingham, Nottingham NG7 2UH, UK.

Peter F Currie MRCP,
British Heart Foundation Junior Research Fellow, Department of Cardiology, the Royal Infirmary of Edinburgh, Edinburgh EH3 9YW, UK.

Henry J Dargie FRCP FESC,
Professor and Co-Director of the Clinical Research Initiative in Heart Failure, University of Glasgow, and Consultant Cardiologist, Western Infirmary, Glasgow G11 6NT, UK.

Neil C Davidson BSc MB MRCP,
Research Fellow, Department of Clinical Pharmacology, University of Dundee, and Ninewells Hospital, Dundee DD1 9SY, UK.

Andrew P Davie MB ChB MRCP,
Registrar in Cardiology, Department of Cardiology, Western General Hospital, Edinburgh EH4 2XU, UK.

Robert Doughty MB MRCP,
Clinical Research Fellow, Department of Medicine, University of Auckland School of Medicine, Auckland, New Zealand.

Henry Eriksson MD PhD,
Section of Preventive Medicine, Department of Medicine, Östra Hospital, S-416 85 Göteborg, Sweden.

Alun Evans MD FRCP FFPHM,
Professor of Epidemiology, Department of Epidemiology and Public Health, The Queen's University of Belfast, Mulhouse, Belfast BT12 6BJ, UK.

Frank Kee BSc MD MRCP MFPHM,
Honorary Senior Lecturer, Department of Epidemiology and Public Health, The Queen's University of Belfast, Mulhouse, Belfast BT12 6BJ, UK.

Michael P Love MB ChB MRCP,
Bristol-Myers Squibb Cardiovascular Fellow, Department of Cardiology, Western General Hospital, Edinburgh EH4 2XU, UK.

Michael D W Lye MD FRCP,
Professor and Head, Department of Geriatric Medicine, Royal Liverpool University Hospital, Liverpool L69 3BX, UK.

Stephen MacMahon PhD FACC,
Associate Professor, Department of Medicine, University of Auckland School of Medicine, Auckland, New Zealand.

Adrian Morley-Davies MB ChB MRCP,
Department of Cardiology, University of Glasgow G12 8QQ, UK.

Jim Nolan MB ChB MRCP,
Senior Registrar, Department of Cardiology, Leeds General Infirmary, Leeds LS1 3EX, UK.

Shaun T O'Keeffe MB MRCPI,
Lecturer, Department of Geriatric Medicine, Royal Liverpool University Hospital, Liverpool L69 3BX, UK.

Philip A Poole-Wilson MD FRCP FESC,
President of the European Society of Cardiology, Simon Marks Professor of Cardiology, National Heart & Lung Institute, University of London, and Honorary Consultant Physician, National Heart & Chest Hospital, London SW3 6LY, UK.

Sundeep Puri MB MRCP,
British Heart Foundation Junior Research Fellow, Department of Medicine (Clinical Cardiology), Royal Postgraduate Medical School, Hammersmith Hospital, London SW12 0HS, UK.

Andrew C Rankin MD MRCP,
Senior Lecturer in Medical Cardiology, Department of Medical Cardiology, Royal Infirmary, Glasgow G31 2ER, UK.

Norman Sharpe MD FRACP FACC,
Professor, Department of Medicine, University of Auckland School of Medicine, Auckland, New Zealand.

Axel Sigurdsson MD PhD,
Associate Director, Division of Cardiology, Department of Medicine, Östra University Hospital, S-416 85 Göteborg, Sweden.

Iain Squire MB ChB MRCP,
Department of Medicine and Therapeutics, University of Leicester, Robert Kilpatrick Clinical Sciences Building, Leicester Royal Infirmary, Leicester LE2 7LX, UK.

Allan D Struthers BSc MD FRCP FESC,
Professor, Department of Clinical Pharmacology, University of Dundee, and Consultant Physician, Ninewells Hospital, Dundee DD1 9SY, UK.

Karl Swedberg MD PhD,
Associate Professor of Medicine and Head, Department of Medicine, Östra University Hospital, S-416 85 Göteborg, Sweden.

Foreword

The cardiac muscle cells with which we start life cannot be renewed. Not surprisingly cardiac damage is a major predictor of prognosis. However, with many compensatory mechanisms available such damage may be insidious, manifesting as 'clinical heart failure' only at an advanced stage. Considerable strides have been made in the past decade in our understanding of heart failure in terms of its early recognition, economic impact, effect on the well-being of individuals, and in establishing treatments which extend the life of patients with this malignant condition.

To deal with such a large and diverse subject presents a challenge. The editors of this book have selected internationally-recognized research workers and clinicians in the field, who have produced an informative and topical account which is particularly relevant to clinical practice. Areas of certainty, of controversy, and of future research are addressed. Some highly relevant but often neglected topics in heart failure are included, such as old age and lung function. Each chapter is complete in its own right and includes an invaluable up-to-date reference list. Taken together, they represent a comprehensive review of heart failure.

Stephen G Ball MA PhD FRCP
British Heart Foundation
Professor of Cardiology
University of Leeds

Preface

Heart failure afflicts one to two per cent of the population, with twice as many people again suffering from its precursor, asymptomatic left ventricular dysfunction. As the incidence and prevalence of other cardiovascular problems such as stroke and myocardial infarction are declining, those of heart failure are increasing. The burden of illness caused by this ever-increasing problem is enormous, both in personal terms for patients and in financial terms for healthcare systems. Though angiotensin converting enzyme inhibitors have been an enormous therapeutic advance for heart failure, morbidity and mortality remain high. The problem of sudden death in particular remains to be even partially resolved. A better understanding of the aetiology, epidemiology, diagnosis, and pathophysiology of heart failure, with a view to improving patient care, is now a public health imperative throughout the world. In this book, experts from many different countries address these important issues and look forward to new developments in this rapidly changing field.

Acknowledgments

We wish to thank the contributors to this book for finding time in their busy schedules to help-with this project. We also wish to acknowledge the unflagging assistance of our secretaries Brenda and Iris. Finally, *Heart Failure in Clinical Practice* would not exist but for the patience and perseverance of Alan Burgess and Ian Mellor of Martin Dunitz Ltd.

Heart failure: a historical context

Adrian Morley-Davies, Jim Nolan

Introduction

> "There is a dead medical literature and a live one. The dead is not all ancient, and the live is not all modern."
>
> Oliver Wendell Holmes

Heart failure is a common disorder characterized by fatigue, breathlessness and exercise intolerance. It is not a separate disease entity, but a complex clinical syndrome with an adverse prognosis. Epidemiological data document its increasing importance as a major cause of cardiovascular morbidity and mortality in developed countries. However, it has been described and studied since the earliest civilizations. This article reviews the development of concepts and ideas about heart failure, placing them in their overall historical context.

Prehistory

The study of fossilized remains of primitive humans reveals that they suffered a wide variety of degenerative and infectious diseases.[1] The oldest humanoid form, the Java Man, lived in the Pleistocene epoch of 500 000 years ago, and examination of this fossil reveals exostoses. An elbow specimen of a Neanderthal man of some 40 000 years ago shows traumatic arthritis, but there is little surviving evidence of cardiovascular disease from these time periods.

The ancient civilizations

Communities capable of social organization, art and literature first appeared about 4000 years ago in the Middle East, China, South America and India. These civilizations have been extensively studied, providing information on the ancients' concepts of disease and their treatments.

The first ever recorded medical text is a Sumerian tablet from around 4000 BC, commenting on various medicinal cures, and suggesting the addition of potassium nitrate to a number of them.[2] The *Edwin Smith Surgical Papyrus* (circa 3000 BC) was probably written by the Egyptian priest Imhotep. It is clear from this document that the Egyptians' knowledge of anatomy was gained from embalming and mummification as the dissection of cadavers for medical purposes was proscribed by religious law. Considering that embalming procedures were carried out through a semicircular incision above the left iliac crest, the knowledge of the Egyptians is remarkable. Although the ancient Greeks are often credited with first describing and counting the pulse, the following quotation from the papyrus suggests that the Egyptians antedated them by twelve centuries:

> "Now if the priests of Sekhmet or any physician put his hands . . . upon the two hands, upon the pulse, upon the two feet he measures the heart, because its ves-

> sels are in the back of the head and in the pulse; and because its pulsation is in every vessel of every member"[3]

Perhaps the most important ancient text is the *Ebers Papyrus*. Although this dates from around 1600 BC, over 300 years before Moses was found in the bullrushes, it is probably a copy of an older work.[4] It was bought by G Ebers in Thebes in 1872–73, and was subsequently donated to the Leipzig University Library. It measures 30 cm high by 20.23 metres long and the text is divided into 110 pages, although some are missing. It contains a passage almost identical to that above, stating:

> "the heart . . . speaks out of the vessels of every limb"

It is also thought to contain the first description of angina:

> "when you examine a man for illness in his cardia, he has pains in his arm, in his breast, on the side of the cardia . . . it is death which approaches him"

Other passages state:

> "The heart is tired; this means that the heart does not speak or the vessels of the heart are mute"
> "When there is inundation of the heart, the saliva [sputum?] is in excess; therefore the body is weak."[5]

This may be the first recorded description of the clinical syndrome of heart failure!

The relief of a tomb from the Sixth Dynasty (2624–2475 BC) suggests that sudden death was a problem in those times, although whether this was due to coronary disease is debatable.[6]

Paleopathology, and particularly the study of Egyptian mummies, provides extensive information on the diseases of this time. The first studied, that of Menephtah (circa 1280–1211 BC), the probable 'Pharaoh of the Hebrew Exodus', had severe atherosclerosis.[7] Although many specimens show evidence of aortic or peripheral vascular atherosclerosis, only one has documented coronary disease with evidence of myocardial infarction.[8]

Medicine at this time was practised by priests, because diseases were thought to be due to the influence of evil spirits or demons. The only treatments available were herbal remedies, spells, prayers, and bleeding. The Egyptians did believe that dyspnoea was due to a blockage in the flow of blood, and employed bleeding as a treatment. This may represent the first use of preload reduction by venesection in the treatment of heart failure.

The ancient Greeks

Greek civilization flourished from 2000 BC to 100 BC, making lasting contributions to medical knowledge. Before the fifth century BC, ancient Greece had physician–seers who combined magic and drug treatments, wound healers adept at battlefield trauma and practitioners of medical dietetics, principally for athletes. They believed that the seat of the human spirit was the heart, while the seat of the human soul was the head. 'Vital spirit' (human life) derived from the 'Universal spirit' (divine life) present in the air, and by breathing this substance was introduced into the body. After mixing with the blood in the liver, 'natural spirit' was formed which was then carried by the ebb and flow of the blood, natural spirit being converted into 'vital spirit' in the heart and 'animal spirit' in the brain. This vital spirit was seen as the foundation of the spirit and soul, while animal spirit animated the body.[9]

Empedocles (496–430 BC) first developed the Humoral Theory of disease. This explained disease as being due to an imbalance of four humours: phlegm, blood, black bile and yellow bile. Hippocrates (460–377 BC) believed that human temperaments and physiques depended on the humours, being phlegmatic, sanguine, melancholic or choleric, respectively. Plato (427–347 BC) also supported this view and even today, some 23 centuries later, we still refer to these descriptions. Hippocrates' commentaries are said to describe cardiac pain:

> "frequent recurrence of cardialgia, in an elderly person, announces sudden death"

and venesection as a cure

> ". . . or if there be heaviness in the breast, or above the diaphragm, one should open the inner vein at the elbow . . ."

However, one should remember that Greek medicine did not envisage organic disease, but imbalances between the humours or between the soul and body.

Following the death of Alexander the Great in 323 BC Alexandria became famous for its library and museum, and dissection of human cadavers was permitted from 400–100 BC. Erasistratus (330–250 BC) carried out many systematic human dissections, and indeed was said to have dissected criminals alive. He recognized that the heart provided the motive power for the circulation. Praxagoras of Cos (circa 340 BC) is first credited with using the pulse in diagnosis, and his pupil Herophilus (circa 300 BC) is credited with recognizing that the plusc was synchronous with the heartbeat. He taught that the pulse had four important characteristics: size, frequency, strength and rhythm, and was the first to count the rate, using a clepsydra, or water-clock.[10] Thus, although the ancient Greeks made great advances in organizing medicine and in the methods of clinical observation, they did not advance knowledge of heart failure beyond that of the Egyptians.

The Romans

From 100 BC to 476 AD Roman civilization dominated the Western World, and improvements in public health through advances in sanitation is one of their permanent legacies. Healing was a widely practised skill but most healers had no particular training. This, combined with the lack of regulation, lead to a general mistrust of physicians.

Celsus (53 BC–7 AD), a Roman author but not physician, wrote the first published textbook of general medicine. In it he describes a condition he terms "Kardiakon":

> ". . . excessive weakness of the body . . . (which) wastes away through immoderate sweating . . . it may be recognized by the weak pulsation of the blood vessels, while sweat . . . breaks out . . . the feet and legs remaining more dry and cold . . ."[3]

Some authorities have taken this to represent myocardial infarction, but it may describe the cardiac cachexia, sympathetic overactivity and peripheral vasoconstriction seen in heart failure.

Treatments of this time often took the form of poultices, or herbal concoctions. A large pharmacopeia produced by Scribonius Largus (circa 50 AD) suggested scylla glycosides and opium for the treatment of breathlessness, being particularly useful ". . . when the patient has a bloody sputum."[5] Examination of a female Chinese corpse from a similar time period,[11] reveals that she died of a left anterior descending coronary artery occlusion. Herbal remedies found in her tomb contain cinnamon, magnolia bark and peppercorns, which are still prescribed today by traditional Chinese doctors for the treatment of angina.

However, the most influential Roman physician was undoubtedly Claudius Galen of Pergammon, who lived from 138–201 AD. He wrote numerous treatises on various diseases, based on his experiences as a surgeon to the gladiators, and his animal dissections. Unfortunately, although an excellent anatomist, he was a bad physiologist, and he developed an erroneous theory of the circulation. He thought that blood ebbed and flowed throughout the body, and that it passed from the right to left ventricle through interventricular septal pores. The lungs exhaled impurities from the body, while 'vital spirit' passed from the lungs to the blood, with nutrients from food entering the blood through the liver. This erroneous belief, based on the ancient Greek assumption of a supreme being ('universal spirit') was subsequently adopted and revered by the Jewish, Christian and Moslem traditions. This exerted a profoundly negative influence on medical thinking for the next 1500 years, during which time it was considered heretical to even doubt Galen's beliefs.

The Middle Ages

Following the collapse of the Holy Roman Empire European medicine declined, and healing became an act of Christian charity which was a divine gift from God. In Byzantium, Christian religious healing flourished along with earlier Greco-Roman medicine. The early Christian church created shelters for the poor called *xenones*, and for the sick called *nosokomeia*, among the first being an inn built around 375 AD in Caesarea by Bishop Basil. In Western Europe, Benedictine monasteries cared for the sick and the cathedral schools became the repository of Western medical knowledge.

The Arabic speaking peoples of North Africa maintained and added to Greco-Roman medical knowledge, principally at Jundishapur in Persia and Alexandria in Egypt. Islam's political supremacy in the Mediterranean basin and Indian subcontinent allowed the collection of many medical texts and medicinal herbs. During this period, many ancient Greek texts were translated into Arabic.

At-Tabari (circa 900 AD) wrote *The Paradise of Wisdom*, synthesizing Greek, Roman and Hindu medicine. His pupil, Rhazes (865–925 AD) was a gifted observer, recognizing the importance of the heart in prognosis. Avicenna (Ibn Sina, 980–1037 AD), a Persian called the 'Prince of Physicians', wrote a five-volume influential *Canon of Medicine*, which was reprinted more than fifteen times and remained a standard medical text until the seventeenth century.[12] In the third volume he describes dyspnoea and orthopnoea, ascribed to imbalance of the humours,[13] and also the effects of pericardial effusions,[4] the surgery of which Galen had described ten centuries earlier.[14] Another possible description of heart failure dates from this time, along with realization of its grim prognosis:

> "dyscrasia [i.e. heart disease] stops the circulation inside the arteries, helping retention of fluids and leading to death."

In the eleventh century, Abu al-Biruni wrote a pharmacopoeia, and subsequent expansion lead to the craft of pharmacy. Abraham Ibn Ezra (an eleventh century Hebrew author) suggested that "anguish of the heart" be treated with opium and rue, the latter also being used in Anglo-Saxon Britain for heartache, pain or tightness in the chest.

Islam significantly influenced hospital development, the first *bimaristan* or 'house of the sick' being established in 803 AD by Ibn Barmak, based on Byzantine models. They were staffed with a director, physicians, a pharmacist and servants, often having their own libraries for apprentice students. The traditional Islamic *hisbah* codes and regulations extended to medicine, and physicians were licensed by the Caliphs.

The first clear description of heart failure occurs in an account of the illness of Alexius I, ruler of the Byzantine Empire from 1081–1118 AD.[15] His daughter describes his illness:

> "felt his pulse and found all sorts of irregularities . . . his heart, they said, was inflamed . . . every day it grew worse, attacking him no longer at intervals, but relentlessly, with no interruption. He was unable to lie on either side, so weak that every breath involved great effort . . . his condition was serious, for never for one moment could he breath freely. He was forced to sit upright to breathe at all . . . but when his stomach was visibly enlarged to a great size and his feet also swelled up and fever laid him low, some of the doctors with scant regard for the fever, had recourse to cauterization."

Further descriptions of heart failure are given by Avenzoar (1113–1162) describing a patient with a pericardial effusion, and Montagena (1422–1441) describing a patient with breathlessness and an irregular pulse.

As the middle ages progressed, a number of universities were founded, particularly important being the University at Salerno (built 1100–1300 AD), and subsequently at Montpelier and Paris in France and Bologna in Italy. Gradually, medical education passed from the Church to these institutions, consolidated by a licensing system for physicians introduced by Frederick I (ruler of the Holy Roman Empire from 1215–1250 AD). At this time, medieval medical education stressed theory, rhetoric and philosophy, while surgery was excluded. Human dissection was introduced, initially in Bologna; the first *post mortem* was performed for legal reasons in 1302 by Varignana, and more widespread dissection was allowed from about 1316 onwards. The first modern treatise on anatomy was authored by Mondino de Luzzi, a professor at Bologna. However, all anatomical works illustrated the descriptions of Galen, even when they were manifestly incorrect.

It was, therefore, the declining power of the Church and the establishment of the universities that opened the door for medical knowledge to be based on empirical evidence rather than mystical beliefs. Interestingly, a similar debate had taken place between the ancient Greeks some thirteen centuries previously. Despite this, Roger Bacon was imprisoned in the thirteenth century for stating:

> "the truth can only be found through experimentation."[16]

The Renaissance

The fall of Constantinople meant that many scholars migrated to Europe, and the development of the Gutemberg printing press facilitated the dissemination of this knowledge. Human dissection was finally authorized by Pope Sixtus IV in the late fifteenth century and this led directly to the rise of the great anatomists who ultimately refuted Galenic teachings.

Andreus Vesalius (1514–1564), Professor of Anatomy at Padua, published the first great anatomical work *De Humani Corporis Fabrica* in 1543. Leonardo da Vinci had produced similar, perhaps even more accurate, illustrations decades earlier but these were in private collections (now in Windsor Castle, England) and would not have been known to him. Vesalius could not demonstrate Galen's interventricular pores, although he did not deny their existence. In this text he also describes tracheostomy, artificial respiration and resuscitation. However, it was still unclear how blood passed from the right to left ventricle. The first discovery of the pulmonary circulation is attributed to the Arabic physician Ibn an-Nafis (1210–1288) although his work remained undiscovered for many centuries. The first European to suggest that blood flowed from the right to left ventricles through the lungs was Michael Servetus, who published *Christianismi Restitutio* in 1553.[17] Only three of the original 500 copies survive. Following the publication of this text Servetus was burnt at the stake for hereticism, although it seems more likely that this was due to his listing of 60 reasons why the Pope was the Antichrist, rather than his anatomical discoveries.[16] *De Re Anatomica*, written by Realdus Columbus, Vesalius' successor at Padua, was published posthumously in 1559. In it he argued for the existence of the pulmonary circulation and the function of the heart valves, and described the timing of the pulse in relation to systole and diastole,[17] refuting accepted Galenic wisdom.

Despite these significant advances, the concept of heart failure remained poorly understood, as knowledge of the circulation of the blood awaited Harvey's great work.

However, the Renaissance marked the start of intellectual freedom in medicine, facilitating a sceptical re-examination of the theories espoused by Empedocles, Hippocrates and Galen.

The seventeenth century

The classical concepts of humoralism were challenged throughout this century. Some argued that the vital functions of life were purely chemical and mechanical (Descartes, 1596–1650), or chemical but governed by an internal alchemist (Phillipus von Hohenheim, or 'Paracelsus').[12] Modernists believed in empiricism and experimentation, freeing medical thought from the straitjacket of dogma and superstition. This revolution in attitudes was rebuked by Shakespeare:

> "There are more things in heaven and earth, Horatio, than are dreamt of in your philosophy."

The death knell of traditionalism was supplied by William Harvey (1578–1657). He studied at Cambridge and then Padua. After returning to London he became attending physician at St Bartholomew's Hospital and Lumleian Lecturer to the College of Physicians. His duties involved teaching anatomy to surgeons, by reading Latin anatomical texts and dissecting the bodies of felons. His lectures began the year that Shakespeare died. In 1628, aged fifty, Harvey published *Exercitatio Anatomica de Motu Cordis et Sanguinus in Animalibus* or *The Movement of the Heart and Blood in Animals*.[18] This was based on extensive experimentation and many human and animal dissections. Indeed he dissected over 100 species of animals, including his own pet parrot and monkey, and even assisted at the dissections of his father, brother and sister.[19] Harvey concluded that the heart, rather than the arteries, propelled the blood and, in agreement with Colombus, that the apex beat and pulse coincided with ventricular systole. In this he was aided by the remarkable case of the eldest son of the Viscount Montgomery who had suffered a fall as a child, and as the wound had failed to heal, the heart could be seen.[20] Harvey directly denied the existence of interventricular pores, and he reasoned that the blood passed through

> "the invisible porosities of the lungs and the minute cavities of their vessels."

Capillaries were subsequently visualized and described by Malpighi (1628–1694) using the microscope in 1661. Later, Harvey clearly describes angina as a cause of "dropsy" or heart failure in a letter to Riolan:

> "Sir Robert Darcy . . . about the middle period of his life, made frequent complaint

> of a certain distressing pain in the chest. The disease going from bad to worse, he by-and-by became cachectic and dropsical . . ."[21]

There are a number of descriptions of heart failure throughout this period. Bartoletti (1576–1630) gives a description in *Methodus in Dyspnoeam*[22] of

> "characteristic dyspnoea from which sudden death can be predicted, where the patients had suffered for a long time from respiratory difficulties when walking and they are forced to stop because they experience the sensation of suffocation . . .".

Following Harvey's discovery, four founding members of The Royal Society confirmed that the lungs oxygenated blood. Boyle (1627–1692) and Hooke (1653–1703) demonstrated that movement of air in and out of the lungs was necessary for life, principally by vivisection of cocks. Lower (1631–1691), a Cornish doctor, took the lungs from freshly slaughtered animals, and poured blue venous blood into the pulmonary artery. Observing that it ran bright red from the pulmonary veins, he thus demonstrated that it was air in the lungs which caused this change.[23] His colleague, Mayow (1643–1679) identified that the gas obtained from nitrates, oxygen, was responsible for the change.

Thus, as scientific knowledge increased, it became clear that disease of the heart caused anasarca and dropsy. Boerhave (1668–1738), professor at Leyden, is credited with first attributing 'anasarca' to cardiac causes,[5] but perhaps the first definition of heart failure was produced by Lower in his textbook of 1669 *Tractatus de Cordis*:[24]

> ". . . but when the parenchyma of the heart has been harmed by various diseases its motion is necessarily much altered; for if the parenchyma of the heart is burdened with too much fat, labours under inflammation, abscess or wound, so that it cannot vibrate or contract without great trouble or difficulty, it soon gives up its motion, whence the movement of the blood also to the same degree becomes weak and languid."

He also described the effect of pericardial constriction and tamponade in the same work.[25]

Mayow and Bonet (1620–1689) produced detailed clinico-pathological studies of valvular heart disease, linking the changes in the heart and lungs with pre-morbid symptoms of dyspnoea and oedema.

Consequently, by the end of the seventeenth century, the concept of the hydropic state was related to heart disease, and the initial steps towards defining and understanding the syndrome of heart failure were made.

The eighteenth century

During this century, acceptance of Harvey's beliefs allowed clinical observations to be correlated with morbid anatomy so that great advances were made in the concept of heart failure. Scotland became the principal centre of progress, based on the establishments of the Edinburgh School of Surgery (founded in 1505), the Royal College of Physicians of Edinburgh (founded 1681), and the Royal Infirmary of Edinburgh, which opened in 1741. The College of Physicians and Surgeons of Glasgow was founded in 1599, and William Cullen founded the Glasgow School of Medicine. Alexander Munro and his heirs taught anatomy at the medical school in Edinburgh for 126 years, while William and John Hunter, of Hunterian Gallery and Museum fame, were initially educated in Scotland. The latter eventually died of a myocardial infarct precipitated by an argument in 1793, his *post mortem* providing proof that coronary disease caused angina.

The pace of discovery increased: Albertini (1662–1738) described dyspnoea due to pulmonary oedema, stressing the importance of cardiac enlargement; Lancisi (1655–1720), a Papal physician who studied sudden death, described its association with cardiac dilatation; while Senac (1693–1770) published in 1749 the most comprehensive manual of heart disease, *Traite sur la Structure du Coeur, de son Action et de ses Maladies*. In it he wrote that dilation of the cardiac chambers could lead to orthopnoea, oedema and cardiac asthma, and that medicine had few remedies for heart disease. Perhaps the most outstanding work of this century was Morgagni's (1682–1771) *The Seats and Causes of Diseases Investigated by Anatomy*,[26] published in 1761 and translated into English in 1769. Among many other diseases he gave lucid descriptions of anginal syndromes, cardiac rupture, pericardial tamponade and constriction and cardiac dilatation associated with

> "serous fluid in the thorax . . . then hydrops; afterwards jaundice, dyspnoea, throbbing of the jugular vessels . . ."

and was credited with coining the term 'cor bovinum'.

Clinical observation was also advancing, and in 1761 the Viennese physician Auenbrugger described percussion in his monograph *Inventum Novum*. He felt that he could diagnose

> "from the testimony of my own senses"

and recognized

> "hydrops of the chest" with a percussion note "as flat as if you percussed a piece of meat"

also noting that such patients had to sleep sitting up.[25] Although Heberden (1710–1801) is well known for his classical description of angina in 1768,[27] he also emphasized the importance of counting the pulse rate in cardiac disease, first suggested by Herophilus, but redisovered by Floyer using a 'pulse watch' with a second hand in 1707.[28]

The first breakthrough in the drug treatment of heart failure occurred in 1785, when Withering published the first work of clinical pharmacology.[29] Although glycosides had been used for many centuries,[30] Withering discovered that the active ingredient of a herbal remedy for dropsy was the foxglove, *Digitalis purpurea*. He conducted careful pharmacological experiments with the drug, defining its therapeutic and toxic dose. He believed that digitalis was a diuretic, but future workers realised that its primary site of action was the heart. Ferriar (1761–1815) of Manchester felt that

> "it furnishes a means of regulating the pulse to our wish"

whilst in 1799 Beddoes wrote

> "digitalis . . . increases the organic action of the contractile fibres."[31]

Unfortunately, much of Withering's advice was ignored, and digitalis was used rather indiscriminately – both for tuberculosis and for 'nervous afflictions'. It is thought that the latter may have played a role in Van Gogh's vivid colourings, as a portrait of his physician Dr Gachet reveals him holding a foxglove![32] Controversy over its usage raged, and the debate regarding its role in heart failure is still unresolved. However, before Withering's work treatment had involved rest, fluid restriction and weak herbal diuretics, so digitalis was a great step forward.

The nineteenth century

If the fifteenth and sixteenth centuries belonged to the anatomists, and the seventeenth to the pathologists, then the nineteenth century belonged to the clinicians and the physiologists. Bedside diagnosis was advanced by the popularization of percussion by Corvisart (1755–1821), and the development of the stethoscope by Laennec (1781–1826). Although Harvey had compared heart sounds with the noise of a horse drinking water in 1628, little further was mentioned until Laennec's work in 1819.[33] As the social mores of the time proscribed direct auscultation of the female chest, in 1816, while examining a young woman with cardiac disease, Laennec rolled a sheaf of paper into a cylinder and through this makeshift instrument heard the heart sounds.[34] He named the stethoscope after the Greek *stethos*, or breast, and *skopein*, to view. He then spent three years at the Necker Hospital in Paris, correlating auscultatory findings with autopsies that he performed. Rouanet published his thesis in 1832, and by using heart specimens into which he suddenly squeezed fluid, was able to define the origin of the heart sounds. Although there was initial suspicion, the invention rapidly gained acceptance throughout Europe, and in America through the pioneering influence of Flint.[35]

A multitude of eponymous syndromes describing the symptoms and signs of valvular heart disease were described, too many to mention here. However, further advances in the physiology of heart failure were provided by Potain (1825–1901), who correctly elucidated that gallop rhythms were due to reduced ventricular compliance or contractility. Cheyne (1777–1836) and Stokes (1804–1878) described periodic breathing and Traube (1818–1876) described pulsus paradoxus in patients with heart failure. Bright (1789–1858) was the first to differentiate congestion due to renal causes from those of cardiac cause. A unifying hypothesis for the pathophysiology of heart failure was propounded by Hope in 1832.[36] This 'back-pressure' theory considered the symptoms to be caused by increasing pressure behind the failing valve or ventricle.

Later in the century, the concept of coronary disease as a cause of heart failure was gradually accepted. As far back as 1776 Fothergill (1712–1780) had described the association of acute cardiac failure with death due to angina, but did not comprehend the link. In 1835 Williams, Professor of Medicine at University College, had described myocardial scarring associated with coronary sclerosis. In 1850, Quain (who was based at the Brompton Hospital) described 83 cases of 'fatty degeneration', noting the close link with coronary 'ossification'.[37] In 1874 Fagge (1838–1883) described heart failure associated with localized thinned, fibrotic areas of myocardium, and in 1884 von Leyden (1832–1910) described chronic diffuse coronary disease leading to 'cardiac asthma and dropsy'. Thus, by the end of this period, ishaemic heart disease was recognized as a cause of heart failure, even though angina and myocardial infarction had not, as yet, been differentiated.

However, despite these advances, treatment options remained limited. Venesection, purgation and the misuse of digitalis were widespread. Pre-load reduction using tourniquets had been described by Parry in 1795, and fluid restriction by Hope in 1831. Direct drainage of the oedema by incision of the skin or insertion of Southey's tubes, developed in 1877 by Southey (1835–1899), were popular measures. Brunton (1844–1916), who first described the therapeutic use of amyl nitrate for angina in 1867,[38] stated in 1888:

> "there are several diseases in which it is desirable to relax the blood vessels . . . in cases of the failing heart where the enfeebled ventricle is barely able to overcome the resistance of the arterial walls and force the blood onwards, we require a drug which will produce a prolonged dilatation of the vessels."[39]

Unfortunately, this suggestion for after-load reduction was ignored for the next 70 years.

However, therapeutic nihilism was still common, as expressed by Oliver Wendell Holmes in 1860:

> "with the exception of opium, anesthetics and wine . . . if the whole materia medica, as now used, could be sunk to the bottom of the sea, it would be all the better for mankind, and all the worse for the fishes."[40]

The twentieth century

The twentieth century might be said to belong to the 'technologists'. Roentgen had discovered X-rays in 1895,[41] the X-ray of his wife's hand being reproduced in publications across the world. The public avidly bought X-ray images of their loved ones, and the Queen of Portugal had radiographs made of all the members of her court![34] Within one month of the initial discovery, cardiac and respiratory motion was observed directly, such that the pioneering American radiologist Williams could state:

> "We may now look where we have previously been able to listen and sometimes to hear but imperfectly."

Waller had produced the first human ECG in 1887, by photographing the movement of a mercury column, but Einthoven's string galvanometer revolutionized the development of electrocardiography, initially being used to facilitate the study of arrhythmias.[42] However, in 1912 Herrick proposed his theory of non-fatal coronary obstruction,[43] and his student published the first ECG of myocardial infarction in the dog in 1918. Starling (1866–1927) determined the effects of different loading conditions on cardiac function in 1914, enabling the modern concepts of pre- and after-load manipulation to emerge.

With the advent of cardiac catheterization haemodynamic measurements could be performed, leading to a greater understanding of cardiac function in health and disease.[44] Direct measurement of the arterial pressure of a horse had been performed by Hales (1677–1761), an English clergyman, in 1733.[45] He estimated cardiac output by bleeding it to death, pouring melted beeswax into the heart via the catheter and then multiplying the volume of remelted wax by the heart rate to determine the cardiac output. Cardiac catheterization was first performed in humans when Forsmann introduced a ureteral catheter into his own right atrium in 1929. Sones introduced selective coronary angiography in 1962, finally allowing the definite *ante-mortem* diagnosis of heart failure secondary to coronary disease to be made.

In 1913, the Scottish physician Sir James MacKenzie had challenged the established 'back-pressure' theory, explaining heart failure in terms of decreased cardiac output, or 'forward failure'. Only more recently, with the advent of these advanced techniques, has it been established that any single patient may exhibit all these syndromes at different times.

The twentieth century also saw great advances in therapeutics. Mercurial diuretics were discovered serendipitously in 1919 in Wenckebach's clinic, when mercury treatments for syphilis were noted to cause diuresis in a young girl.[46] Interestingly, mercury had been used as a diuretic by Stokes (1804–1878) over a century before. Subsequently, thiazides and loop diuretics dramatically changed the treatment of acute and chronic heart failure.[47] Despite this, the prognosis of patients with heart failure remained poor, with suggested treatments including thyroid ablation, inferior vena caval ligation[48] and even rib resection to allow the heart more space.[49] Direct acting vasodilators were introduced in the 1970s, when large trials demonstrated their ability to produce prolonged symptomatic and haemodynamic benefit[50] by changing loading conditions, something Brunton had suggested 100 years before. In the 1980s, the angiotensin converting enzyme (ACE) inhibitors were introduced, and have now been shown to improve symptoms and mortality in severe,[51] moderate,[52] and 'asymptomatic' heart failure.[53] Neurohumoral antagonism has now become a therapeutic target in heart failure, with endothelin and angiotensin II inhibitors being currently evaluated. Over 200 years after its introduction, the debate over digoxin carries on. Newer inotropic agents have failed to impress because of improved symptoms at the expense of increased mortality.[54]

Conclusion

For over 5000 years, cardiovascular function has been studied in health and disease. Although the Egyptians, ancient Greeks and Romans developed the concept of the heart as the organ circulating the blood, even describing the symptoms and treatment of heart failure, their pathophysiological understanding did not allow them to identify the heart as its basis. Traditionalist Galenic dogma was finally refuted by Harvey in the seventeenth century, allowing the concept of empiricism to flourish. Continuing advances in anatomy, pathology and physiology allowed the identification of the heart as the cause of heart failure, and the introduction of digitalis, the first effective pharmacological agent, in the eighteenth century sparked the beginning of therapeutic optimism. Progress in clinical examination in the nineteenth century and the advent of technology, including radiology, electrocardiography, cardiac catheterization and echocardiography, in the twentieth century advanced the understanding of this highly lethal condition. The introduction of diuretics, direct-acting vasodilators, ACE inhibitors and surgical techniques such as transplantation and cardiomyoplasty enable us to relieve symptoms and decrease mortality in patients with heart failure. Despite these advances, the incidence and prevalence of heart failure continues to rise in industrialized countries,[55] it remains difficult to diagnose and treat, and still has a worse overall prognosis than neoplastic disease.

References

1 Karsh RS, McCarthy JD. Archeology and arthritis. *Arch Intern Med* 1960;**105**:640–644.

2 Kramer SN, Levey M. The oldest medical text in man's history: a Sumerian physicians prescription book of 4000 years ago. *Illustrated London News* 1955;**226**:370.

3 Horine EF. An epitome of ancient pulse lore. *Bull Hist Med* 1941;**10**:209–249.

4 Leibowitz JO. Antiquity and the Middle Ages. In: The History of Coronary Heart Disease, 1st edn. William Clowes and Sons, London and Beccles, 1970:15–48.

5 Dalla Volta S. A short historical survey of heart failure. *Clin Invest* 1993;**71**:S167–S176.

6 Bruetsch WL. The earliest record of sudden death possibly due to atherosclerotic coronary occlusion. *Circulation* 1959;**20**:438–441.

7 Shattock SG. A report on the pathological condition of the aorta of King Menephtah, traditionally regarded as the Pharaoh of the Exodus. *Proc Roy Soc Med, Path Sect* 1909;**2**:122–127.

8 Sandison AT. Degenerative vascular disease in the Egyptian mummy. *Med Hist* 1962;**6**:77–81.

9 McGirr EM. A matter of principle: the Vital Spirit. *Scott Med J* 1992;**37**:87–89.

10 Fye WB. Disorders of the heartbeat: a historical overview from antiquity to the mid-20th century. *Am J Cardiol* 1993;**72**:1055–1070.

11 Cheng TO. Glimpses of the past from the recently unearthed ancient corpses in China. *Ann Intern Med* 1984;**101**:714–715.

12 McGirr EM, Stoddart W. Changing theories in 18th-century medicine: the inheritance and legacy of William Cullen. *Scott Med J* 1991; **36**:23–26.

13 Nolan J. A historical review of heart failure. *Scott Med J* 1993;**38**:53–57.

14 Siegel RE. Galen on surgery of the pericardium: an early record of therapy based on anatomic and experimental studies. *Am J Cardiol* 1970; **26**:524–527.

15 Lutz JE. A XII century description of congestive heart failure. *Am J Cardiol* 1988;**61**:494–495.

16 Boyle IT. William Harvey – a man of his time? *Scott Med J* 1991;**36**:187–189.

17 Whitteridge G. The discoveries of Realdus Columbus and their importance for Harvey. In: *William Harvey and the Circulation of the Blood*, 1st edn. Macdonald & Co. (Publishers) Ltd, London, 1971:41–77.

18 Harvey W. *Exercitatio Anatamica de Motu Cordis et Sanguinis in Animalibus*, 1st edn. Guiliemia Fitzieri, Frankfurt, 1628.

19 Boyle IT. A social and personal history of William Harvey, 1578–1657. *Scott Med J* 1994;**39**:53–57.

20 Whitteridge G. De generatione animalum and the final assessment. In: *William Harvey and the Circulation of the Blood*, 1st edn. Macdonald & Co. (Publishers) Ltd, London, 1971:210–236.

21 Leibowitz JO. The Renaissance and the seventeenth century. In: *The History of Coronary Heart Disease*, 1st edn. William Clowes and Sons, London and Beccles, 1970:49–61.

22 Bartoletti F. *Methodus in Dyspnoeam.* Bologna: Tebaldini for the Heirs of Dozza, 1663.

23 Dock W. Medical research from Harvey to Harrison. *Arch Intern Med* 1959;**104**:323–329.

24 Lower R. *Tractatus de Corde, Item de Motu, et Colore Sanguinis et Chyli in Sum Transiti*, 1st edn. J Allestry, London, 1669.

25 Spodick DH. Medical history of the pericardium. The hairy hearts of hoary heroes. *Am J Cardiol* 1970;**26**:447–454.

26 Morgagni JB. *De Sedibus et Causis Morborem per Anatomen Indigatis*, 1st edn. Typographica Academica, Louvain, 1761.

27 Heberden W. Some account of a disorder of the breast. *Med Trans Coll Phys Lond* 1772;**2**:59–67.

28 Townsend GL. Sir John Floyer (1649–1734) and his study of the pulse and respiration. *J Hist Med Allied Sci* 1967;**22**:286–316.

29 Withering W: *An Account of the Foxglove and Some of its Medical Uses – Practical Remarks*

on Dropsy and other Diseases, 1st edn. M Swinney, Birmingham, 1785.

30 Somberg J, Greenfield BA, Tepper D. Digitalis: 200 years in perspective. *Am Heart J* 1986;**111**:615–620.

31 Somberg J, Greenfield BA, Tepper D. Digitalis: 200 years in perspective. *Am Heart J* 1986;**111**:615–620.

32 Lee TC. Van Gogh vision, digitalis intoxication? *JAMA* 1981;**245**:727.

33 Laennec RTH. *Traite de l'Auscultation Mediate et des Maladies du Poumon en de Coeur*, 1st edn. JA Brosson and JS Chaude, Paris, 1819.

34 Reiser SJ. The medical influence of the stethoscope. *Sci Am* 1979;**240**:114–122.

35 Smith DC. Austin Flint and auscultation in America. *J Hist Med Allied Sci* 1978;**33**:129–149.

36 Hope J. *A Treatise on the Diseases of the Heart and Great Vessels, Comprising a New View of the Heart's Action*, 1st edn. W Kidd, London, 1832.

37 Fye WB. The delayed diagnosis of myocardial infarction: it took half a century. *Circulation* 1985;**72**:262–271.

38 Brunton TL. On the use of amyl nitrate in angina pectoris. *Lancet* 1867;**ii**:97–98.

39 Fye WB. T. Lauder Brunton and amyl nitrate: a Victorian vasodilator. *Circulation* 1986; **74**:222–229.

40 Fye WB. Cardiology in 1885. *Circulation* 1985; **72**:21–26.

41 Nolan DJ. 100 years of X-rays. *Br Med J Clin Res Ed* 1995;**310**:614–615.

42 Gottlieb LS. Willem Einthoven, M.D., Ph.D., 1860–1927. *Arch Intern Med* 1961;**107**:447–449.

43 Herrick JB. Clinical features of sudden obstruction of the coronary arteries. *JAMA* 1912; **59**:2015–2020.

44 Cournand A. The history of cardiac catheterisation. *Acta Med Scand* 1975;(suppl 579):8–32.

45 Hales S. Statical essays, containing haemostaticks: or, an account of some hydraulick and hydrostatical experiments made on the blood vessels of animals. 1st edn. Innys and Manby, London, 1733.

46 Vogl A. The discovery of the organic mercurial diuretics. *Am Heart J* 1950;**39**:881.

47 Novello FC, Sprague JM. Benzothiadiazine dioxides as novel diuretics. *J Am Chem Soc* 1957;**79**:2028.

48 Wood PD: Heart failure. In: *Diseases of the Heart and Circulation*, 3rd edn. Eyre and Spottiswoode, London, 1968:291–325.

49 White PD. Congestive heart failure. In: *Heart Disease*, 1st edn. The Macmillan Co. New York, 1931,564–598.

50 Cohn JN, Archibald DG, Ziesche S, et al. Effect of vasodilator therapy on mortality in chronic congestive heart failure. Results of a Veterans Administration Cooperative Study. *N Engl J Med* 1986;**314**:1547–1552.

51 The Consensus Study Group. Effects of enalapril on mortality in severe congestive heart failure: results of the Cooperative North Scandinavian Enalapril Study Group. *N Engl J Med* 1987;**316**:1429–1435.

52 The SOLVD Investigators. Effect of enalapril on survival in patients with reduced left ventricular ejection fractions and congestive heart failure. *N Engl J Med* 1991;**325**:293–302.

53 The SOLVD Investigators. Effect of enalapril on mortality and the development of heart failure in asymptomatic patients with reduced left ventricular ejection fractions. *N Engl J Med* 1992;**327**:685–691.

54 Cohn JN. Inotropic therapy for heart failure: Paradise postponed. *N Engl J Med* 1992; **327**:729–731.

55 McFate Smith W. Epidemiology of congestive heart failure. *Am J Cardiol* 1985;**55**:3A–8A.

SECTION I

EPIDEMIOLOGY

1

What is heart failure?

Henry J Dargie

Introduction

The term 'heart failure' seems simple enough, even self-explanatory. Why, therefore, in 1995 are we questioning what it is? The answer is quite simple – heart failure has become interesting again.

There can be little doubt that the reason for the heightened interest in chronic heart failure is the demonstration in recent years of the improvements in well-being at a clinical level, and on survival in clinical trials brought about by the group of drugs known as ACE inhibitors. The earliest reports of substantial survival benefit in CONSENSUS I,[1] a trial of patients with severe heart failure, have been followed by a succession of trials in progressively less severely affected patients. These trials have consistently shown benefit across the whole spectrum of left ventricular systolic dysfunction, from less severe clinical heart failure (SOLVD Treatment,[2] V-HeFT II[3]) through post-myocardial infarction (SAVE,[4] AIRE,[5] GISSI-3,[6] ISIS-4[7]), and even in patients with none of the symptoms that we currently associate with heart failure (SOLVD Prevention[8]). This success has prompted further studies aimed at preventing left ventricular dysfunction by reducing coronary ischaemic events.

These major trials in patients with symptomatic heart failure have led to a quest to identify and treat all those patients in the community who have characteristics similar to those treated in the trials, i.e. left ventricular systolic dysfunction. In turn, this has led to the exposure of some anomalies in clinical practice concerning heart failure. Specifically, examination of medical records for patients on loop diuretics for presumed heart failure showed that, while a respectable 70% or so of men had left ventricular systolic dysfunction on echocardiography and should, therefore, be candidates for ACE inhibition, only 40% of women had left ventricular dysfunction. Thus it would appear that, on clinical grounds at least, only about 50% of all patients in the community being treated for heart failure actually seem to have evidence of the type of heart disease for which ACE inhibitors would be appropriate, or indeed any significant heart disease at all.[9,10] Even in hospital practice, elucidation of the underlying cause of heart failure is by no means universal.[11]

Given the poor prognosis that epidemiologists have told us attends a diagnosis even of mild heart failure,[12] the search for heart failure amenable to treatment with ACE inhibitors has stimulated interest in all the other heart diseases that can cause the heart to 'fail', some of which are potentially correctable. The intriguing notion that left ventricular dysfunction might be reversible has reawakened interest in ischaemic left ventricular dysfunction and the concept of 'hibernating myocardium'. Increasing interest in the diastolic properties of the myocardium has led to renewed interest in left ventricular hypertrophy and dysfunction associated with ageing, hypertension and valve disease.

This chapter will discuss:

- What is currently understood by the term 'heart failure'.
- What is already known about the epidemiology of heart failure.
- The new European Society of Cardiology guidelines.
- Why the precursors of heart failure, particularly left ventricular dysfunction, are important.
- How patients with asymptomatic left ventricular dysfunction might be identified.
- A proposal for a modern definition of heart failure.

What is currently understood by the term 'heart failure'?

Whatever heart failure is, it is not a simple diagnosis. Heart failure, in pathophysiological terms, is a "state in which an abnormality of cardiac function is responsible for failure of the heart to pump blood at a rate commensurate with the requirements of the metabolizing tissues or to do so only from an elevated filling pressure".[13] While this is useful for the physiologist, the clinician requires a more pragmatic approach, and it is at this point that problems of definition begin to emerge.

The difficulty in defining heart failure, clinically, stems from the fact that heart failure is not a diagnosis *per se* but a clinical syndrome consisting of a constellation of symptoms and signs attributable, ultimately, to cardiac dysfunction. As such it represents the ultimate expression of most serious forms of heart disease.[14] It should, therefore, be borne in mind that, when heart failure can be detected on clinical grounds, an advanced stage has been reached. Contained within the definition (Table 1.1) is a wide spectrum of pathophysiological states varying from those caused by rapid impairment of pump function, e.g. massive myocardial infarction, or tachy or brady arrhythmias, to the progressive and gradual impairment of myocardial function observed in a patient whose heart is subjected to pressure or volume overload or an intrinsic disorder of heart muscle for a prolonged period. While these difficulties do exist in the recognition of acute heart failure, the major diagnostic problem is in chronic heart failure (CHF).

The commonest causes of chronic heart failure

CHF is most commonly caused by myocardial or ventricular dysfunction (mostly left but occasionally right) and valvular stenosis or incompetence; hypertension is now an increasingly uncommon cause of heart failure, possibly as a result of earlier detection and more effective treatment. Non-cardiac causes of heart failure, such as anaemia, thyroid disease, and arteriovenous fistulae are distinctly uncommon though important because they are correctable.

As currently recognized, the most characteristic symptoms of heart failure are breathlessness and fatigue while the signs are usually those of fluid retention, most commonly ankle swelling. As is obvious, these are rather nonspecific features of which more common causes are obesity and venous insufficiency.

Cardiologists vary considerably in their faith in the time-honoured cardiac signs of heart failure, such as tachycardia, raised jugular venous pressure (JVP), and a third heart sound. That most would agree to disagree on the relative sensitivity and specificity of these signs is symptomatic of the problem of definition we face, not only in the presence of these signs but especially in their absence.

Criteria 1 and 2 should be fulfilled in all cases
1. Symptoms of heart failure (at rest or during exercise)
and
2. Objective evidence of cardiac dysfunction (at rest)
and
3. Response to treatment directed towards heart failure (in cases where the diagnosis is in doubt)

Table 1.1
Definition of heart failure.

So what do we mean by chronic heart failure?

For one answer to this we can look at how CHF was defined in the large epidemiological studies aimed at determining how common it is. The Framingham Study, in which cohorts of men and women were recruited who had a subsequently high mortality, showed that heart failure worthy of treatment can be recognized on the basis of clinical features supported by a chest X-ray.[12] Similarly, clinical trials, such as the AIRE study,[5] show that cohorts of men and women after myocardial infarction who benefit from ACE inhibitor treatment can also be recruited on the basis of clinical signs (tachycardia, S3 and bi-basular rates), again supported by a chest X-ray. However, when the sensitivity and specificity of standard clinical features have been assessed, sensitivity has been found to be poor and the specific signs or symptoms are usually quite insensitive (Table 1.2).

	Sensitivity (%)	Specificity (%)	Positive* predictive value (%)
Symptom			
Dyspnoea	66	52	23
Orthopnoea	21	81	2
Paroxysmal nocturnal dyspnoea	33	76	26
History of oedema	23	80	22
Sign			
Heart rate >100/minute at rest	7	99	6
Pulmonary crackles	13	91	27
Oedema by examination	10	93	3
Third heart sound	31	95	61
Jugular venous distension	10	97	2

**proportion of patients in whom heart failure was correctly diagnosed.*

Table 1.2
Diagnosis of heart failure[14a].

Correctly recognizing the presence of heart failure is important for three reasons:

- as an indicator of the presence of significant underlying cardiac disease which must be investigated to ensure correct management.
- to prevent unnecessary and potentially harmful treatment being administered on a life-long basis.
- because, as it is likely that symptomatic heart failure represents only the tip of an iceberg of cardiac disease, and given its poor prognosis, early identification of such patients could have important implications for prevention.

What is already known about the epidemiology of heart failure?

Eriksson and coworkers[15] used evidence from symptoms and signs and the prescription of digoxin and/or diuretics to conclude that 'manifest' heart failure was present in 2.1% of men at age 50, 2.4% at 54, 4.3% at 60, and 10.3% at 67. No women were studied. In the National Health and Nutrition Survey in the United States the overall prevalence of heart failure in subjects aged 25–74 was 2%.[16] This lower overall prevalence could perhaps be explained by the additional specificity conferred by the inclusion of a chest X-ray in the selection process. These data are similar to the older Framingham Study in which the steep increase in prevalence among older people was particularly evident[12].

Examination of general practitioner records gives information on patients presenting in the course of ordinary clinical practice. In the United States, Gibson et al[17] studied practices in two different rural counties and noted remarkably similar prevalence rates – 0.9 and 1%. Parameshwar,[10] in a study of general practice records in London, concluded that heart failure was present in 0.06% of those under 65 and 2.77% in those over 65. It is quite clear from these studies that estimates of the prevalence of heart failure by various clinical definitions, with or without a chest X-ray, vary widely.

Thus, all existing epidemiological studies have relied on clinical criteria for a 'diagnosis' of heart failure. The symptoms and some of the signs of heart failure are notoriously non-specific and recent studies have shown that one-third to one-half of patients thought to have heart failure may have been incorrectly classified.[9,18] We do not know for certain, therefore, how common true heart failure is in the population. In addition, the clinical criteria used do not permit any assessment of the underlying cause of heart failure. Furthermore, the type of myocardial failure ('systolic' or 'diastolic') could not be determined in these studies, yet the prognosis and treatment of these may be very different.

Guidelines of the European Society of Cardiology

What should be our yardstick for inferring the presence of heart failure? The European Society of Cardiology (ESC) has recently produced guidelines for the diagnosis of heart failure.[19] According to the ESC guidelines, heart failure can diagnosed in a patient with the appropriate symptoms in the presence of appropriate underlying heart disease. Thus, a view has been taken that, for a patient to have 'heart failure', they must have symptoms, the essential components of which are breathlessness or fatigue.

The relationships between cardiac dysfunction, heart failure, heart failure rendered asymptomatic by treatment, and transient heart failure are shown in Fig. 1.1. The ESC Working Party that produced these guidelines

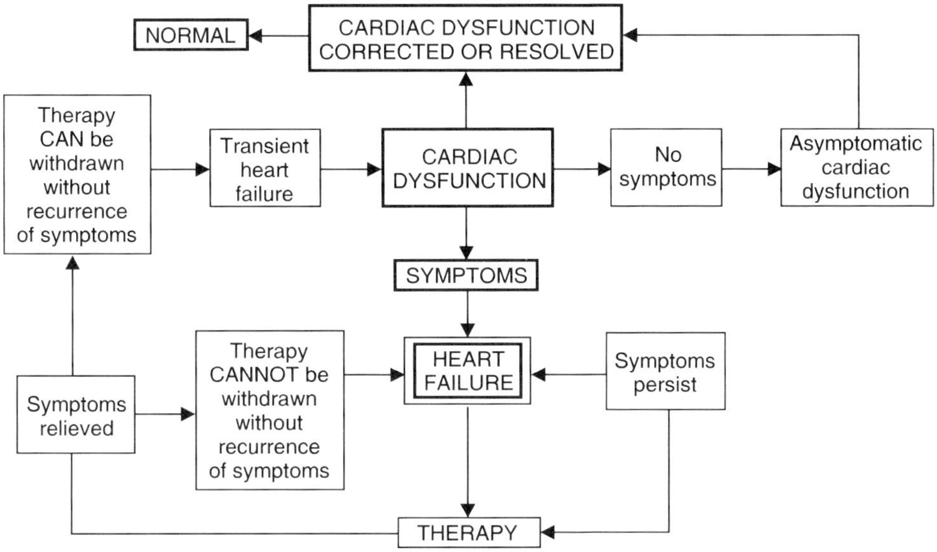

Fig. 1.1
Cardiac dysfunction, heart failure, and heart failure rendered asymptomatic.

has also recognized the importance of asymptomatic left ventricular dysfunction – not only that which is rendered 'asymptomatic' as a result of treatment, but also *de novo* left ventricular dysfunction without symptoms. Importantly, the ESC guidelines state implicitly that objective evidence of heart disease is intrinsic to the diagnosis of heart failure. The mainstay for providing evidence of the type and severity of heart disease is echocardiography, which is the best allround technique for detecting myocardial, valvular and pericardial disease. Many hospitals are now providing 'open' or 'rapid' access to echocardiography to facilitate the management of patients with symptoms conducive with heart failure.[20] These initiatives are showing that many patients seem not to have obvious causes for their symptoms in terms of myocardial structural or functional abnormalities or valve disease. Although criteria for establishing the presence of left ventricular dysfunction are not standardized, there are a number of accepted criteria, including by ejection fraction, internal dimensions, shortening fraction or wall motion; in contrast, the criteria for diastolic dysfunction are insufficiently accepted at the moment to allow a confident diagnosis of this elusive condition.

Serious left ventricular dysfunction or valvular disease is readily identifiable on echocardiography but milder degrees of abnormalities give rise to much difficulty. Therefore echocardiography cannot be regarded as a 'gold standard' for the diagnosis of the presence of heart failure. It is certain, however, that echocardiography should be used much more widely to confirm or exclude the presence of heart disease in patients with symptoms of heart failure; and the ESC guidelines will, inevitably, lead to an increased demand for echocardiograms (ECGs).

The guidelines also make clear, however, that the standard 12-lead ECG is also important in excluding heart disease. The ECG cannot be used to diagnose heart failure but a convincingly absolutely normal ECG as decided by a validated computer programme will render the diagnosis of heart failure unlikely. In the CASS Registry, only 0.6% of patients with a normal ECG by Minnesota coding had a reduced left ventricular ejection fraction ($\leqslant$35%).[21,21a] Thus the simple ECG could greatly improve the specificity of the initial diagnosis.

Why asymptomatic left ventricular dysfunction should come under the heart failure umbrella

Recent clinical trials have shown that treatment with ACE inhibitors can improve both symptoms and survival in all grades of highly selected groups of patients with heart failure. The absolute benefit of therapy is, however, disappointingly modest. For example, in the CONSENSUS I study,[1] one-year mortality in New York Heart Association (NYHA) Class IV ('severe') patients was reduced from 52% in the placebo group to 36% in the intervention (ACE inhibitor) group. Similarly, in NYHA Class II–III ('mild–moderate'), patients in the treatment arm of SOLVD,[2] the placebo mortality after four years of follow-up was 40% compared to 35% in the intervention (ACE inhibitor) group.

The findings of these clinical trials reinforce the belief that overt heart failure represents an advanced and irreversible condition. Therefore detection and treatment of 'asymptomatic' left ventricular dysfunction (where annual mortality is 4%) represents the strategy most likely to reduce the burden of illness and death, ultimately attributable to heart failure, in the population. Our present approach to heart failure, which involves the treatment of an advanced stage of a disease that has symptomatically declared itself, is analagous to that of treating malignant hypertension. The modern and successful management of hypertension involves the detection and treatment of the asymptomatic precursor. A recent clinical trial suggests the same may be true for heart failure. In the prevention arm of SOLVD,[8] patients with 'asymptomatic' left ventricular dysfunction (the precursor of heart failure) were randomized to treatment with placebo or an ACE inhibitor. The reduction in the risk of developing heart failure was 37% in the active treatment group. In this group there was a 36% reduction in the risk of first hospitalization for heart failure and a 20% reduction in the risk of death or development of heart failure. Epidemiological studies laid the foundation of the appreciation of the size of the problem of hypertension in the population, and its under-detection and under-treatment. The results of the SOLVD prevention arm suggest that this same approach should be applied to left ventricular dysfunction/heart failure.[8]

Ventricular dysfunction post-myocardial infarction

Myocardial infarction is a major risk factor for the development of heart failure. The widespread use of thrombolytic therapy and aspirin has resulted in many more patients per thousand surviving acute myocardial infarction.[22] It can be argued that thrombolysis 'salvages' the myocardium and preserves ventricular function. Several studies, however, have shown that mean left ventricular ejection fraction in patients who have received thrombolysis is little different from that of controls. It can also be argued that it is the patients with the greatest degree of left ventricular damage, who might otherwise have died, who gain the greatest survival benefit from thrombolysis. More patients may therefore be surviving to be at risk of developing substantial left ventricular dysfunction in the 'thrombolytic era'.

Although some patients develop transient left ventricular failure in the acute phase of myocardial infarction and some develop heart failure, the great majority do not, appearing to recover satisfactorily despite electrocardiographic and enzyme evidence of substantial, even extensive, infarction.[23,24] Many patients, therefore, may survive myocardial infarction to be left with 'asymptomatic' left ventricular dysfunction.

How many patients are left with left ventricular dysfunction following myocardial infarction and what subsequently happens to them has never been accurately documented. In the Framingham Study, 15% of patients who had a myocardial infarction developed overt heart failure within five years of diagnosis, a ten-year age-adjusted risk of heart failure 10–20 times that of the general population.[12] Why these patients develop heart failure is not completely understood. Some may develop recurrent myocardial infarction but many appear to progress to heart failure without further infarction; in these patients, the size of the initial myocardial injury is probably the main determinant of progression.[25] Other possible risk factors are the neuroendocrine, vascular and renal responses that occur in an individual, but the nature of these responses and their relationship to subsequent outcome have not been studied in a discrete population.[26,27] 'Asymptomatic' left ventricular dysfunction, therefore, represents the least well understood of the stages of the development of heart failure. It prevalence and incidence in the population are unknown. Its natural history in the modern era of myocardial infarction management is not known (other than in highly selected patient groups). The pathophysiological responses to left ventricular dysfunction and the role that these responses may play in the subsequent natural history of left ventricular dysfunction remain to be fully elucidated.

Heart failure appears to be the final expression of the sequence outlined in Fig. 1.2. Prevention (i.e. prevention of 'progression' from ventricular dysfunction to heart failure) is the ultimate aim of any therapeutic strategy in this area. It is important because the occurrence of myocardial infarction is the best opportunity we have of identifying patients with the most common form of left ventricular dysfunction.

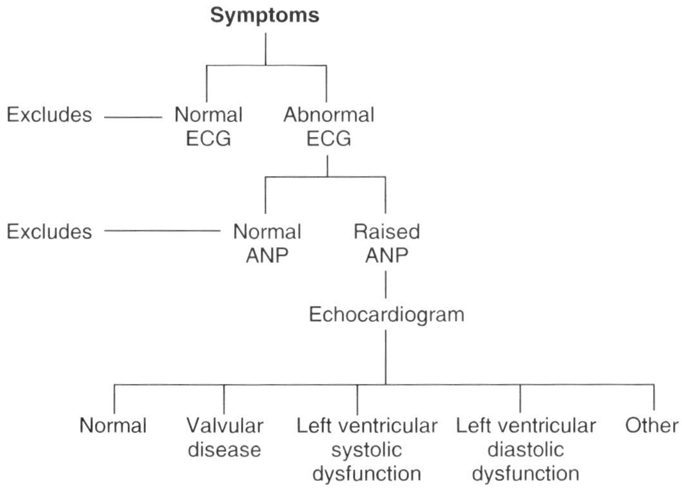

Fig. 1.2
Clinical algorithm for detecting heart failure in untreated patients.

Could there be a 'blood test' for heart failure?

Considerable evidence has now accumulated supporting the concept of utilizing one or more components of the neuroendocrine response to cardiac dysfunction to infer the presence of heart failure. Currently the two major contenders for the blood test approach are N-terminal ANP or BNP, the former because it is stable and probably reflects the adequacy of the circulation over time, and the latter because it is more specific for ventricular dysfunction.[28,29] In an untreated patient, therefore, an elevated N-ANP would seem to be a marker for circulatory insufficiency in as much as it suggests the presence of an elevated filling pressure.

The precise relationships between left ventricular dysfunction, natriuretic peptides, and heart failure remain to be determined in populations of unselected subjects, which would enable the true value of a blood test to be assessed in relation to other diagnostic criteria. It seems likely that no single clinical modality will emerge as 'the test'; rather a hierarchical algorithmic approach is much more plausible.

Putting it all together

There is no accepted 'gold standard' for the presence of heart failure (and certainly no single non-haemodynamic parameter). Recognition of the presence of heart failure in the future, therefore, is likely to require some metabolic indicator of circulatory dysfunction to complement the clinical features, ECG and echocardiogram in situations where clinical doubt persists.

A clinical algorithm in *untreated* patients could be constructed on present knowledge as shown in Fig. 1.2.

Looking to the future

It is a matter of frequent clinical observation that the relationship between symptoms and disease severity is tenuous. Many patients with severe pathology have few symptoms and vice versa. For example, in aortic stenosis the first symptoms may present late in life when the gradient across the aortic valve is approaching or even greater than 100 mmHg. Similarly patients with moderate and occasionally severe left ventricular dysfunction complain of no limitation (perhaps as a result of their sedentary lifestyle).

If symptomatic or clinical heart failure has a prevalence of 1–2% then its main precursors, especially left ventricular dysfunction, must be considerably more prevalent.

If we take as an example the situation after acute myocardial infarction, we know that approximately 40% of patients have 'significant' left ventricular dysfunction, i.e. may have a left ventricular ejection fraction $\leqslant$40%, yet heart failure will be overt in only a minority of these patients. Should such patients with ventricular dysfunction be regarded as not having heart failure simply on the basis that they do not volunteer symptoms of breathlessness and fatigue or show signs of fluid retention?

A proposal for a modern definition of heart failure

As we have seen, doctors diagnose heart failure when fatigue, dyspnoea or oedema develop in patients whom they suspect have heart disease. By these standards, this clinical syndrome is a terminal state because its annual mortality, in severe cases, may exceed 50%. Physiologists define heart failure as an inability of the heart to deliver sufficient oxygen to meet the needs of the body. In favour of this approach is the recent demonstration that, among patients with substantial left ventricular dysfunction, the majority may have no symptoms of heart failure. However, evidence of insufficient oxygen delivery could be inferred from their impaired functional capacity on exercise testing; and, during follow-up, many more of those who remained untreated went on to develop the clinical syndrome of heart failure than did those who were treated with an ACE inhibitor. Thus physiologists would classify as having heart failure patients within a much broader spectrum of cardiac disease, whose clinical expression might vary from apparent normality to serious impairment of the quality and, potentially, the length of life.

This poses a problem of definition, the solution to which lies in accepting that the term 'heart failure' is insufficiently descriptive and inadequately specific to be an acceptable label for all patients who might benefit from earlier identification and treatment. However, so engrained is this term in the clinical consciousness that to abandon it completely would serve only to confuse matters further. It is sensible, therefore, to retain 'heart failure' as the term for the syndrome recognized by doctors on the basis of symptoms and signs with objective evidence of underlying heart disease; but we should focus more on diagnosing the precise cause of the symptoms. Left ventricular dysfunction can be used as one of the generic terms that would encompass both heart failure and its clinically important precursors. Both clinical features and modern cardiological investigation would be used to sub-categorize all patients within this generic classification. This proposed classification may be applied to all diseases of the heart – pericardial, myocardial, endocardial or valvular – that have the potential to cause what doctors recognize as 'heart failure'. This broader, physiologists' definition is the basis of a modern definition for heart failure.

'Clinical' heart failure is merely the ominous result of the progression of a number of heart diseases to an advanced and often irreversible stage. It should be regarded as health care failure since most of its causes are detectable at a much earlier stage. Early detection is the challenge for modern cardiology.

References

1 The CONSENSUS Trial Study Group. Effects of enalapril on mortality in severe congestive heart failure. *N Engl J Med* 1987;**316**:1429–1435.

2 The SOLVD Investigators. Effect of enalapril on survival in patients with reduced left ventricular ejection fractions and congestive heart failure. *N Engl J Med* 1991;**325**:293–302.

3 Cohn JN, Johnson G, Ziesche S, et al. A comparison of enalapril with hydralazine-isosorbide dinitrate in the treatment of chronic congestive heart failure. *N Engl J Med* 1991;**325**:303–310.

4 Pfeffer MA, Braunwald E, Moye LA, et al. Effect of captopril on mortality and morbidity in patients with left ventricular dysfunction after myocardial infarction: results of the Survival and Ventricular Enlargement Trial. *N Engl J Med* 1992;**327**:669–677.

5 The Acute Infarction Ramipril Efficacy (AIRE) Study Investigators. Effect of ramipril on mortality and morbidity of survivors of acute myocardial infarction with clinical evidence of heart failure. *Lancet* 1993;**342**:821–828.

6 GISSI-3 – Gruppo Italiano per lo Studio della Sopravvivenza nell'Infarto Miocardico. GISSI-3 study protocol on the effects of lisinopril, of nitrates, and of their association in patients with acute myocardial infarction. *Am J Cardiol* 1992;**70(Suppl)**:62C–69C.

7 ISIS-4 Collaborative Group. Fourth International Study of Infarct Survival: protocol for a large sample study of the effects of oral mononitrate, of oral captopril, and of intravenous magnesium. *Am J Cardiol* 1991;**68** (**Suppl**):87D–100D.

8 The SOLVD Investigators. Effect of enalapril on mortality and the development of heart failure in asymptomatic patients with reduced left ventricular ejection fractions. *N Engl J Med* 1992;**327**:685–691.

9 Remes J, Miettinen H, Reunanen A, Pyorale K. Validity of clinical diagnosis of heart failure in primary health care. *Eur Heart J* 1991;**12**:315–321.

10 Parameshwar J, Shackell MM, Richardson A, Poole-Wilson PA, Sutton GC. Prevalence of heart failure in three general practices in north west London. *Br J Gen Pract* 1992;**42**:287–289.

11 Clarke KW, Gray D, Hampton JR. Evidence of inadequate investigation and treatment of patients with heart failure. *Br Heart J* 1994;**71**:584–587.

12 Kannel WB, Sorlie P, McNamara PM. Prognosis after initial myocardial infarction: the Framingham study. *Am J Cardiol* 1979;**44**:53–59.

13 Braunwald E, Grossman W. Clinical aspects of heart failure. In: Braunwald E, ed. *Heart Disease* 4th edn (W B Saunders 1992): 444.

14 Lenfant C. Report of the task force on research in heart failure. *Circulation* 1994;**90**:1118–1123.

14a McMurray J. The signs and symptoms of heart failure. In: Ball SG, Campbell RWF, Frances GS. *International Handbook of Heart Failure*. Euromed Communications Ltd, 1994: 5–12.

15 Eriksson H, Svardsudd K, Larsson B, et al. Risk factors for heart failure in the general population: the study of men born in 1913. *Eur Heart J* 1989;**10**:647–656.

16 Schocken DD, Arrieta MI, Leaverton PE, Ross EA. Prevalence and mortality rate of congestive heart failure in the United States. *J Am Coll Cardiol* 1992;**20**:301–306.

17 Gibson TC, White KL, Klainer LM. The prevalence of congestive heart failure in two rural communities. *J Chronic Dis* 1966;**19**:141–152.

18 Wheeldon NM, MacDonald TM, Flucker CJ, McKendrick AD, McDevitt DG, Struthers AD. Echocardiography in chronic heart failure in the community. *Q J Med* 1993;**86**:17–23.

19 The Task Force on Heart Failure of the European Society of Cardiology. Guidelines for the diagnosis of heart failure. *Eur Heart J* 1995;**16**:741–751.

20 Francis CM, Caruana L, Kearney P, et al. Open access echocardiography in management of heart failure in the community. *BMJ* 1995;**10**:634–636.
21 Rihal CS, Davis KB, Kennedy JW, Gersh BJ. The utility of clinical, electrocardiographic, and roentgenographic variables in the prediction of left ventricular function. *Am J Cardiol* 1995;**75**:220–223.
21a Francis CM, Davie A, Love MP, et al. The value of the electrocardiogram in identifying patients with heart failure due to left ventricular systolic dysfunction. *BMJ* 1995 (in press).
22 Fibrinolytic Therapy Trialists (FTT) Collaborative Group. Indications for fibrinolytic therapy in suspected acute myocardial infarction: collaborative overview of early mortality and major morbidity results from all randomised trials of more than 1000 patients. *Lancet* 1994;**343**:311–322.
23 Gottlieb S, Moss AJ, McDermott M, Eberly S. Interrelation of left ventricular ejection fraction, pulmonary congestion and outcome in acute myocardial infarction. *Am J Cardiol* 1992; **69**:977–984.
24 Moye LA, Pfeffer MA, Braunwald E. Rationale, design and baseline characteristics of the survival and ventricular enlargement trial. *Am J Cardiol* 1991;**68**:70D–79D.
25 Greene HL, Richardson DW, Hallstrom AP, et al. Congestive heart failure after acute myocardial infarction in patients receiving antiarrhythmic agents for ventricular premature complexes (Cardiac Arrhythmia Pilot Study). *Am J Cardiol* 1989;**63**:393–398.
26 McAlpine HM, Morton JJ, Leckie B, Rumley A, Gillen G, Dargie HJ. Neuroendocrine activation after acute myocardial infarction. *Br Heart J* 1988;**60**:117–124.
27 Sussex BA, Arnold JMO, Parker JO, et al. Independent and interactive prognostic information of neurohormones and echocardiogram in high risk post-MI patients. *J Am Coll Cardiol* 1992;**19**:205A (abstract).
28 Lerman A, Gibbons RJ, Rodeheffer RJ, et al. Circulating N-terminal atrial natriuretic peptide as a marker for symptomless left ventricular dysfunction. *Lancet* 1993;**341**:1105–1109.
29 Wei CM, Kao PC, Lin JT, Heublein DM, Schaff HV, Burnett JC Jr. Circulating beta-atrial natriuretic factor in congestive heart failure in humans. *Circulation* 1993;**88**:1016–1020.

2

How common and how much of a problem is heart failure?

Henry Eriksson

Introduction

Over the past few decades decreasing mortality rates from cardiovascular disease (i.e. myocardial infarction and stroke) have been reported.[1–3] However, despite the declining trends for cardiovascular disease mortality, there are increasing rates of morbidity and mortality from congestive heart failure (CHF), especially in the elderly.[4–6] There may be several reasons for this development. Changes in the levels of cardiovascular risk factors in the population, aggressive treatment of hypertension, and improved treatment regimes for coronary heart disease and stroke partly account for these declining trends.[7]

It is likely that antihypertensive treatment may not actually prevent heart failure, but rather postpone its development.[8] Furthermore, the ageing of the population, improved survival after myocardial infarction due to coronary care units, the life-saving benefits of thrombolytic therapy, and greater awareness and improved diagnostic techniques for the detection of heart failure may all be reasons for increasing rates of heart failure in the population.

The definition of heart failure

When studying how much of a problem CHF represents in the community, the most crucial question is how to formulate an up-to-date working definition of heart failure. Because of its insidious onset, early heart failure is not readily apparent. It is only in the advanced stages that specific signs and symptoms are evident generally. Numerous definitions have been proposed but none is generally agreed upon.[9]

The ultimate goal must be prevention and detection of the early stages of heart failure before irreversible damage has occurred. For screening of large population samples, a useful definition must be simple and reproducible and must not require equipment that is too complicated.

Heart failure has been termed 'the end-stage of heart disease that ensues after the myocardium has exhausted all its reserve capacity and compensatory mechanisms'.[10] This definition reflects the stringent criteria that characterized heart failure (mostly severe) in the Framingham Study (Table 2.1). In contrast, the Study of Men Born in 1913 used a broader definition that included dyspnoea (cardiac origin) as a symptom of mild to moderate CHF (see Table 2.1).

In medical practice, a diagnosis of heart failure must be based on patient history, clinical findings, and a limited number of investigations. A range of symptoms, signs, and non-invasive tests are needed for a definite diagnosis. The choice of which symptoms and signs to be included in the definition will

The Framingham Heart Study	*The Study of Men Born in 1913*		*The Boston scale criteria*
Major criteria paroxysmal nocturnal dyspnoea neck vein distension râles cardiomegaly acute pulmonary oedema S3-gallop increased venous pressure (>16 cm water) circulation time $\geq$ 25 sec. hepato-jugular reflux	**Cardiac scores** heart disease angina pectoris swollen legs (evenings) dyspnoea at night râles atrial fibrillation	**Pulmonary scores** bronchitis/asthma cough, phlegm, wheezing rhonchi	**Category I:** history rest dyspnoea (4 points) orthopnoea (4 points) paroxysmal nocturnal dyspnoea (3 points) dyspnoea on walking on level (2 points) dyspnoea on climbing (1 point) **Category II:** physical examination heart rate: 91–110 (1 point); > 110 (2 points) jugular venous pressure elevation (if > 6 cm H_2O (2 points); if > 6 cm H_2O plus hepatomegaly or leg oedema (3 points) lung râles – basilar (1 point); more than basilar (2 points) wheezing (3 points) third heart sound (3 points)
Minor criteria ankle oedema night cough hepatomegaly pleural effusion vital capacity reduced by one third from maximum tachycardia ($\geq$ 120)	**Stages of CHF** 1. Cardiac scores only 2. Cardiac score and dyspnoea or cardiac score and treatment for CHF 3. Cardiac score, dyspnoea and treatment for CHF 4. Deceased with or due to CHF		**Category III:** chest radiography alveolar pulmonary oedema (4 points) interstitial pulmonary oedema (3 points) bilateral pleural effusion (3 points) cardiothoracic ratio $\geq$ 0.50 (3 points) upper zone flow redistribution (2 points)
Major or minor criterion weight loss of more than 4.5 kg over 5 days in response to treatment			(Point value within parentheses and no more than 4 points from each category allowed. Hence a maximum possible of 12 points.)
Definite CHF: 2 major criteria or 1 major and 2 minor criteria	**'Latent' CHF**: stage 1 **'Manifest' CHF**: stage 2 and 3 (4)		**'Definite' CHF**: 8–12 points **'Possible' CHF**: 5–7 points

Table 2.1
Criteria for heart failure in the Framingham study,[15] the Study of Men Born in 1913,[16] and according to the Boston scale.[17,23]

determine the stage of the syndrome identified and will very much influence both prevalence rates and prognosis. Clearly, CHF is not a single condition but a complex of symptoms and signs that develop as a compensatory response to some underlying cardiac abnormality (e.g. a mechanical disorder, myocardial dysfunction, or some disturbance in cardiac rhythm).

Prevalence of heart failure

Most earlier studies of CHF, whether in hospital or in the community, have been performed on selected populations, which are often inadequately described and give little or no information on the population at risk. Hence these data have to be taken with caution for epidemiological analyses of the problem of CHF in the community as a whole.[11]

According to the US National Data, about 35 000 people die each year with CHF as the primary cause of death. This is probably an underestimate of the real prevalence. As a whole, the number of deaths due to CHF in the US increased more than four-fold during the period 1955 to 1983. There was a parallel increase in the number of deaths in which CHF was considered a contributing cause. Furthermore, the age-adjusted death rates showed a two-fold increase for CHF as the underlying cause of death. During the period 1968 to 1978, CHF mortality declined in the younger age group, whereas in the older age groups (65 year and older) an increase could be seen.[8] However, a specific aetiology of heart failure mortality is often not available in a death certificate, and in more than 85% of the certificates, CHF was not given as the underlying cause of death but rather as a contributing cause.

Morbidity studies undertaken by general practitioners in England and Wales (1958) showed a prevalence rate of 0.2% in the age group 45–64 years and 1.9% in those 65 years and older.[12] Six-month prevalence rates of CHF in the corresponding age groups found in the Two Counties Survey (1962) in the USA were 1.0% and 6.5% respectively.[13]

In 1988, an estimation was done in north-west London based on practice records of patients with heart failure who were given a prescription for diuretic medication.[14] In this study, CHF was considered present when there was evidence of heart disease together with past or present fluid retention, breathlessness or fatigue, or relief of symptoms with diuretics. The overall prevalence rate was 0.4%. Below 65 years of age, the prevalence rate was 0.06% but it increased to 2.8% for those 65 years and older.

In summary, the older studies on CHF indicate that about 1% of the population has been or is in heart failure. However, mortality and morbidity data are derived from observations based on different methods, in different circumstances, on different populations, and at different times. Prevalence rates for all CHF in the general population cannot be estimated from such data.

Only a few epidemiological studies based on random population samples, using strictly defined criteria for CHF, have been undertaken. The Framingham Heart Study was the first population study reporting epidemiological data on heart failure.[15] In that study, a number of 'major' and 'minor' criteria were used to define CHF (see Table 2.1). This definition mostly includes severe heart failure. At entry into the Framingham study, 17 out of 5209 men and women had CHF, giving a prevalence rate of 0.3%, though no subject was older than 62 years. At the 34-year follow-up a prevalence rate (men and women) of 0.8% at ages 50–59 and as high as 9.1% in the age group 80 years and older was estimated (Table 2.2).[10] Even higher prevalence rates would probably have

Reference	Sex	Age groups (yrs) 50–59	60–69	70–79	≥ 80
Framingham[10]	M + F	0.8	2.3	4.9	9.1
Study of Men Born in 1913[16]	M	2.1	4.3*	13.0**	—
Swedish[19]	M	—	—	11#	—
	F	—	—	8#	—
	M	—	—	17##	—
	F	—	—	11##	—
NHANES–I[20]	M	0.8^{+}	4.5^{++}	4.8^{+++}	—
	F	1.3^{+}	3.0^{++}	4.3^{+++}	—
West London[14]	M + F	0.06¤	2.8¤¤	—	—

Table 2.2
*Prevalence rates (%) in five epidemiological studies in relation to different age groups. (M – male; F – female; * – age 60 yrs; ** – age 67 yrs; # – age 70 yrs; ## – age 75 yrs; + – age 25–54 yrs; ++ – age 55–64 yrs; +++ – age 65–74 yrs; ¤ – age < 65 yrs; ¤¤ – age ≥ 65 yrs.)*

been found if milder forms of CHF had also been included.

In Sweden, the Study of Men Born in 1913 examined a random third of all men born in the same year in Gothenburg. These men were studied between 1963 and 1980. Samples were drawn using the same criteria at ages 50, 54 and 67.[16] The prevalence rates are shown in Table 2.2. Prevalence rate of CHF increased with age, as in the Framingham study, with a steeper increase after the age of 60. In the Study of Men Born in 1913, the definition of CHF was based on criteria such that the early stages of the syndrome would also be included (see Table 2.1). The prevalence rate increased from 2% at age 50 to 13% at age 67 years (see Table 2.2). If 'latent' forms of CHF were also included, the prevalence rate in 67-year-old men increased to over 20%. However, in these very early stages of CHF, most patients are asymptomatic and further diagnostic tests are needed to confirm the presence of myocardial dysfunction. Furthermore, the rate of false-positive diagnosis of heart failure seem to be as high as 30–50% when the diagnosis is made on only clinical findings.[17,18]

Another Swedish population study of both men and women reported prevalence rates of 11–17% among men and 8–11% among women at ages 70 and 75 years (see Table 2.2).[19] In this study, the definition of heart failure included symptoms, signs, and chest X-ray.

Whereas the Framingham data represent a semiurban American community, prevalence data from the National Health and Nutritional Examination survey (NHANES-I) correlate the trends for the nation as a whole (see Table 2.2).[20] The prevalence of CHF based on clinical criteria was 2%, suggesting that 1–2 million adults are affected in the USA.

Incidence of heart failure

Surveys by physicians in two counties of the USA estimated that the incidence of CHF in the population ranges between 3.8 and 5.0 per

	Age groups (yrs)									
	≤ 54		55–64		65–74		75–84		≥ 85	
Reference	Men	Women	Men	Women	Men	Women	Men	Women	Men	Women
Framingham[10]	2	1	4	3	8	5	14	13	54	85
Study of Men Born in 1913[16]	1.5	—	4.3*	—	10.2**	—	—	—	—	—
Finnish[22]	1.9	—	3.1	1.5	8.2	2.0	—	—	—	—
(includes possible CHF)	2.3	1.2	3.8	2.5	9.1	4.3	—	—	—	—

Table 2.3
Annual incidence rates of CHF per 1000 in three population-based studies. (– age group 55–60 yrs; ** – age group 61–67 yrs.)*

1000 per year.[13] Furthermore, data from these two rural communities were used to estimate that the prevalence of CHF (in the age group 45 and over) in the USA was almost 2 million in 1980. In the same way it was estimated that the incidence of CHF increased from 200 000 new cases per year in 1960 to 300 000 in 1980.[21]

Estimations of the incidence rate of CHF in the general population are almost entirely based on the Framingham study and the Study of Men

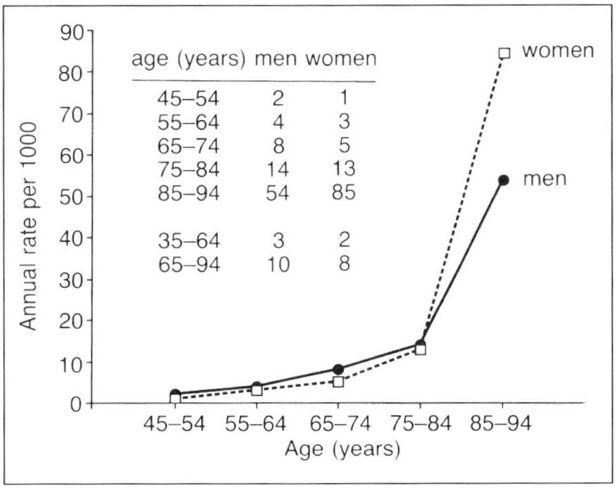

Fig. 2.1
Incidence of heart failure by age and sex: 30-year follow-up in the Framingham study.[10]

Born in 1913 (Table 2.3). In both these studies, the incidence rate increased with age, especially in the highest age groups (Fig. 2.1). It should also be noted that the incidence rates and the prevalence rate in the Framingham study are probably underestimations, as stated by the authors, since the criteria did not include the milder forms of heart failure.[15] However, milder forms of CHF were included in the Study of Men Born in 1913 giving an average annual incidence rate of 1.5 per 1000 per year in the age group 50–54 years; this increased to 10.2 per 1000 per year at ages 61–67 (see Table 2.3). If latent or asymptomatic forms were also included these incidence rates almost doubled.[16]

In a study from Finland the age-adjusted incidence rates of all 'definite' heart failure were 4.0 per 1000 per year in men and 1.0 per 1000 per year for women.[22] This population-based surveillance study used the Boston criteria[17,23] for defining CHF (see Table 2.1). If both 'definite' and 'possible' CHF were included the incidence rates of all CHF increased to 4.7 per 1000 in men and 2.4 per 1000 in women. The Finnish study found similar incidence rates whether the Boston criteria or the Framingham criteria were used, indicating that more advanced forms of

CHF were selected. In various age groups the rates of CHF were similar to those found in the Framingham and the Gothenburg study (see Table 2.3).

Socioeconomic consequences of heart failure

Throughout much of the industrialized world, escalating healthcare costs constitute a serious burden on various systems of financing health care – some countries spend more than 10% of their gross national product on healthcare.[24]

The prevalence rate of CHF, according to the American Heart Association, is 2.3–3 million cases in the US alone.[25] In the Federal Republic of Germany, 1.9 million people, representing more than 3% of the population, suffer from CHF. The costs associated with CHF amounted to almost 6.8 million German Marks (DM) in 1985.[26]

Hospital care is a significant part of the economic burden of CHF, and the hospitalization rates for CHF have steadily increased.[5,27] In the USA, the rates of discharges with a first-listed diagnosis of CHF have increased over 100% during 1970 and 1985 for the age group 45 years and above.[6]

Most of these figures represent discharges, not individuals (i.e. one CHF patient may have been admitted more than once during the same year). However, in Gothenburg, Sweden, the age-adjusted hospital rates of discharges for heart failure (first-listed diagnosis and counting only one admission per year) supported the hospital data from the US and Scotland.[27,28]

The SOLVD study estimated that 35% of all CHF patients were admitted to hospital each year.[29] In the USA between 1973 and 1986, hospital discharges for CHF rose by 99% and 118% for white and non-white men respectively, and by 27% and 43%, for white and non-white women respectively.[5]

According to the US National Center for Health Statistics, 722 000 discharges were related to CHF as the first-listed diagnosis, requiring more than 5.7 million days at hospital. CHF was the most prevalent diagnosis for patients aged 65 and older (1.4 times that of myocardial infarction). Only childbirth and psychoses accounted for more inpatient days.[30] Furthermore, the length of hospitalization for heart failure is often prolonged, especially for the elderly.[27]

Similar data has been reported by the Swedish National Board of Health and Welfare.[31] In Sweden, 20% of all discharges and over 30% of the number of days in hospital (for heart disease) were related to CHF. Men and women over 65 years of age accounted for more than 95% of all discharges for CHF. In the United Kingdom, it has been estimated that 100 000 to 120 000 cases of CHF were admitted annually to hospital.[32]

For a small part of the CHF population, heart transplantation may prolong survival and improve quality of life. However, the high costs of transplantation exclude a significant segment of the population.[33]

There are also less direct socioeconomic costs. Patients with milder forms of CHF, as in the Study of Men Born in 1913, reported less energy, lower levels of fitness, fewer spare-time activities, and more physical complaints compared to the non-CHF males in the population.[34]

Prognosis of heart failure

Regardless of the underlying cause, CHF always is a serious condition indicating a poor prognosis.[15,16,35–39] CHF is a highly lethal disease, as lethal as several common malignancies (Fig. 2.2). With more advanced heart failure, as studied in the Framingham study, 37% of the men and 38% of the women died within 2 years,

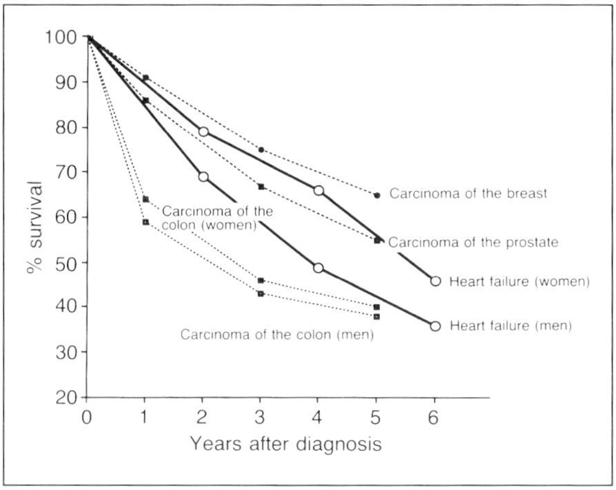

Fig. 2.2
Survival curves for heart failure and various forms of cancer among males and females aged 55–74 years. (Data from the Framingham Study[40] and the Norwegian Cancer Registry, Oslo, 1980.)

and within 6 years 82% of men and 67% of women had died.[10] In addition, congestive heart failure remains highly lethal, with a median survival time of 1.7 years in men and 3.2 years in women.[41]

The Finnish study (Boston criteria for definition of CHF) recently reported a 5–7-year follow-up of possible and definite CHF. Mortality rates were found to be 17% and 65% for possible and definite heart failure compared to 9% in the non-CHF men and women.[42]

Comparative 5-year mortality in mild to moderate CHF (as in the Study of Men Born in 1913) was 26% compared to 8% in non-CHF men.[16]

In the NHANES-I Epidemiologic Follow-up Study (1982 to 1984), overall 10-year mortality due to heart failure (men and women, aged 25–74 years) was 43% in those with self-reported heart failure and 38% in those with heart failure defined by a clinical score. The mortality rate was three to five times higher than in those without heart failure.[20]

For those with heart failure who are admitted to hospital, the in-hospital mortality rate is as high as 20–30%.[27,32]

Despite changes in the strategy of treating heart failure during a 40-year follow-up in the Framingham study, a 5-year death rate of more than 50% has remained stable with conventional therapy over this period.[43] However, it is too early to evaluate the global importance of ACE inhibitors on CHF in the community.

Not only mortality but also morbidity represents a significant component of the tragedy of heart failure. Within 6 years of initial diagnosis, more than 60% of men and women will experience one or more recurrences of overt heart failure. Moreover, those with CHF will have a four-fold higher risk of stroke and 2.5–5 times greater likelihood of myocardial infarction than the general population.[44] The association of left ventricular dysfunction and overt heart failure with increased risk of ischaemic manifestations was demonstrated in findings of the SOLVD studies. In the two SOLVD studies combined, placebo-treated patients had a 22% greater risk of myocardial infarction and unstable angina, compared to patients treated with an ACE-inhibitor.[45]

Conclusion

The similarity of the prognosis of CHF to that of several malignancies, together with increasing prevalence and incidence of CHF, suggests that heart failure will be one of our greatest public health problems in the future. Therefore, heart failure has to be taken seriously. Whether modern treatment strategies, including ACE inhibitors, will alter such an increasing public health problem has to be studied further. As the 20th century draws to a close, the challenge will be to arrest the progression of heart failure at an early stage, before prognosis becomes poor. Consequently, identification of early symptoms of CHF, proper diagnosis and treatment of heart diseases as well as intervention on risk factors for the underlying heart diseases are clearly desirable objectives in the future.

Acknowledgements

This review was supported by grants from the Swedish Medical Research Council (B95-27X-06276-14C), King Gustav V and Queen Victoria's Foundation, the Swedish Heart and Lung Foundation, the Gothenburg Medical Association, and the University of Gothenburg.

References

1 Gillum, RF, Folsom AR, Blackburn H. The decline in coronary heart disease mortality. Old questions and new facts. *Am J Med* 1984; **76**:1055–1065.

2 Wilhelmsen L, Johansson S, Ulvenstam G, et al. CHD in Sweden: mortality, incidence and risk factors over 20 years in Gothenburg. *Int J Epidemiol* 1989;18(suppl 1):S101–S108.

3 Sytkowski PA, Kannel WB, D'Agostino RB. Changes in risk factors and the decline in mortality from cardiovascular disease. *N Engl J Med* 1990;**322**:1635–1641.

4 Ghali JK, Cooper R, Ford E. Trends in hospitalization rates for heart failure in the United States 1973–1986: evidence for increasing population prevalence. *Arch Intern Med* 1990; **150**:769–773.

5 Gillum RF. Heart failure in the United States 1970–1985. *Am Heart J* 1987;**113**:1043–1045.

6 Gillum RF. Epidemiology of heart failure in the United States. *Am Heart J* 1993;126:1042–1047.

7 Levy RI. Causes of the decreases in cardiovascular mortality. *Am J Cardiol* 1984;**54**:7C–13C.

8 Yusuf S, Thom T, Abbott RD. Changes in hypertension treatment and in congestive heart failure mortality in United States. *Hypertension* 1989;**13(suppl I)**: I74–I79.

9 Denolin H, Kuhn H, Krayenbuel AP, et al. The definition of heart failure. *Eur Heart J* 1983; **4**:445–448.

10 Kannel WB, Belanger, AJ. Epidemiology of heart failure. *Am Heart J* 1991;**121**:951–957.

11 Klainer LM, Gibson TC, White KL. The epidemiology of cardiac failure. *J Chron Dis* 1965; **18:797–814.**

12 Logan WPD, Cushion AA. *Morbidity statistics from general practice*, volume 1. Studies on medical and population subjects (no 14). HMSO, London, 1958.

13 Gibson TC, White KL, Klainer LM. The prevalence of congestive heart failure in two rural communities. *J Chron Dis* 1966;**19**:141–152.

14 Parameshwar J, Shackell MM, Richardson A, et al. Prevalence of heart failure in three general practices in North West London. *Br J Gen Pract* 1992;**42**:287–289.

15 McKee PA, Castelli WP, McNamara PM, et al. The natural history of congestive heart failure: the Framingham Study. *N Engl J Med* 1971;**285**:1441–1446.

16 Eriksson H, Svärdsudd K, Larsson B, et al. Risk factors for heart failure in the general population. The study of men born in 1913. *Eur Heart J* 1989;**10**:647–656.

17 Remes J, Miettinen H, Reunanen A, Pyörälä K. Validity of clinical diagnosis of heart failure in primary health care. *Eur Heart J* 1991;**12**:315–321.

18 Wheeldon NM, MacDonald TM, Flucker CJ, McKendrick AD, McDevitt DG, Struthers AD. Echocardiography in chronic heart failure in the community. *Q J Med* 1993;**86**:17–23.

19 Landahl S, Svanborg A, Åstrand K. Heart volume and the prevalence of certain common cardiovascular disorders at 70 and 75 years of age. *Eur Heart J* 1984;**5**:326–331.

20 Schocken DD, Arrieta MI, Leaverton PE, et al. Prevalence and mortality rate of congestive heart failure in the United States. *J Am Coll Cardiol* 1992;**20**:301–306.

21 McFate Smith M. Epidemiology of congestive heart failure. *Am J Cardiol* 1985;**55**:3A–8A.

22 Remes J, Reunanen A, Aromaa A, et al. Incidence of heart failure in eastern Finland: a population-based surveillance study. *Eur Heart J* 1992;**13**:588–593.

23 Carlson KJ, Lee DCL, Goroll AH, et al. An analysis of physicians' reasons for prescribing long-term digitalis therapay in outpatients. *J Chron Dis* 1985;**38**:733–739.

24 Abel-Smith B. Global perspective on health service financing. *Soc Sci Med* 1985;**21**:957–963.

25 American Heart Association. Heart and Stroke Facts and Statistics. American Heart Association, Dallas, 1992.

26 Dinkel R, Büchner K, Holtz J. Chronic heart failure. Socioeconomic relevance in the Federal Republic of Germany. *Munch Med Wochenschr* 1989;**131**:686–689.
27 McMurray J, McDonagh T, Morrison CE, et al. Trends in hospitalization for heart failure in Scotland 1980–1990. *Eur Heart J* 1993; **14**:1158–1162.
28 Eriksson H, Wilhelmsen L, Caidahl K, et al. Epidemiology and prognosis of heart failure. *Z Kardiol* 1991;**80(suppl 8)**:1–6.
29 The SOLVD Investigators. Effect of enalapril on survival in patients with reduced left ventricular ejection fractions and congestive heart failure. *N Engl J Med* 1991;**325**:293–302.
30 Graves EJ. Detailed diagnosis and procedures: National Hospital Discharge Survey, 1990. National Center for Health Statistics. *Vital Health Statistics* 1992;**13**:113.
31 Eriksson H. Heart failure – a major public health problem. In: *Workshop: Pharmacological Treatment of Heart Failure*. Medical Products Agency 1993 (2):**7–19**.
32 Sutton GC. Epidemiological aspects of heart failure. *Am Heart J* 1990; **120**:1538–1540.
33 Copeland JG, Emery RW, Levinson MM, et al. Selection of patients for cardiac transplantation. *Circulation* 1987;**75**:2–9.
34 Eriksson H, Svärdsudd K, Larsson B, et al. Quality of life in early heart failure. The Study of Men Born in 1913. *Scand J Prim Health Care* 1988;**6**:161–167.
35 Massie BM, Conway M. Survival of patients with congestive heart failure: past, present and future prospects. *Circulation* 1987;**75(suppl IV)**:IV11–IV19.
36 Franciosa JA, Wilen M, Ziesche S, et al. Survival in men with severe chronic congestive heart failure due to coronary heart disease or dilated cardiomyopathy. *Am J Cardiol* 1983;**51**:831–836.
37 Califf RM, Bounous P, Harrell FE, et al. The prognosis in the presence of coronary artery disease. In: Braunwald E, Mock MB, Watson J, eds. *Congestive Heart Failure, Current Researches and Clinical Applications*. Grune and Stratton, New York, 1982.
38 Franciosa JA. Epidemiological patterns, clinical evaluation, and long term prognosis in chronic congestive heart failure. *Am J Med* 1986; **80(suppl 22)**:14–21.
39 Firth BG, Yancy CW Jr. Survival in congestive heart failure: have we made a difference? *Am J Med* 1990;**88(1N)**:3N–8N.
40 Kannel WB, Saveage D, Castelli WP. Cardiac failure in the Framingham Study: twenty-year follow-up. In: Braunwald E, Mock MB, Watson J, eds. *Congestive Heart Failure: Current Research and Clinical Applications*. Grune and Stratton, New York, 1982.
41 Ho KKL, Pinski JL, Kannel WB, et al. The epidemiology of heart failure: The Framingham Study. *J Am Coll Cardiol* 1993;**22(suppl A)**:6A–13A.
42 Remes J, Laitinen M, Reunanen A, et al. Mortality of patients with suspected heart failure can be predicted by using clinical observations. *Eur Heart J* 1994;**15(abstract suppl)**:539.
43 Ho KKL, Andersen KM, Kannel WB, et al. Survival after the onset of congestive heart failure in Framingham Heart Study subjects. *Circulation* 1993;**88**:107–115.
44 Kannel WB. Epidemiological aspects of heart failure. *Cardiol Clin* 1989;**7**:1–9.
45 Yusuf S, Pepine CJ, Garces C, et al. Effect of enalapril on myocardial infarction and unstable angina in patients with low ejection fractions. *Lancet* 1992;**340**:1173–1178.

3

The economic effects of ACE inhibitors

Andrew P Davie, John JV McMurray

Introduction

Angiotensin converting enzyme (ACE) inhibitors are the treatment of choice for chronic heart failure (CHF) secondary to left ventricular systolic dysfunction, which is itself secondary to ischaemic heart disease (IHD) or other aetiologies. However, it is estimated that less than 10% of CHF patients receive the treatment they require.[1]

One possible reason for this discrepancy is that ACE inhibitors are perceived as being expensive drugs. In fact, a number of formal economic analyses have shown that ACE inhibitors are extremely cost-effective. Whilst it is fairly easy to establish that ACE inhibitors may improve symptoms and prolong life, it is less readily apparent that ACE inhibitors may prevent hospitalization and save money. However, it follows that any treatment that improves symptoms has the potential to prevent hospitalization, and any treatment that has the potential to prevent hospitalization has the potential to save money, because of the high cost of hospitalization relative to the costs of treatment (for example, the cost of 1 or 2 days of hospitalization is equivalent to the cost of 1 year's treatment). ACE inhibitors do indeed have the desired effects, so that their benefits outweight their costs to the extent of greater cost-effectiveness, overall cost-neutrality, or even net cost savings. It is the effect of ACE inhibitors on hospitalization that is causal in this phenomenon, so a consideration of the economic effects of ACE inhibitors must first consider the effects of ACE inhibitors on hospitalization.

Effect of ACE inhibitors on hospitalization

At least seven major randomized double-blind placebo-controlled trials have included data on the effect of ACE inhibitors on hospitalization – the Cooperative North Scandinavian Enalapril Survival Study (CONSENSUS),[2,3] the Vasodilator-Heart Failure Trial (VHeFT II),[4,5] the Captopril-Digoxin Multicentre Research Group (CDMRG),[6] the treatment trial of the Studies of Left Ventricular Dysfunction (SOLVD-t),[7] the Munich Mild Heart Failure Trial (MHFT),[8,9] the prevention trial of the Studies of Left Ventricular Dysfunction (SOLVD-p),[10,11] and the Survival and Ventricular Enlargement Trial (SAVE).[12] The only exception to the rule that ACE inhibitors reduce rates of hospitalization for CHF was in VHeFT II which found no difference between ACE inhibitor and hydralazine–nitrate (VHeFT I having found no difference between hydralazine–nitrate and placebo). The results of the other six trials can be compared one against another if they are expressed in terms of hospitalizations per 100 patient years (Fig. 3.1).

There are a number of ways in which the comparisons implied in Fig. 3.1 are between groups that are not strictly comparable. The figures for CONSENSUS, SOLVD-t, SOLVD-p

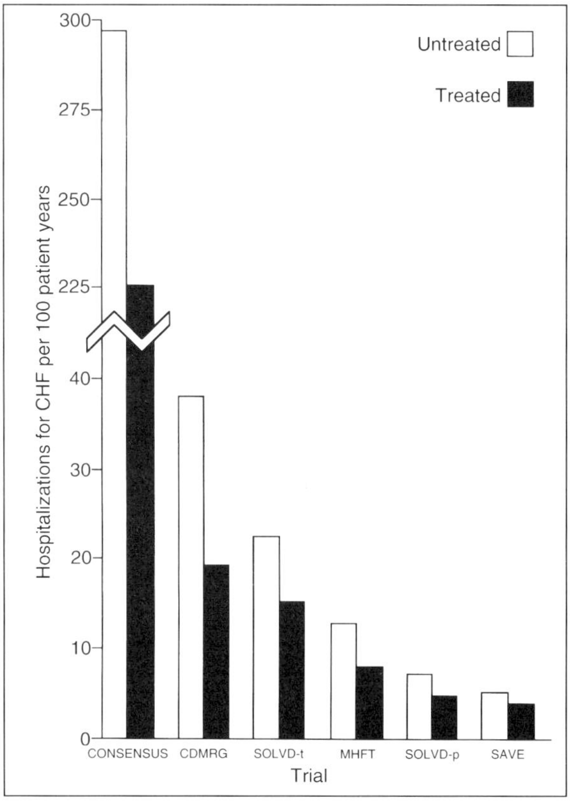

Fig. 3.1
Hospitalizations for CHF per 100 patient-years.

and SAVE are corrected for differential survival between treatment groups (otherwise treatment effects might be underestimated), but the figures for CDMRG and MHFT are not, because these shortest and smallest trials (respectively) did not find a significant difference in mortality. The figures for CDMRG, MHFT and SAVE are underestimates, as they represent numbers hospitalized rather than numbers of hospitalizations (which ignores the extra contribution of patients admitted more than once). The figures for all but CONSENSUS are for hospitalization for CHF as opposed to all hospitalizations although it is likely that most hospitalizations of the severely ill patients in CONSENSUS were directly or indirectly related to CHF in any case.

The trials in Fig. 3.1 are ranked in order of magnitude of the hospitalization problem (from 296 hospitalizations per 100 patient years for untreated patients in CONSENSUS to 3.9 per 100 patient years for treated patients in SAVE). This is an inalienable consequence of the fact that they are similarly ranked in order of severity of CHF (from exclusively NYHA class IV in CONSENSUS to exclusively NYHA class I in SAVE). It is also no coincidence that they are ranked in chronological order (from CONSENSUS in 1987 to SAVE in 1992), the clinical profile of ACE inhibitors having evolved through that time towards ever greater use ever earlier in the natural history of CHF.

It is a notable feature of Fig. 3.1 that there is a relatively constant treatment effect. Although the absolute number of hospitalizations saved with treatment depends on the underlying rate of hospitalization, the proportional reduction in hospitalization with treatment is of the same order of magnitude irrespective of the underlying rate of hospitalization (around one third, ranging from one fifth to one half). This is despite a significant dilutional effect, as all trials were analysed on an intention-to-treat basis, yet all trials had a significant rate of default in the treatment group (between 2.9% and 29% of treated patients) and all except CONSENSUS allowed open label active treatment in the placebo group (between 15% and 23% of untreated patients).

One of the most completely satisfactory of all the ACE inhibitor trials was SOLVD-t. It was one of the larger trials (only SAVE was larger) with a representative patient population (mainly NYHA classes II and III), a good length of follow-up (only VHeFT and SAVE were longer) and hospitalization for CHF was a predefined endpoint, with significant rates of hospitalization in both control and treatment groups, and a significant difference between the two. Formal analyses of the economic effects of ACE inhibitors have varied in their assumptions, design, application, results and sensitivity analyses, but SOLVD-t has been the premise for all but one.

German study[13]

The one economic analysis not based on SOLVD-t was based on MHFT; indeed it was a development of the original trial to include cost data on the majority of the original trial population over the length of the trial. It was thus possible to make a direct comparison of costs in the treated group with costs in the untreated group. Furthermore, the observed reduction in progression of CHF with treatment combined with the observed greater cost of progressive CHF implies that there were cost savings with treatment. These cost savings were not enough to lead to a net cost saving, but they did offset the cost of treatment by almost three-quarters (from DM76 per patient per month to DM20 per patient per month). As the analysis was based on actual costs there was no sensitivity analysis and, as there was no significant difference in mortality in MHFT, it was impossible to calculate an incremental cost-effectiveness ratio (that is, cost per life year gained).

Netherlands study[14,15]

The Institute for Medical Technology Assessment addressed the question: "What would be the costs and effects of using ACE inhibitors as first line pharmacotherapy for heart failure, in the Netherlands?". An epidemiological mode was developed to simulate the baseline scenario (current practice of only modest deployment of ACE inhibitors). The effect of ACE inhibitors as well as a number of sensitivity analyses was then examined by adjusting the appropriate input parameters. The model necessarily involved a number of assumptions, many of which were somewhat questionable, although the doubtfulness of some of these was addressed by the sensitivity analysis.

The analysis found that net costs decrease (Fig. 3.2) across a wide range of sensitivity analyses, despite a substantial benefit in terms of life years gained (Fig. 3.3), that is, costs decrease

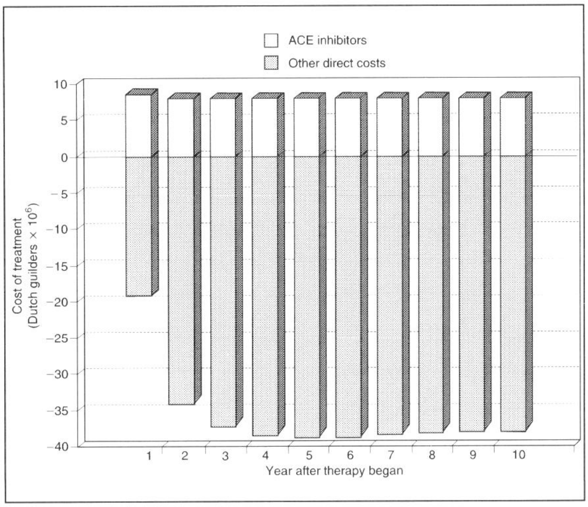

Fig. 3.2
Annual projected changes in costs of treatment of heart failure.

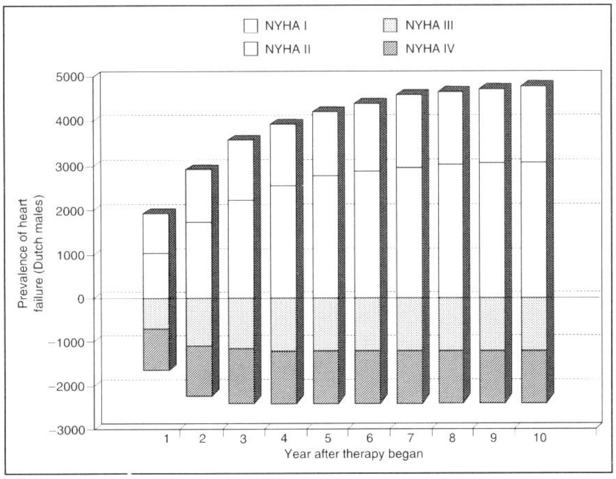

Fig. 3.3
Modelled changes in prevalence of heart failure.

and benefits increase. It would thus be highly misleading to express the results in terms of an incremental cost-effectiveness ratio, which assumes a directly proportional relationship between costs and benefits (that is, costs increase and benefits increase).

USA study[16]

A similar modelling approach was used by a group in the USA, though with a different set of assumptions and methods. It is hardly surprising, therefore, that they came to a different conclusion. Although the model was based on SOLVD-t, much of the sensitivity analysis (including two-way sensitivity analysis contour plots of incremental cost-effectiveness ratio) was concerned with the balance of difference between SOLVD-t, VHeFT I, and VHeFT II, perhaps because this analysis considered the effects of hydralazine–nitrate as well as ACE inhibitors. Indeed the result was a cheaper incremental cost-effectiveness ratio for hydralazine–nitrate compared with standard therapy (i.e. diuretics and digoxin) (US$5600 per life year gained) than for ACE inhibitors compared with hydralazine–nitrate (US$9700 per life year gained). This was qualified, however, with the proviso that ACE inhibitors are a more efficacious treatment (and their greater efficacy may exceed their more expensive cost-effectiveness, even though their greater efficacy is exceeded by their greater cost) and their cost-effectiveness compares favourably with standard therapies.

UK study[17]

A straightforward cost-benefit equation was used to examine the application of SOLVD-t to the UK. This derived estimates of lives saved and hospitalizations prevented from SOLVD-t and combined them with estimates of hospitalization costs, drug costs, blood chemistry costs, out-patient costs and general practice costs[18] to calculate an incremental cost-effectiveness ratio under various conditions of initiation and follow-up. This study was the only one to consider the effects of the extra costs of initiation of treatment in its sensitivity analysis, yet this was found to be a potent determinant of cost-effectiveness. Proposed initiation scenarios ranged from all patients admitted to hospital for 3 days,[19] to all patients admitted to hospital for 1 day, to 40% of patients admitted to hospital for 1 day,[20] to all patients initiated in the community. Most practitioners would probably adopt an approach somewhere in the middle of these in terms of cost-effectiveness (for example, the majority of patients admitted to hospital as a day case). The range of cost-effectiveness was wide, from £2508 per life year gained of £747 per life year gained to £251 per life year gained to a net cost saving of £11 per patient treated, for the above scenarios. These figures can be converted to cost-quality-adjusted-life-year (QALY) by giving CHF life years gained a quality-adjusted value of 0.5.[21] This gives a cost/QALY of £502 for treating CHF with ACE inhibitors assuming 40% of patients admitted to hospital for 1 day for initiation. This compares favourably with other widely quoted examples of cost-effective treatments (Table 3.1).[22]

SOLVD study[23]

The SOLVD investigators themselves have supplied an economic analysis of the consequences of their findings. This combined trial data on survival and events, including hospitalization, with estimates of costs in order to examine the economic effects of ACE inhibitors over the lifetime of the trial. A model was also developed to extrapolate these findings over the patient lifetime, specifically addressing the question of whether or not ACE inhibitors save costs or

	Cost/QALY
ACE inhibitor for CHF	£502
Pacemaker implantation	£1100
Aortic valve replacement	£1140
Hip replacement	£1180
CABG (left main stem stenosis)	£2090
Kidney transplant	£4710
Breast cancer screening	£5780
Heart transplant	£7840
CABG (single vessel disease)	£18 830
Renal haemodialysis	£21 970

Table 3.1
Cost per quality-adjusted-life-year (QALY), 1990 prices.

merely postpone them. A net cost saving of US$691 over 4 years mainly in the first 16 months was sustained although contained to $71 over a lifetime. This is at least consistent with the US sensitivity analysis which found that the overall cost-effectiveness of ACE inhibitors is relatively insensitive to whether or not their efficacy lasts indefinitely.

Costs and sensitivity analyses

These economic analyses differ widely in their methods. That they differ in their results arises not least because apart from making different assumptions, they consider different costs and apply different sensitivity analyses. It is no surprise that they all consider hospitalization costs and drug costs, as these are the main variables in the cost–benefit equation. Only the Netherlands and UK studies considered general practice costs, only the Netherlands study considered nursing home and district nursing costs, and only the UK study considered initiation costs, monitoring costs, and outpatient costs. Only the Netherlands study considered indirect costs (those due to production losses) although it was somewhat dismissive of their effects (covering them under a 'friction costs' approach). Only the SOLVD study considered the direct costs of death and none of the studies considered the indirect costs of death.

With respect to sensitivity analysis, the Netherlands, US and UK studies considered the effect of varying the proposed efficacy of treatment with ACE inhibitors and found the economic analysis to be sensitive to this variable, especially in the Netherlands study. The US, UK and SOLVD studies considered the effect of varying hospitalization costs and found the economic analysis to be sensitive to this variable, which is hardly surprising. It is similarly unsurprising that the US study found their economic analysis to be sensitive to drug costs. The US and UK studies considered the effect of a discount rate and found the economic analysis to be relatively insensitive to this variable. The US study found greater sensitivity to varying mortality than the Netherlands study. Other factors considered included initiation and follow-up strategies in the UK study, dose regime in the SOLVD study, and duration of efficacy in the US study.

Conclusion

It is not difficult to conclude from the major ACE inhibitor trials that ACE inhibitors prevent hospitalization for CHF. It follows from this that cost-savings will accrue to set against the cost of treatment, though these savings may or may not be enough to result in net cost savings. They will at least result in a more cost-effective treatment. The German study found just that, the Netherlands study proposed that benefits increase and costs decrease, the US study proposed a moderately cost-effective treatment, the UK study proposed a net cost saving in certain scenarios and the SOLVD study proposed a net cost saving, even over the entire lifetime of a patient.

These may seem to be a diverse set of conclusions but there is a consensus of opinion. ACE inhibitors are not only more cost-effective than they at first appear to be, in fact they are highly cost-effective compared with other therapies. That is the most conservative interpretation of the available economic analyses. A more radical reading of the situation, however, suggests that treatment of CHF with ACE inhibitors may represent a scenario in which benefits increase and costs decrease. Treatment of patients with ACE inhibitors in whom it is clinically indicated may be verging on economic necessity.

References

1 Editorial. Failure to treat heart failure. *Lancet* 1992;**329**:278–279.

2 The CONSENSUS Trial Study Group. Effects of enalapril on mortality in severe congestive heart failure. *N Engl J Med* 1987;**316**:1429–1435.

3 Kjekshus JD, Swedberg K. Tolerability of enalapril in congestive heart failure. *Am J Cardiol* 1988;**62**(**Suppl A**):67A–72A.

4 Cohn JN, Johnson G, Ziesche S, et al. A comparison of enalapril with hydralazine-isosorbide dinitrate in the treatment of chronic congestive heart failure. *N Engl J Med* 1991;**325**:303–310.

5 Loeb HS, Johnson MS, Henrick A, et al. Effect of enalapril, hydralazine plus isosorbide dinitrate, and prazosin on hospitalization in patients with chronic congestive heart failure. *Circulation* 1992;**87**(Suppl VI):V178–V187.

6 The Captopril-Digoxin Multicenter Research Group. Comparative effects of therapy with captopril and digoxin in patients with mild to moderate heart failure. *JAMA* 1988;**259**:539–544.

7 The SOLVD Investigators. Effect of enalapril on survival in patients with reduced left ventricular ejection fractions and congestive heart failure. *N Engl J Med* 1991;**325**:293–302.

8 Kleber FX, Niemoller L, Doering W. Impact of converting enzyme inhibition on progression of chronic heart failure. *Br Heart J* 1992;**67**:289–296.

9 Kleber FX. Socioeconomic aspects of ACE inhibition in the secondary prevention of cardiovascular diseases. *Am J Hypertens* 1994;**7**:112S–116S.

10 Pfeffer MA, Braunwald E, Moye LA, et al. Effect of captopril on mortality and morbidity in patients with left ventricular dysfunction after myocardial infarction. *N Engl J Med* 1992;**327**:669–677.

11 The SOLVD Investigators. Effect on enalapril on mortality and the development of heart failure in asymptomatic patients with reduced left ventricular ejection fractions. *N Engl J Med* 1992;**327**:685–691.

12 Cohn JN, Archibald DG, Ziesche S, et al. Effect of vasodilator therapy in chronic congestive heart failure. *N Engl J Med* 1986;**314**:1547–1552.

13 Kleber FX, Niemoller L, Rohrbacher R. Socioeconomic significance of ACE inhibitors in early forms of cardiac insufficiency. *Munch Med Wschr* 1992;**134**:749–752.

14 van Hout BA, Wielink G, Bonsel GJ, Rutten FFH. Effects of ACE inhibitors on heart failure in the Netherlands. *PharmacoEconomics* 1993;**3**:387–397.

15 van Hout BA, Wielink G, Bonsel GJ, Rutten FFH. Heart failure and ACE inhibitors. *iMTA* Report number 92.13. Erasmus University, Rotterdam, 1992.

16 Paul SD, Kuntz KM, Eagle KA, Weinstein MC. Costs and effectiveness of angiotensin converting enzyme inhibition in patients with congestive heart failure. *Arch Intern Med* 1994;**154**:1143–1149.

17 Hart W, Rhodes G, McMurray JJV. The cost effectiveness of enalapril in the treatment of chronic heart failure. *Br J Med Economics* 1993;**6**:91–98.

18 McMurray JJV, Hart W, Rhodes G. An evaluation of the cost of heart failure to the National Health Service in the UK. *Br J Med Economics* 1993;**6**:99–110.

19 McMurray JJV, Lang C, Struthers AD, et al. Current practice in the use of angiotensin converting enzyme inhibitors by Scottish physicians in the treatment of chronic heart failure. *Scot Med J* 1989;**34**:428–430.

20 Hood WB, Youngblood M, Ghali JK, et al. Initial blood pressure response to enalapril in hospitalized patients. *Am J Cardiol* 1991;**68**:1465–1568.

21 Euroquol 1990.

22 Mason J, Drummond M, Torrance G. Some guidelines on the use of cost effectiveness league tables. *BMJ* 1993;**306**:570–572.

23 Gerth WC. Personal communication.

4

Heart failure in the elderly: the same syndrome as the clinical trials?

Shaun T O'Keeffe, Michael DW Lye

Ageing and the cardiovascular system

For convenience, people older than 65 years are often grouped together as 'the elderly'. Indeed, this convention will be followed in this chapter. Nevertheless, it must be recognized that people of 65 years and more are the most heterogenous group within the population. Also, there are immense differences in physiological and pathological states between those aged 65 to 75 years and those aged more than 75 years. Age-related changes in physiological capacity frequently interact with pathological changes, and many changes that are considered 'age-related' may in fact be due to subclinical disease. A distinction can be drawn between 'successful ageing', in which changes in functional capacity with advancing age are solely physiological, and 'usual ageing', in which the effects of prevalent diseases and adverse environmental and lifestyle factors are combined with true 'age-related' changes. Unfortunately, successful ageing is relatively uncommon.

The wide variability in results of studies dealing with cardiac function and ageing is in part related to the high prevalence of occult coronary heart disease in elderly people. For example, approximately 50% of people aged 60 years and more have severe coronary artery narrowing, but only 50% of these have clinical symptoms and signs.[1] Rigorous screening of elderly subjects in studies on ageing to exclude coronary artery disease is a relatively recent development.

Additionally, the sedentary lifestyle of many older people results in physical deconditioning, which adversely effects exercise capacity and cardiovascular performance.

Structural changes

Systolic and, to a lesser extent, diastolic blood pressure increase with age. Changes in the architecture of peripheral arteries increase the stiffness of vessel walls; these changes include increased calcification, changes in the cross-linking of collagen, loss of elastin, and thickening of the smooth muscle layers in the media.[2] However, arterial stiffness is related, at least in part, to salt consumption and so may not be a true intrinsic age-related change.[3] Changes in the structure of the vessel wall cannot be explained on the basis of atherosclerosis.

Increased stiffness of the ascending aorta and a fall in the total cross-sectional area of the peripheral vasculature increases the impedance to left ventricular ejection. This is one reason for the slightly increased left ventricular wall thickness observed in normotensive elderly subjects. This increase in thickness is attributed chiefly to an increase in myocyte size, although myocyte hyperplasia may also be important.[4] There is a progressive age-related decrease in myocyte number and in the number of cells in the sinus node. In general, the overall size of the heart does not change grossly with age, although increased left atrial size with age has been reported even in subjects carefully screened to exclude disease.[5]

Resting systolic function

Data from animal models suggest that contractile force production of the myocyte is preserved with age, although the velocity of tension development is slowed.[6] Although afterload increases with age, the increase in left ventricular mass acts to normalize wall tension, and ejection fraction and end-systolic volumes are maintained at rest in healthy elderly subjects.[7]

Resting heart rate does not change with age, although spontaneous variation in heart rate over 24 hours does decrease.[8] A moderate age-related decrease in cardiac output has been reported in cross-sectional studies.[9] However, in healthy active subjects screened by exercise testing and thallium scintigraphy to exclude coronary artery disease, resting cardiac output remains virtually unchanged with age.[10] In this study of highly selected people, the decrease in heart rate seen with increased age was offset by an increase in stroke volume.

Diastolic function

Left ventricular diastolic function is altered by increasing age, and this has major implications for the pattern of heart failure in the elderly. Many echocardiographic and radionuclide studies have shown age-related decreases in the rate and extent of early diastolic rapid filling.[11,12] Although similar changes occur in patients with systemic hypertension and coronary artery disease,[13] changes in diastolic function with increasing age have been confirmed in subjects screened to exclude coronary artery disease and in subjects matched for potentially confounding haemodynamic variables.[14]

Two factors contribute to impaired diastolic function in the elderly:

- structural changes, including increased left ventricular mass and increased myocardial collagen, which decrease ventricular compliance; and
- cellular mechanisms involved in ventricular filling, which alter with age.

Early ventricular filling is an active, energy-requiring process directed at removing calcium from myocardial cells into the sarcoplasmic reticulum. Depressed function of the sodium–calcium trans-sarcoplasmic exchange pump and of the calcium pump in the sarcoplasmic reticulum result in relative intracellular calcium overload and prolonged interaction of the contractile proteins.[6,15] Recent evidence that short-term verapamil treatment can improve ventricular filling in healthy elderly subjects emphasizes the importance of these dynamic cellular mechanisms in determining age-related diastolic dysfunction.[16] Vigorous atrial contraction compensates for the decline in early diastolic ventricular filling, and there is no reduction in end-diastolic volume in healthy subjects.[17] However, the pressure–volume relationship is shifted to the right as a result of diastolic changes, and the same volume of blood is accommodated at a higher left ventricular end-diastolic pressure.[18]

Exercise capacity

Maximal physical work capacity decreases with age. Decline in maximum oxygen consumption rate (VO_{2max}) with ageing has been documented in cross-sectional and longitudinal studies.[19,20] However, it remains unclear to what extent this can be attributed to a decline in cardiac reserve.

There is little direct evidence that limitation of cardiac output limits peak work capacity in elderly people screened to exclude occult disease.[15] In healthy elderly subjects who participated in the Baltimore Longitudinal Study on Aging, ejection fraction still increased with exercise, although less than in younger subjects.[10] At a given work load, exercise-induced increase in heart rate is attenuated in elderly subjects. Hence, the increase in stroke volume during exercise is accomplished by an increase (which may be as high as 30%) in end-diastolic volume – that is, by reliance on the Frank–Starling mechanism.[10] Young subjects, in contrast, increase stroke volume by a decrease in end-systolic volume, probably as a result of beta-adrenergic stimulation. The haemodynamic profile in older patients resembles that seen in healthy young subjects who are given propranolol before exercise. Thus, decreased responsiveness to beta-adrenergic stimulation may partly explain age-related changes in the cardiac response to exercise.[21]

Peripheral circulatory factors probably contribute to the decline in maximal oxygen consumption with age. Peak arteriovenous oxygen difference has been reported to decline with age.[19] However, correction of peak arteriovenous oxygen difference for muscle mass greatly attenuates the age-related decline.[22] Also, a sedentary lifestyle may account for much of the decline in VO_{2max}; exercise training may significantly increase VO_2 in elderly subjects.[23]

Diagnosis of heart failure in the elderly

There are a number of difficulties in performing and analysing research into heart failure in the elderly. The clinical diagnosis of heart failure is frequently inaccurate or unsubstantiated by objective tests.[24,25] In a study of 500 patients in Nottinghamshire who were treated with loop diuretics by their general practitioner, only 56% satisfied quite broad diagnostic criteria for heart failure, and less than half were referred to hospital; elderly patients (median age 80) were least likely to be referred to hospital.[26]

Even the use of formal clinical scoring systems to diagnose heart failure, as for example in the Framingham study, does not necessarily guarantee diagnostic accuracy in older patients.[27–29] The specificity of many of the classical symptoms and signs of heart failure is poor in older patients.[30] Pulmonary crackles and peripheral oedema occur in many healthy elderly people and in many people with diseases other than heart failure. Left ventricular fourth heart sound is also common in healthy elderly people.[31] Respiratory disease and physical deconditioning are common causes of dyspnoea in the elderly. Failure to appreciate these facts might lead to overdiagnosis of heart failure in the elderly.

Underdiagnosis is also possible since heart failure may present in later life with non-cardiac symptoms such as delirium, immobility or anorexia. Cognitive impairment often makes it difficult to obtain a reliable history. Finally, as with other clinical signs, the reproducibility of cardiac signs is often relatively poor, even for experienced examiners;[32] it is likely that this is even more of a problem with elderly patients.

Diagnosis and monitoring of mild congestive heart failure is particularly difficult. Exercise testing, for example a 6-minute walk or the use of a self-powered treadmill, has been used in this setting.[33,34] While this approach may be valuable in selected elderly people, neurological and musculoskeletal problems limit its value in many. Additionally, the discriminant and prognostic value of exercise testing is least in patients with mild heart failure.[33] Recently, Hausdorf and colleagues have reported that increased step rate variability during walking is characteristic of elderly people with heart failure and may be a better discriminant of normal elderly from elderly people with heart failure than either step rate or distance walked.[35]

There has been considerable recent interest in the use of natriuretic peptides to diagnose mild heart failure and asymptomatic left ventricular systolic dysfunction.[36] In a study of frail nursing home residents, high atrial natriuretic peptide levels at baseline were an independent predictor of risk for developing clinical heart failure during the following year.[37] Further work is needed to confirm this finding.

Epidemiology of heart failure in the elderly

The difficulties described above mean that the scarce data from different studies regarding the epidemiology of heart failure in the elderly are hard to compare.

In the Framingham study, the average incidence rates for development of the first episode of clinical heart failure increased from 1–2 per 1000 between the ages of 45 and 54 to 13 per 1000 at 75–84 years, and to more than 50 per 1000 at 85–94 years.[27] Framingham prevalence figures for heart failure also show a substantial increase with age, from 0.8% in people 50–59 years of age to 2.3% at ages 60–69, 4.9% at ages 70–79, and 9.1% in those over 75 years.[28] The criteria used in the Framingham studies are strict, and the real frequency of heart failure may be underestimated.

In a longitudinal population study in Gothenburg, Sweden, the prevalence in men of 'manifest heart failure', defined as cardiac disease in association with dyspnoea, increased from 2% at 50 years of age to 13% at 67 years of age.[38] Another report from Gothenburg identified heart failure in 11% of women and 17% of men aged 75 years.[39]

In a study of general practices in the London area, Sutton studied the records of patients taking diuretics and noted a prevalence of heart failure of 0.06% in those under 65 years and 2.8% in those aged more than 65 years.[25] The overall prevalence of 0.4% in this study is substantially lower than the 1% prevalence figure for the USA calculated by Smith by extrapolating the Framingham data to the 1981 USA census data.[40] However, a study in Dundee, Scotland, estimated that the prevalence across all adult age ranges of systolic dysfunction is 0.8%;[41] since systolic dysfunction may account for two thirds of clinical heart failure,[2] this suggests an overall prevalence of about 1.2%, which is compatible with the USA data.

Systolic versus diastolic heart failure

In recent years it has become apparent that a substantial proportion of people with clinical heart failure due to various aetiologies have normal systolic function by echocardiography or radionuclide scanning (Table 4.1). Heart failure patients who have normal non-invasive indices of systolic function are usually presumed to have abnormal diastolic function – hence the widespread use of the term 'diastolic heart failure' even in studies where no attempt has been made to assess diastolic function. Proof of diastolic impairment requires invasive studies to document an increase in filling pressure of the left ventricle. Non-invasive indirect techniques such as doppler echocardiography and radionuclide scanning are frequently used to assess filling indices of the ventricle. However, these indices are influenced by preload, afterload, and heart rate.[13] Salt retention or reflex vasoconstriction may improve the pressure gradient between the left atrium and left ventricle and 'normalize' the non-invasive filling indices.[53] Thus, diastolic filling indices were normal in

Reference	No. of patients	Age (years)	Systolic function: Definition	Systolic function: % normal
Takarada et al[42]	62	≤65	ef ≥45, echo	12
	110	≥65		30
Wong et al[43]	17	≤60	echo*	6
	28	61–70		21
	54	>70		41
Soufer et al[44]	74	not stated	ef ≥45, radionuclide scan	42
Echeverria et al[45]	50	56	ef ≥50, echo	40
Cohn and Johnson[46]	623	59	ef ≥45, radionuclide scan	13
Dougherty et al[47]	188	63	ef ≥45, radionuclide scan	36
Aguirre et al[48]	151	69	ef ≥55, echo	34
Taffet et al[49]	94	83	ef ≥45, radionuclide scan/echo	43
Aronow et al[50]	247	82	ef ≥50, echo	47
Luchi et al[51]	12	86	ef ≥45, radionuclide scan	58
Forman et al[52]	47	87	ef ≥50, echo	74

Table 4.1
*Heart failure with normal systolic function. (ef – ejection fraction. *Normal systolic function was defined here as the absence of regional or global wall motion abnormality on 2-dimensional echocardiography.)*

the majority of patients with presumed diastolic heart failure in two series.[44,48]

Data from hospital series suggest that heart failure with normal systolic function is commoner in older patients. Because of the additional effects of age-related changes in diastolic filling, it is not surprising that heart failure due to diastolic dysfunction is seen most frequently in elderly subjects. However, it is also possible that heart failure is being overdiagnosed in elderly patients. Age-related changes in filling patterns impede interpretation of the indices of diastolic filling in the elderly. Nevertheless, recent work has confirmed the reproducibility of doppler-derived diastolic indices in most elderly subjects.[54] Data from the Framingham study have provided reference values in healthy subjects for different age groups, and this will assist interpretation of future studies.[55]

It has been suggested that patients with systolic dysfunction tend to have gradually worsening daytime symptoms and paroxysmal nocturnal dyspnoea, whereas acute rapid deterioration is characteristic of diastolic impairment.[49,56] However, other reports have failed to confirm these findings and, in general, clinical features are not helpful in distinguishing between systolic and diastolic impairment (Table 4.2).

Aetiology of heart failure in the elderly

The main causes of heart failure in the elderly are similar to those in younger patients, namely coronary artery disease and hypertension. However, as with other conditions, heart failure in elderly patients is characterized by multiple aetiologies and precipitating factors and by the interaction of pathology with the age-related changes discussed earlier. For example, elderly subjects rely on atrial contraction to

	Normal systolic function (%)	Abnormal systolic function (%)
Jugular venous distension	39	48
Third heart sound gallop	36	53
Fourth heart sound gallop	47	49
Crackles (râles)	59	56
Peripheral oedema	39	51

Table 4.2
Clinical features in heart failure patients with and without systolic impairment. Data are mean percentages derived from three studies.[45,47,48]

compensate for impaired early diastolic filling, and the development of atrial fibrillation, which occurs in up to 4% of patients over 70 years, may readily precipitate clinical heart failure.[57]

Coronary artery disease

Ischaemic heart disease is probably now the most important cause of cardiac failure in the elderly.[2,58] In the Framingham study, the prevalence of pre-existing coronary heart disease among heart failure patients increased from 22% in the 1950s to 67% in the 1980s.[59] Other studies have reported similar findings,[60,61] Coronary artery disease can have adverse effects on both systolic and diastolic function. Myocardial ischaemia induced by rapid atrial pacing reversibly depresses diastolic function to a greater extent than systolic performance.[62] In 1948, Dodek and colleagues used the term 'stiff heart syndrome' to describe a heart condition in which recurrent episodes of pulmonary oedema occurred in patients with coronary artery disease who had no clinical or radiological evidence of cardiomegaly.[63] Recent studies have confirmed that isolated coronary artery disease is a common cause of diastolic heart failure, although some of these patients also have intermittent systolic dysfunction.[46–49]

Hypertension

In the Framingham study, hypertension preceded heart failure in 75% of cases.[28] Some writers have suggested that better detection and treatment of hypertension may have resulted in a shift in the aetiology of heart failure from hypertension to coronary artery disease.[58,64] Nevertheless, hypertension is still probably the commonest cause of diastolic heart failure. For example, Dougherty and colleagues reported that hypertension was a contributing factor in 65% of heart failure patients with normal systolic function and 23% of patients with abnormal systolic function;[47] other reports have noted similar findings.[42,65] Heart failure with normal systolic function in hypertensive patients is usually attributed to the effects on ventricular filling of myocardial hypertrophy. However, impaired left ventricular filling has been noted in hypertensive patients without hypertrophy.[18] Also, exercise-induced hypertrophy in athletes is not associated with abnormal diastolic filling.[66] Recent research has established that regional myocardial ischaemia, often due to coronary artery disease, is also an important aetiology of heart failure in hypertensive patients.[67]

Valvular heart disease

Heart murmurs occur in up to 7% of healthy elderly people.[68] Furthermore, mild, clinically inaudible valvular regurgitation can be detected using doppler echocardiography in almost all patients aged 80 years and over.[69] Clinically significant valvular heart disease increases in frequency with old age, chiefly owing to the effects of degenerative changes and ischaemic heart disease; rheumatic heart disease is now a relatively uncommon cause of heart failure.[27]

The commonest valve disorder in the elderly is calcific aortic stenosis. Using echocardiography, Aronow and Kronson identified mild calcific aortic stenosis in 9.4% and moderate or severe stenosis in 8.7% of almost 800 unselected long-stay patients with a mean age of 82 years.[70] Physical signs of aortic stenosis may not be obvious in elderly subjects with reduced cardiac output or increased stiffness of major arteries, and the severity of aortic stenosis cannot be determined reliably by clinical findings alone.[71] Heart failure is a late finding in aortic stenosis and is associated with a poor prognosis. Mitral regurgitation due to papillary muscle dysfunction from ischaemic heart disease or to degenerative changes of the annulus or leaflets is also an important common cause of heart failure in the elderly.[48] Surprisingly, severe mitral regurgitation causing heart failure may not be obvious on auscultation.[72]

Heart failure with normal systolic function but without an intrinsic abnormality of ventricular diastolic performance can be secondary to valvular disease. Heart failure has been attributed to aortic stenosis or mitral regurgitation in 8–30% of patients with normal systolic function.[44–48]

Cardiomyopathies

Cardiomyopathies are often thought of as diseases of younger people. However, it has become apparent in recent years that cardiomyopathies are significant causes of heart failure in the elderly. Hypertrophic and restrictive cardiomyopathies occur in 5–20% of elderly patients with heart failure who have normal systolic function,[44,47] while idiopathic dilated cardiomyopathy occurs in up to one third of elderly patients with abnormal systolic function.[42,45,47] In a population-based study in Minnesota, USA, the highest incidence and prevalence rates for both dilated cardiomyopathy and hypertrophic cardiomyopathy were in people over 75 years.[73] Although advanced age is an independent predictor of a poor outcome in dilated cardiomyopathy, elderly patients with hypertrophic cardiomyopathy have a relatively benign prognosis.[74]

There is an overlap between hypertensive heart disease and hypertrophic cardiomyopathy in the elderly. Topol and colleagues have described the entity of 'hypertensive hypertrophic cardiomyopathy of the elderly', which includes severe concentric hypertrophy, small left ventricular cavity, and supernormal indices of systolic function.[65] However, in the series of 134 elderly patients with hypertrophic cardiomyopathy described by Lewis and Maron, one third had relatively mild hypertension, and left ventricular hypertrophy was mild and localized compared with that commonly found in younger patients.[75] These authors also noted genetic transmission in 11% of the elderly patients. Although myosin gene mutations have not yet been documented in elderly hypertrophic cardiomyopathy patients, it is possible that hypertension can precipitate hypertrophic cardiomyopathy in genetically predisposed patients.[74,76]

Distinction of restrictive cardiomyopathy and age-related diastolic impairment is particularly difficult. The prototype of restrictive cardiomyopathy is amyloid heart disease, which is a common cause of death in patients with amyloidosis associated with immunocyte disorders. Although senile amyloid deposits are commonly found at *post mortem* in the very old, this is often thought to be a clinically insignificant finding. Nevertheless, cardiac amyloid was recorded as the cause of death in up to 10% of patients and was believed to have caused significant cardiac dysfunction in between one quarter and one half of patients in two series of autopsies in nonagenarians.[77,78]

Atrial fibrillation

The atrial contribution to ventricular filling is particularly important in patients with diastolic impairment. Wong and colleagues reported atrial fibrillation in 22% of elderly heart failure patients with decreased systolic function and in 54% of subjects with normal systolic function.[43]

Prognosis of heart failure in the elderly

Heart failure has a poor prognosis regardless of age. In the Framingham study, 2-year mortality was 37% in men and 38% in women;[27] the 6-year mortality was 82% in men and 67% in women, which is four to eight times higher than in the general population.[28] About 60% of patients with new-onset heart failure in the Framingham series had an underlying serious illness or chronic disease.

In a study in the 1950s, Bedford and Caird reported a 3-year mortality of 80% in men aged 65 years and more with heart failure.[79] They noted that patients who survived the first year after presentation with heart failure had a life expectancy 'at least equal to the normal'. A more recent study of veterans 75 years and older has confirmed this finding: Taffet and colleagues noted 28% of patients died within 1 year of their first documented episode of heart failure; after that, the slope of the survival curve did not differ from that of an age-matched control group.[49] Although some reports suggest that age is an important determinant of survival in heart failure,[80] analysis of data from the Veterans Affairs Heart Failure Trials (V-HeFT) suggested that age was not an independent predictor of survival in patients less than 75 years (Fig. 4.1).[81]

The prognosis of patients with heart failure caused by diastolic dysfunction is not as poor as in patients with abnormal systolic function. In the V-HeFT studies, the annual mortality in patients with heart failure and a normal ejection fraction was 8% compared with 18% in the low ejection fraction group.[46] Aronow and colleagues used a stepwise proportional hazards model to estimate that patients with coronary artery disease and a low ejection fraction had a

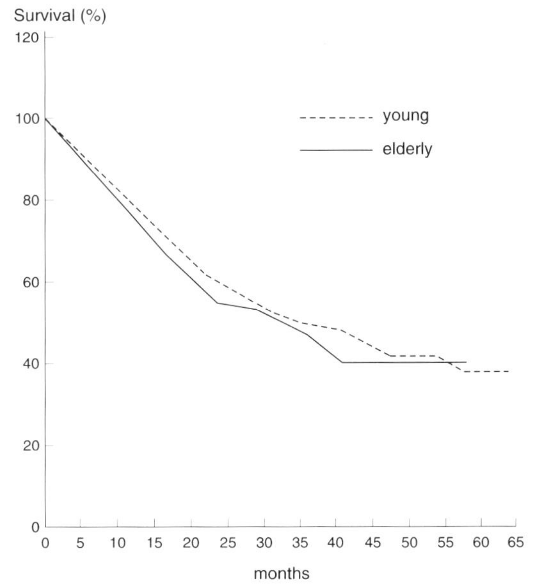

Fig. 4.1
Survival curves by age group in V-HeFT study. (From Reference 81.)

mortality rate 2.3 times higher than those with a normal ejection fraction.[50] Follow-up of 284 patients from the Coronary Artery Surgery Study registry data base who had moderate to severe heart failure symptoms but a normal left ventricular ejection fraction revealed a 6-year survival of 82%.[80] One reason why patients with diastolic heart failure could have a relatively good prognosis may be the relative absence of neurohormonal activation compared with patients with systolic heart failure,[82] although this could also be interpreted as indicating that the diagnosis of heart failure was incorrect.

A number of reports suggest that in older patients, the differences in mortality between systolic and diastolic heart failure may be less marked: Setaro and colleagues reported cardiovascular mortality of 46% at 7 years in patients with diastolic heart failure,[83] while Taffet and colleagues noted no difference in outcome between the two forms of heart failure at a minimum follow-up of 3 years.[49]

Heart failure is associated with considerable morbidity. Data from Hillingdon District General Hospital in London suggests that heart failure accounts for about 5% of adult medical and geriatric hospital admissions in the UK.[24] The average duration of hospital stay with heart failure ranges from 8–17 days in different reports.[20,80] Heart failure also accounts for a sizeable proportion of the workload of general practitioners.[41] In spite of the relatively good survival reported in several studies, morbidity from recurrent episodes of decompensation is also substantial in patients with diastolic heart failure.[85] This is not surprising since exercise incapacity may be more strongly related to diastolic impairment than to systolic impairment.[86]

Treatment of heart failure in the elderly

Systolic heart failure

Diuretics

Diuretics remain the cornerstone of the treatment of heart failure in the elderly. They alleviate the sodium retention that is characteristic of heart failure, thereby reducing ventricular and blood vessel wall stress and improving the symptoms of dyspnoea and oedema. The effects of diuretics on mortality in heart failure patients are unknown. In many patients with heart failure, diuretics alone are insufficient to maintain long-term symptomatic control, possibly because they increase neurohormonal activation.[87] Also, electrolyte depletion may be troublesome in some patients.

Patients with mild heart failure may be adequately controlled with treatment by thiazide diuretics.[88,89] However, thiazide diuretics, with the exception of metolazone, are not effective when glomerular filtration rate (GFR) falls below 30 ml/minute.[87] Loop diuretics produce a greater natriuresis and are effective until GFR falls to 5 ml/minute. Metabolic problems are less common with these agents than with thiazide diuretics. Urinary incontinence can be a significant problem when loop diuretics are used in elderly patients. This results from the reduced renal clearance and increased elimination half-life of these agents.

Angiotensin converting enzyme inhibitors

A series of large trials have established that angiotensin converting enzyme (ACE) inhibitors prolong survival and reduce progression of heart failure in patients with heart failure or asymptomatic systolic dysfunction. There is also evidence that ACE inhibitors may prevent development of heart failure when given to patients after myocardial infarction.

Are these results applicable to elderly people with heart failure? The CONSENSUS trial studied patients with severe heart failure (NYHA IV) and found improved cardiovascular and all-cause mortality in patients treated with enalapril compared with patients given placebo.[90] The mean age of patients in this study was 71 years, so these results are applicable at least to the 'young' elderly. Unfortunately, the SOLVD (treatment) and V-HeFT 2 trials which showed the benefits of ACE inhibitor treatment in patients with mild to moderate heart failure excluded patients older than 80 and 75 years respectively;[91,92] the mean age of patients in these studies was about 60 years. Furthermore, only patients with a reduced ejection fraction were included in these studies.

The SAVE and SOLVD (prevention) trials, which showed the value of ACE inhibition in preventing morbidity and mortality in patients with an asymptomatic reduction in ejection fraction, excluded patients older than 80 years, and the mean age of patients in both studies was only 59 years.[93,94] In the SAVE study, 15% of patients were 70 years or older, and a proportional hazards model showed that the effect of captopril in reducing mortality was independent of age.[93] The AIRE study randomized patients with clinical evidence of heart failure (transient or sustained) at any time after acute myocardial infarction to receive ramipril or placebo; all causes mortality was significantly reduced (17% *vs* 23%) in patients receiving ramipril.[95] There was no upper age limit in this study, and the mean age of the study population was 65(±11) years. Subgroup analysis confirmed the benefit with ramipril in patients older than 65 years.

Two studies in which ACE inhibitors were given to all patients after myocardial infarction have provided contrasting results. In the CONSENSUS 2 study, 6090 patients were randomized to receive either placebo or an intravenous infusion of enalapril within 24 hours of myocardial infarction.[96] The mean age of patients was 66 years, and 42% were aged 70 years or older. There was no significant difference in outcome between the treatment and the placebo groups. Furthermore, in a planned subgroup analysis, mortality was slightly higher in patients aged 70 years or older who were given enalapril (17% *vs* 15%, $p = 0.07$). Of the patients given enalapril, those who developed first-dose hypotension had a higher mortality rate (17% *vs* 9%), but the incidence of hypotension was similar in patients younger than 70 years and those aged 70 years or older. The GISSI-3 study randomized 18 895 patients, 27% of whom were aged 70 years or older, to receive oral lisinopril or placebo within 24 hours of infarction.[97] Treatment with lisinopril was associated with a significant reduction in mortality and a significant reduction in total adverse outcomes. The reduction in combined adverse outcomes was 12% for patients aged 70 years and older and 4% for those less than 70 years.

In general, the studies discussed above support the value of ACE inhibitors in elderly patients with symptomatic heart failure, and provide some evidence for treating elderly patients with ACE inhibitors after myocardial infarction. However, caution needs to be exercised. Because of the restricted age range of some of the large trials, it is not yet clear that the benefits of ACE inhibition can be extrapolated to patients aged 80 years or more, especially if heart failure is mild to moderate in severity. Hypotension and renal insufficiency due to ACE inhibitors are more common and less well tolerated in the older patient.[98] Impaired baroreceptor reflex sensitivity, use of other hypotensive medications, and the high frequency of extensive atheromatous disease in the elderly increase the risk of ACE-inhibitor-induced hypotension. Pre-existing renal impairment or renal artery stenosis, the high frequency of diabetes mellitus, and the use of non-steroidal anti-inflammatory agents increase the likelihood of ACE inhibitor-induced renal dysfunction. Cody and colleagues have demonstrated that age-related impairments in baroreceptor and renal function are superimposed on the changes associated with heart failure;[99] in their study, mean GFR in elderly (mean 72 years) patients with mild to moderate heart failure was only 35 ml/minute.

The three ACE inhibitors in widespread use at present – captopril, enalapril, and lisinopril – are excreted by glomerular filtration; delayed excretion, higher serum concentrations and more prolonged duration of action have been reported using these agents in the elderly.[100–103] The risk of serious adverse effects is likely to be highest in the very old; for example, O'Neill and colleagues gave a maximum of 2.5 mg of enalapril to 33 patients ranging in age from 72–93 years; 17 patients (52%) suffered adverse reactions, including 'dramatic' reduction in renal function in four patients and mesenteric ischaemia in four patients.[104] On the other hand, Murphy and colleagues reported no major renal impairment or hypotension in 30 heart failure patients with a mean age of 82 years who were given captopril, although 40% of patients failed to complete the 3-month study.[105]

For these reasons, considerable care should be exercised when starting ACE inhibitors in the elderly. Starting doses should be low and the dose increased slowly; renal function must be monitored carefully. First dose hypotension sometimes occurs later after the first dose in the elderly because of the altered pharmacokinetics of ACE inhibitors in the elderly. The authors' preference is to start treatment with 6.25 mg captopril twice daily and titrate the dose slowly upwards to 25 mg three times daily or 50 mg twice daily, then switch to a longer-acting agent to assist compliance.

Digoxin

The role of digoxin in treating heart failure patients with atrial fibrillation is well established; the role of digoxin in patients in sinus rhythm is more controversial. A meta-analysis of high-quality double-blind controlled trials concluded that digoxin was of benefit in 12% (95% confidence interval 3–20%) of patients with heart failure and sinus rhythm; predictors of benefit from digoxin were the presence of a third heart sound and increased severity and duration of heart failure.[106] Digoxin may also improve symptoms of cardiac failure even in patients receiving an optimal dose of ACE inhibitor.[107]

However, another analysis of the literature concluded that the benefits from digoxin in patients in sinus rhythm are at best modest, and there is even a question as to whether digoxin may worsen outcome during the year after a myocardial infarction.[108] Furthermore, the results of recent trials of other positive inotropic agents have been very discouraging.[109–111] The ongoing study conducted by the National Institutes of Health in the USA may clarify whether digoxin is beneficial or not.

The mean age of patients studied in the large digoxin trials has been relatively low (61 years), and few studies have specifically examined the risks and benefits of using digoxin in the elderly.[48,108–110] There are a number of reasons for particular caution in this age group:

- there is some evidence that clinical predictors identified in younger patients, such as a third heart sound or cardiomegaly, may be less useful in predicting a beneficial response;[108]
- the pharmacokinetics of digoxin are altered in old age – reduced volume of distribution, as a result of the reduction in lean body mass,

and reduced renal clearance mean that serum levels are generally higher in older patients for a given dose;

- digoxin toxicity is common in elderly patients and may present in an atypical manner;[111]
- side effects such as lassitude, anorexia, and delirium are particularly common in elderly patients and may develop even when serum digoxin levels are within the generally accepted therapeutic range;[112] and
- digoxin-induced cardiac arrhythmias may be particularly troublesome in patients with cardiac amyloidosis.[113]

In general, a maintenance dose of 0.125 mg or less daily is effective in most elderly people.

In conclusion, digoxin may benefit a proportion of elderly patients with severe heart failure that is due to systolic dysfunction. However, this must be set against the increased risk of side effects. In practice, the authors do not use digoxin in patients in sinus rhythm.

Diastolic heart failure

Until recently, therapeutic recommendations for heart failure were concerned solely with systolic dysfunction. The recent recognition that a large proportion of elderly patients have diastolic heart failure with normal systolic function presents a therapeutic problem, because, as yet, there have been no large clinical trials in this population. Furthermore, no agent with specific lusitropic (relaxation-enhancing) activity is available at present.

Treatment of the underlying cause of diastolic heart failure, such as hypertension or ischaemic heart disease, is a logical approach. Medications that lower blood pressure, cause regression of left ventricular hypertrophy, reduce intracellular calcium, reduce myocardial ischaemia, and slow the heart rate might be expected to benefit patients with diastolic dysfunction.

Although there has been much work to evaluate the effects of different agents on diastolic filling indices measured by echocardiography or radionuclide scanning, to date there are relatively little data regarding the long-term outcome of therapy in patients with symptomatic heart failure. Change (or lack of change) in non-invasive filling indices does not necessarily reflect changes in ventricular relaxation, since these indices are highly dependent on loading conditions. Also, changes in filling indices may not correlate well with change in clinical status.[83]

Maintenance of sinus rhythm

Atrial fibrillation is common in patients with clinical diastolic heart failure.[42,43] In such patients, restoration of sinus rhythm frequently increases cardiac output and exercise capacity and also reduces the risk of emboli.[118,119] Attempts to restore sinus rhythm are less often successful in older patients than they are in younger patients, primarily because of the high prevalence of chronic atrial fibrillation and left atrial enlargement in the elderly.[120,121] Nevertheless, in the authors' view, the potential benefits are such that an attempt should be considered, particularly in patients with heart failure. There are no trials in any age group that directly compare different methods of restoring and maintaining sinus rhythm in patients with atrial fibrillation. The authors' preference is to use chemical cardioversion with amiodarone followed by low dose maintenance amiodarone. This therapy is well tolerated in older patients, including those with heart failure.[122–124]

A decision analysis comparing different approaches to management of chronic atrial fibrillation in elderly people concluded that electrical cardioversion followed by low-dose amiodarone offered the lowest 5-year mortality and the best quality-adjusted life-years.[125]

Recent evidence of improved survival in patients with severe heart failure treated with low-dose amiodarone provides additional support for this approach.[126]

The importance of the atrial contribution to diastolic filling in elderly people also suggests that dual chamber pacemakers will benefit those patients in need of pacing, although because of the extra costs and 'ageist' attitudes, some physicians reserve such treatment for younger patients.[127,128] Retrospective non-randomized studies have reported that morbidity – including atrial fibrillation, stroke, and congestive heart failure – and mortality in elderly people are improved by atrial or dual chamber pacemakers.[129–131] In a prospective non-randomized study of patients with heart failure at the time of pacemaker implantation for high-degree atrioventricular block, Alpert and colleagues reported that those who received dual chamber pacemakers had a better 5-year survival than those who received a ventricular pacemaker (75% *vs* 57%, $p < 0.03$).[132] However, it has also been suggested that permanent pacing may accelerate haemodynamic deterioration in patients with severe heart failure.[133]

Treatment of hypertension

The commonest cause of diastolic heart failure is probably hypertension, usually, but not always, associated with left ventricular hypertrophy. Data from the EWPHE and STOP trials suggest that treatment of hypertension in the elderly can reduce the incidence of heart failure.[134,135] Gaasch has suggested that left ventricular hypertrophy can be taken as evidence for left ventricular dysfunction, even when clinical heart failure is mild or absent.[136] Two large meta-analyses have concluded that many antihypertensive agents produce a regression in left ventricular hypertrophy.[137,138] For example, Dahlöf and colleagues reported that ACE inhibitors reduced left ventricular mass by 15%, beta-blockers by 8%, calcium antagonists by 8.5%, and diuretics by 11.3%;[137] methyldopa also promotes regression of left ventricular hypertrophy, whereas vasodilators such as hydalazine have relatively little effect.[138] The mean age of patients in Dahlöf's meta-analysis was 47(±7) years. Relatively few studies have examined regression of hypertrophy in elderly subjects: Frishman and colleagues reported that the beta-blockers dilevalol and atenolol did not reduce left ventricular mass in elderly hypertensive patients;[139] Schulman and colleagues reported that verapamil but not atenolol reduced left ventricular mass;[140] and Nagano and colleagues reported reduced left ventricular mass with both calcium channel blockers and with ACE inhibitors in elderly subjects.[141]

Studies involving ACE inhibitors, beta-blockers, and calcium antagonists have demonstrated an improvement in diastolic filling indices with the reduction in left ventricular mass,[142–146] although there have been some negative reports.[147,148] Since the development of hypertrophy is an adaptive response to an increased workload, there had been concern that regression of hypertrophy might lead to systolic heart failure if antihypertensive medications were stopped and blood pressure returned to pretreatment levels.[149] However, Schulman and colleagues found that regression of left ventricular hypertrophy with improvement in diastolic filling in elderly hypertensives did not impair systolic function at rest or on exertion.[140]

Diuretics

Diuretics are effective in relieving symptoms in patients with heart failure with normal systolic function. Diuretics can improve the left ventricular pressure–volume relationship in heart failure.[150] One possible mechanism is that a reduction in right ventricular filling pressure may reduce the pericardial constraint on the heart. However, volume depletion is a major concern when treating elderly patients with diuretics, and patients with diastolic heart failure are particularly volume sensitive.[151] An excessive diuresis in a patient with impaired diastolic filling may result in a reduction in stroke volume and cardiac output. Thus, low doses of loop diuretics are advisable when commencing diuretics in elderly heart failure patients.

Angiotensin converting enzyme inhibitors
Little is known about the effects of ACE inhibitors in patients with diastolic heart failure. The acute vasodilator actions of ACE inhibitors might be deleterious in patients with stiff ventricles because vasodilatation might reduce stroke volume and cardiac output in such patients. Alternatively, there may be long-term benefits from blood pressure reduction and from regression of left ventricular hypertrophy.[137] Schunkert and colleagues have reported that tissue ACE activity is increased in pressure-overload hypertrophy, and the resulting increased production of angiotensin-II is associated with reduced ventricular relaxation and increased end-diastolic pressure.[152] Short-term inhibition of intracardiac ACE has been noted to improve the compliance of the left ventricle in patients with aortic stenosis and severe left ventricular hypertrophy.[153] The ability of ACE inhibitors to attenuate the coronary vasoconstrictor effects of angiotensin-II may also have benefits for diastolic function.

In an uncontrolled study, Aronow and Kronzon reported improved early ventricular filling and exercise tolerance after 3 months of treatment with enalapril in 10 elderly patients (mean age 80 years) with congestive heart failure due to ischaemic heart disease and a normal left ventricular ejection fraction.[154] However, double-blind controlled studies are needed to confirm this finding.

Digoxin
It is now apparent that digoxin is of little benefit and may even be harmful in patients with normal systolic function.[66] Cardiac muscle in patients with diastolic heart failure are already in a state of relative intracellular calcium overload, and digoxin acts to increase intracellular calcium further. In animal studies, treatment with digoxin increases left ventricular stiffness and left ventricular filling pressures.[155] In clinical studies, discontinuation of digoxin in elderly subjects with normal ejection fractions does not result in deterioration in heart failure.[52] In a randomized crossover trial of digoxin and placebo, Lee and colleagues noted clinical improvement with digoxin in 14 of 19 patients with systolic impairment and in none of six patients without systolic impairment.[156]

Calcium channel blockers
The theoretical benefits of calcium channel blockers in patients with diastolic dysfunction include blood pressure control and regression of left ventricular hypertrophy, reduction in intracellular calcium, and reduction in myocardial ischaemia. Verapamil has been investigated the most thoroughly. In healthy elderly subjects, verapamil improved diastolic filling without any detrimental effect on systolic function.[16] Setaro and colleagues conducted a double-blind placebo-controlled 5-week crossover trial of verapamil in 20 patients with a mean age of 68 years who had heart failure associated with normal ejection fraction and abnormal filling indices; 15 patients had a history of hypertension and five had coronary artery disease.[83] Clinical and radiographic features of heart failure improved with verapamil, but there was no correlation between the improved clinical status and changes in filling indices. Verapamil improves diastolic filling in patients with hypertrophic cardiomyopathy, and this correlates with improved exercise tolerance and reduction

in other symptoms of failure.[157,158] Other reports have suggested a clinical benefit from nifedipine in patients with diastolic heart failure that is due to a variety of causes.[159,160]

While the rationale behind the use of calcium antagonists in diastolic heart failure is appealing and the initial results are encouraging, a note of caution must be sounded. These agents have a negative inotropic action, and deleterious effects have been reported in patients with chronic heart failure, even with nifedipine, which is thought of as having relatively minor cardiodepressant effects.[161] Worsening of heart failure has also been reported when patients with diastolic impairment due to amyloid heart disease are treated with calcium channel blockers.[162] Furthermore, although the theoretical rationale for using calcium channel blockers in patients who have had a myocardial infarction is also appealing, the results of calcium antagonist therapy in this population have proved disappointing to date.[163] Larger and longer-term studies are required before these agents can be recommended for general use in patients with diastolic heart failure.

Beta-blockers

Since $beta_1$-agonists such as noradrenaline improve myocardial relaxation, beta-blockers might be expected to impair diastolic function. However, several studies have documented an improvement in diastolic filling with beta-blockers,[143,144] and Topol and colleagues reported that patients with diastolic heart failure and hypertension benefitted from atenolol or propranolol.[66] To date, improved diastolic filling with beta-blockade has not been convincingly demonstrated in the elderly. The reasons why beta-blockers may be of value in diastolic heart failure include control of blood pressure, regression of left ventricular hypertrophy, reduced myocardial oxygen demand, and slowing of heart rate to allow more time for ventricular filling especially during exercise.[18] Recently, Eichorn and colleagues investigated the effects of 3 months' therapy with bucindolol, a beta-blocker with vasodilator activity, in patients with heart failure from various causes; even at matched atrial pacing rates, bucindolol improved myocardial relaxation, assessed by measuring the time constant of ventricular relaxation.[164]

Like calcium antagonists, beta-blockers have negative inotropic actions. However, unlike calcium antagonists, there is increasing evidence that beta-blockers have beneficial haemodynamic and clinical effects when taken long-term by patients with impaired systolic function,[165,166] and that they improve mortality when taken by postinfarct patients.[167]

At present, beta-blockers are seldom prescribed for elderly patients for two main reasons. Firstly, beta-blockers have many side effects, including postural hypotension, bronchospasm, heart conduction abnormalities, diabetes mellitus, depression, and peripheral vascular insufficiency, and these are more likely to occur and to produce management difficulties in older patients.[98] On the other hand, evidence for an association between beta-blockers and depression and peripheral vascular insufficiency is controversial,[168,169] and diabetic postinfarct patients have been treated successfully with beta-blockers.[170] Secondly, beta-adrenergic responsiveness is reduced in the elderly.[171] However, in studies of patients treated with beta-blockers after myocardial infarction, relative and absolute reductions in mortality have been greater in patients aged 65–75 years than in younger groups.[172,173] More studies are necessary to determine the long-term outcome of beta-blockade in patients with diastolic heart failure, including older patients.

General considerations

The therapeutic objectives in treating heart failure in elderly people depend on the individual patient. In patients with major cognitive impairment or severe cardiac or other illness, symptom control and improvement in quality of life may be more important than prolonging survival. Although improved exercise tolerance is usually the primary therapeutic goal, 'activities of daily living' are of equal importance in older people. For example, reduction in dyspnoea with diuretic therapy must be balanced against the propensity of the agents to cause incontinence and postural dizziness.

Improved exercise capacity and cardiovascular function (including improved early diastolic filling) have been demonstrated with exercise training in elderly people (including people in their nineties) and in younger heart failure patients.[174–176] Although no study of elderly heart failure patients has been reported to date, these data do suggest that elderly people with heart failure should be advised to maintain a reasonable level of exercise.

Potentially reversible factors that may contribute to the development of heart failure in elderly people include atrial fibrillation, anaemia, hyperthyroidism, infection, malnutrition, medications, excessive intravenous fluids, and poor compliance with prescribed treatment. Medications that may cause problems include sodium-retaining medications such as corticosteroids and non-steroidal anti-inflammatory agents, and cardiodepressant agents such as antiarrhythmic, beta-blocking drugs and calcium channel blocking drugs.

A recent American survey revealed that only 10% of elderly people prescribed digoxin filled enough prescriptions to have daily medications for the entire year, and on average, patients were without daily medications for 4 months each year.[178] Although non-compliance is not associated with old age itself, the high frequency of polypharmacy and of cognitive impairment increases the risk of non-compliance among the elderly; patients are most likely to comply with simple drug regimens.

Malnutrition is common in elderly people and can cause bradycardia and decreased cardiac output and contractility.[179] Malnutrition is also a common consequence of heart failure ('cardiac cachexia').[180] Recognition and correction of undernutrition will be of general benefit to most patients. However, there is no evidence to date for a specific improvement in cardiac function, and rapid refeeding may actually precipitate severe heart failure.[181] Thiamine deficiency is also common in elderly people, especially those living in institutional care, and can cause heart failure (beriberi). Many patients with cardiac beriberi do not have the classic features of high-output failure.[182] Thiamine deficiency also occurs as a consequence of heart failure, especially in patients treated with high doses of diuretics. Seligmann and colleagues recently reported thiamine deficiency in 85% of 23 patients (mean age 70 years) treated with frusemide for heart failure; functional class and left ventricular ejection fraction improved in patients treated with intravenous thiamine.[183]

Conclusion

The incidence and prevalence of heart failure increase dramatically with increasing age because of accumulated, age-related changes in the cardiovascular system associated with coronary artery disease with or without coronary hypertension. Atypical presentations of heart failure in old age may contribute to over- and under-diagnosis. Management of heart failure in the elderly must, as always, be tailored to the individual patient. Potentially reversible factors that may contribute to the development of heart failure are common and must be sought as many may be directly treatable. Elderly people are more likely than younger patients to experience adverse drug effects during treatment. ACE inhibitors probably improve survival in elderly patients with heart failure and systolic dysfunction. However, it is uncertain whether patients aged 80 years or more also benefit from this treatment. A large proportion of elderly people with heart failure have normal systolic function. At present, optimal drug treatment of this group of patients remains uncertain.

References

1 Elveback L, Lie JT. Continued high incidence of coronary artery disease in Olmstead County, Minnesota, 1950–1979. *Circulation* 1984; **70**:345–349.

2 Wei JY. Age and the cardiovascular system. *N Engl J Med* 1992;**327**:1735–1739.

3 Avolio AP. Effect of aging on arterial distensibility in populations with high and low prevalence of hypertension: comparison between urban and rural communities in China. *Circulation* 1985;**71**:202–210.

4 Olivetti G, Melissari M, Balbi T, Quaini F, Sonnenblick EH, Anversa P. Myocyte nuclear and possible cellular hyperplasia contribute to ventricular remodeling in the hypertrophic senescent heart in humans. *J Am Coll Cardiol* 1994;**24**:140–149.

5 Lakatta EG. Normal changes of aging. In: Abrams WB, Berkow R, eds. *Merck Manual of Geriatrics*. Merck, West Point, NY, 1990: 310–325.

6 Wei JY, Spurgeon HA, Lakatta EG. Excitation–contraction in rat myocardium: alterations with adult aging. *Am J Physiol* 1984;**246**:H784–H791.

7 Yin FCP, Raizes GS, Guarnieri T, et al. Age-associated decrease in ventricular response to haemodynamic stress during beta-adrenergic blockade. *Br Heart J* 1978;**40**:1349–1355.

8 Kostis JB, Moreyra AE, Amendo MT, Di Pietro J, Cosgrove N, Kuo PT. The effect of age on heart rate in subjects free of heart disease. *Circulation* 1982;**65**:141–145.

9 Brandfonbrener M, Lansdowne M, Shock NW. Changes in cardiac output with age. *Circulation* 1955;**12**:557–577.

10 Rodeheffer RJ, Gerstenblith G, Becker L, Fleg JL, Weisfeldt ML, Lakatta EG. Exercise cardiac output is maintained in healthy human subjects: cardiac dilatation and increased cardiac output compensate for a diminished heart rate. *Circulation* 1984;**69**:203–213.

11 Bryg RJ, Williams GA, Labovitz AJ. Effect of aging on left ventricular filling in normal subjects. *Am J Cardiol* 1987;**59**:971–974.

12 Spirito P, Maron BJ. Influence of aging on Doppler echocardiographic indices of left ventricular diastolic function. *Br Heart J* 1988; **59**:672–679.

13 Harizi RC, Bianco JA, Alpert JS. Diastolic function of the heart in clinical cardiology. *Arch Intern Med* 1988;**148**:99–108.

14 Kitzman DW, Sheikh KH, Beere PA, Philips JL, Higginbotham MB. Age-related alterations of Doppler left ventricular filling indexes in normal subjects are independent of left ventricular mass, heart rate, contractility and loading conditions. *J Am Coll Cardiol* 1991;**18**:1243–1250.

15 Lakatta EG, Yin FCP. Myocardial aging: functional alterations and related cell mechanisms. *Am J Physiol* 1982;**242**:H927–H941.

16 Arrighi JA, Dilsizian V, Perrone-Filardi P, Diodati JG, Bacharach SL, Bonow RO. Improvement of the age-related impairment in left ventricular diastolic filling with verapamil in the normal human heart. *Circulation* 1994; **90**:213–219.

17 Arora RR, Machac J, Goldman HE, Butler RN, Gorlin R, Horowitz SF. Atrial kinetics and left ventricular diastolic filling in the healthy elderly. *J Am Coll Cardiol* 1987;**9**:1255–1260.

18 Bonow RO, Udelson JE. Left ventricular diastolic dysfunction as a cause of congestive cardiac failure. Mechanisms and management. *Ann Intern Med* 1992;**117**:502–510.

19 Julius S, Amery A, Whitlock LS, Conway J. Influence of age on the hemodynamic response to exercise. *Circulation* 1967;**36**:222–230.

20 Higginbotham BM, Morris KG, Williams RS, Coleman RE, Cobb FR. Physiologic basis for the age-related decline in aerobic work capacity. *Am J Cardiol* 1986;**57**:1374–1379.

21 Gerstenblith G, Renlund DG, Lakatta EG. Cardiovascular response to exercise in younger and older men. *Fed Proc* 1987;**46**:1834–1839.

22 Fleg JL, Lakatta EG. Role of muscle loss in the age-associated reduction in Vo_{2max}. *J Appl Physiol* 1988;**65**:1147–1151.
23 Seals DR, Hagberg JM, Hurley BF, Ehsani AA, Holloszy JO. Endurance training in older men and women: 1. Cardiovascular responses to exercise. *J Appl Physiol* 1984;**57**:1024–1029.
24 Parameshwar J, Poole-Wilson PA, Sutton GC. Heart failure in a district general hospital. *J R Coll Phys Lond* 1992;**26**:139–142.
25 Sutton GC. Epidemiologic aspects of heart failure. *Am Heart J* 1990;**120**:1538–1540.
26 Clarke KW, Gray D, Hampton JR. Evidence of inadequate investigation and treatment of patients with heart failure. *Br Heart J* 1994;**71**:584–587.
27 McKee PA, Castelli WP, McNamara PM, Kannel WB. The natural history of congestive heart failure: the Framingham study. *N Engl J Med* 1971;**285**:1441–1446.
28 Kannel WB, Belanger AJ. Epidemiology of heart failure. *Am Heart J* 1991;**12**:951–957.
29 Marantz PR, Tobin JN, Wassertheil-Smoller S, et al. The relationship between left ventricular systolic function and congestive heart failure diagnosed by clinical criteria. *Circulation* 1988;**77**:607–612.
30 Stevenson LW, Perloff JK. The limited reliability of physical signs for estimating haemodynamics in chronic heart failure. *JAMA* 1989; **261**:884–888.
31 Rectra EH, Khan AH, Pigott VM, Spodick DH. Audibility of the fourth heart sound. A prospective, 'blind' auscultatory and polygraphic investigation. *JAMA* 1972;**221**:36–41.
32 Raftery EB, Holland WW. Examination of the heart: an investigation into variation. *Am J Epidemiol* 1967;**85**:438–444.
33 Lipkin DP, Scrivin AL, Crake T, Poole-Wilson PA. Six-minute walking test for assessing exercise capacity in chronic heart failure. *BMJ* 1986;**292**:653–655.
34 Parameshwar J, Dambrink JHE, Sparrow J, et al. A new exercise test for the assessment of heart failure: use of a self-powered treadmill. *Br Heart J* 1989;**61**:421–425.
35 Hausdorff JM, Forman DE, Ladin Z, Goldberger AL, Rigney DR, Wei JY. Increased walking variability in elderly persons with congestive heart failure. *J Am Geriatr Soc* 1994;**42**:1056–1061.
36 Struthers AD. Ten years of natriuretic peptide research: a new dawn for their diagnostic and therapeutic use? *BMJ* 1994;**308**:1615–1619.
37 Davis KM, Fish LC, Elahi D, Clark BA, Minaker KL. Atrial natriuretic peptide levels in the prediction of congestive heart failure risk in frail elderly. *JAMA* 1992;**267**:2625–2629.
38 Eriksson H, Svardsudd K, Larsson B, et al. Risk factors for heart failure in the general population: the study of men born in 1913. *Eur Heart J* 1989;**10**:647–656.
39 Landahl S, Svanborg A, Åstrand K. Heart volume and the prevalence of certain common cardiovascular disorders at 70 and 75 years of age. *Eur Heart J* 1984;**5**:326–321.
40 Smith WM. Epidemiology of congestive heart failure. *Am J Cardiol* 1985;**55**:3A–8A.
41 Wheeldon NM, MacDonald TM, Flucker CJ, McKendrick AD, McDevitt DG, Struthers AD. Ecchocardiography in chronic heart failure in the community. *Q J Med* 1993;**86**:17–23.
42 Takarada A, Kurogane H, Minamiji T, et al. Congestive heart failure in the elderly – echocardiographic insights. *Jpn Circ J* 1992; **56**:527–534.
43 Wong WF, Gold S, Fukuyama O, Blanchette PL. Diastolic dysfunction in elderly patients with congestive heart failure. *Am J Cardiol* 1989;**63**:1526–1528.
44 Soufer R, Wohlgelernter D, Vita NA, et al. Intact systolic left ventricular function in clinical congestive heart failure. *Am J Cardiol* 1985; **55**:1032–1036.
45 Echeverria HH, Bilsker MS, Myerburg RJ, Kessler KM. Congestive heart failure: echocardiographic insights. *Am J Med* 1983;**75**:750–755.
46 Cohn JN, Johnson G. Heart failure with normal ejection fraction. The V-HeFT study. *Circulation* 1990;**81(suppl 3)**:48–53.
47 Dougherty AH, Naccarelli GV, Gray EL, Hicks CH, Goldstein RA. Congestive heart failure with normal systolic function. *Am J Cardiol* 1984;**54**:778–782.
48 Aguirre FV, Pearson AC, Lewen MK, McCluskey M, Labovitz AJ. Usefulness of doppler echocardiography in the diagnosis of

congestive heart failure. *Am J Cardiol* 1989; **63**:1098–1102.
49 Taffet GE, Teasdale TA, Bleyer AJ, Kutka NJ, Luchi RJ. Survival of elderly men with congestive heart failure. *Age Ageing* 1992;**21**:49–55.
50 Aronow WS, Ahn C, Kronzon I. Prognosis of congestive heart failure in elderly patients with normal versus abnormal left ventricular systolic function associated with coronary artery disease. *Am J Cardiol* 1990;**66**:1257–1259.
51 Luchi RJ, Snow E, Luchi JM, Nelson CL, Pircher EJ. Left ventricular function in hospitalized geriatric patients. *J Am Geriatr Soc* 1982; **30**:700–705.
52 Forman DE, Coletta D, Kenny D, et al. Clinical issues related to discontinuing digoxin therapy in elderly nursing home patients. *Arch Intern Med* 1991;**151**:2194–2198.
53 Ishida Y, Meisners JS, Tsujioka K, et al. Left ventricular filling dynamics: influence of left ventricular relaxation and left atrial pressure. *Circulation* 1986;**74**:187–196.
54 Ren JF, Strain J, Lighty GW, et al. Measurement yield and reproducibility of key M-mode and Doppler echocardiographic variables in the elderly. *Cardiol Elderly* 1994; **2**:247–250.
55 Sagie A, Benjamin EJ, Galderisi M, et al. Reference values for doppler indexes of left ventricular diastolic filling in the elderly. *J Am Soc Echocardiogr* 1993;**6**:570–576.
56 Wei JY. Congestive heart failure. In: Abrams WB, Berkow R, eds. *Merck Manual of Geriatrics*. Merck, West Point, NY, 1990:380–386.
57 Kannel WB, Abbot RD, Savage DD, McNamara PM. Epidemiologic features of chronic atrial fibrillation. The Framingham study. *N Engl J Med* 1982;**306**:1018–1022.
58 Teerlink JR, Goldhaber SZ, Pfeffer MA. An overview of contemporary etiologies of congestive heart failure. *Am Heart J* 1991;**121(suppl 6, part 1)**:1852–1853.
59 Ho KKL, Anderson KM, Kannel WB, Grossman W, Levy D. Survival after the onset of congestive heart failure in Framingham heart study subjects. *Circulation* 1993;**88**:107–115.
60 Remes J, Reunanen A, Aromaa A, Pyorala K. Incidence of heart failure in Eastern Finland: a population based surveillance study. *Eur Heart J* 1992;**13**:588–593.
61 Wilhelmsen L, Eriksson H, Svärdsudd K, Cajdahl K. Improving the detection and diagnosis of congestive heart failure. *Eur Heart J* 1989;**10(suppl C)**:13–18.
62 Aroesty JM, McKay RG, Heller GV, Royal HD, Ais AV, Grossman W. Simultaneous assessment of left ventricular systolic and diastolic dysfunction during pacing-induced ischaemia. *Circulation* 1985;**71**:889–900.
63 Dodek A, Kassebaum DG, Bristow JD. Pulmonary edema in coronary-artery disease without cardiomegaly: paradox of the stiff heart. *N Engl J Med* 1972;**286**:1347–1350.
64 Yusuf S, Thom T, Abbot RD. Changes in hypertension treatment and in congestive heart failure mortality in the United States. *Hypertension* 1989;**13(suppl)**:74–79.
65 Topol EJ, Traill TA, Fortuin NJ. Hypertensive hypertrophic cardiomyopathy of the elderly. *N Engl J Med* 1985;**312**:277–283.
66 Granger CB, Karimeddini MK, Smith VE, Shapiro HR, Katz AM, Riba AL. Rapid ventricular filling in left ventricular hypertrophy. 1. Physiologic hypertrophy. *J Am Coll Cardiol* 1985;**5**:862–868.
67 Iriarte M, Murga N, Sagstagoita D, et al. Congestive heart failure from left ventricular diastolic dysfunction in systemic hypertension. *Am J Cardiol* 1993;**71**:308–312.
68 Howell TH. Cardiac murmurs in old age: a clinico-pathological study. *J Am Geriatr Soc* 1967; **20**:509–516.
69 Akasaka T, Yoshikawa J, Yoshida K, et al. Age-related valvular regurgitation: a study by pulsed doppler echocardiography. *Circulation* 1987; **76**:262–265.
70 Aronow WS, Kronzon I. Prevalence and severity of valvular aortic stenosis determined by doppler echocardiography and association with echocardiographic and electrocardiographic left ventricular hypertrophy and physical signs of aortic stenosis in elderly patients. *Am J Cardiol* 1991;**67**:776–777.
71 Lombard JT, Selzer A. Valvular aortic stenosis: a clinical and hemodynamic profile of patients. *Ann Intern Med* 1987;**106**:292–298.

72 Cox, N, McLenachan JM, Corrado OJ. Is an echocardiogram useful in heart failure in the elderly? *Age Ageing* 1994;**23(suppl 4)**:4–5.
73 Codd MB, Sugrue DD, Gersh BJ, Melton LJ. Epidemiology of idiopathic dilated and hypertrophic cardiomyopathy: a population based study in Olmstead County, Minnesota, 1975–1984. *Circulation* 1989;**51**:564–574.
74 Fay WP, Talierio CP, Ilstrup DM, Tajik AJ, Gersh BJ. Natural history of hypertrophic cardiomyopathy in the elderly. *J Am Coll Cardiol* 1990;**16**:821–826.
75 Lewis JF, Maron BJ. Clinical and morphologic expression of hypertrophic cardiomyopathy in patients ≥65 years of age. *Am J Cardiol* 1994; **73**:1105–1111.
76 Watkins H, Rosenzweig A, Hwang DS, et al. Characteristics and prognostic implications of myosin missense mutations in familial hypertrophic cardiomyopathy. *N Engl J Med* 1992; **326**:1108–1114.
77 Lie JT, Hammond PI. Pathology of the senescent heart: anatomic observations on 237 autopsy studies of patients 90 to 105 years old. *Mayo Clin Proc* 1988;**63**:552–564.
78 Roberts WC. Ninety-three hearts ≥90 years of age. *Am Heart J* 1993;**71**:599–601.
79 Bedford PD, Caird FI. Congestive heart failure in the elderly. *Q J Med* 1956;**25**:407–411.
80 Judge KW, Pawitan Y, Caldwell J, Gersh BJ, Kennedy JW. Congestive heart failure symptoms in patients with preserved left ventricular systolic function: analysis of the CASS registry. *J Am Coll Cardiol* 1991;**18**:377–382.
81 Hughes CV, Wong M, Johnson G, Cohn JN. Influence of age on mechanisms and prognosis of heart failure. *Circulation* 1993;**87(suppl 6)**:111–117.
82 Benedict CR, Johnstone DE, Bourassa MG, et al. Neurohormonal responses in patients with diastolic vs systolic left ventricular dysfunction: SOLVD registry study. *Circulation* 1992; **86(suppl I)**:120.
83 Setaro JF, Soufer R, Remetz MS, Perimutter RA, Zarat BL. Long-term outcome in patients with congestive heart failure and intact systolic left ventricular performance. *Am J Cardiol* 1992;**69**:1212–1216.
84 McMurray J, Dargie H. Coronary artery disease. *BMJ* 1991;**303**:1546.
85 Brogan WC, Hillis D, Flores ED, Lange RA. The natural history of isolated left ventricular diastolic dysfunction. *Am J Med* 1992;**92**:627–630.
86 Packer M. Abnormalities of diastolic function as a potential cause of exercise intolerance in chronic heart failure. *Circulation* 1990; **81(suppl 3)**:78–86.
87 Packer M. Treatment of chronic heart failure. *Lancet* 1992;**340**:92–95.
88 Küpper AJ, Fintelman H, Huige MC, Liem KL, Lustermans FA. Cross-over comparison of the fixed combination of hydrochlorthiazide and triamterene and the free combination of furosemide and triamterene in the maintenance treatment of congestive heart failure. *Eur J Clin Pharmacol* 1986;**30**:342–343.
89 Whight C, Morgan T, Carney S, Wilson M. Diuretics, cardiac failure and potassium depletion: a rational approach. *Med J Aust* 1974; **2**:831–833.
90 The CONSENSUS Trial Study Group. Effects of enalapril on mortality in severe congestive heart failure. Results of the Cooperative North Scandanavian Enalapril Survival Study (CONSENSUS). *N Engl J Med* 1987;**316**: 1429–1435.
91 The SOLVD Investigators. Effect of enalapril on survival in patients with reduced left ventricular ejection fractions and congestive heart failure. *N Engl J Med* 1991;**325**:293–302.
92 Cohn JN, Johnson G, Ziesche S, et al. A comparison of enalapril with hydralazine–isosorbide dinitrate in the treatment of chronic congestive heart failure. *N Engl J Med* 1991; **325**:303–310.
93 Pfeffer MA, Braunwald E, Moye LA, et al. Effect of captopril on mortality and morbidity in patients with left ventricular dysfunction after myocardial infarction. Results of the Survival and Ventricular Enlargement Trial. *N Engl J Med* 1992;**327**:669–677.
94 The SOLVD Investigators. Effect of enalapril on mortality and the development of heart failure in asymptomatic patients with reduced left ventricular ejection fraction. *N Engl J Med* 1992;**327**:685–691.
95 The Acute Infarction Ramipril Efficacy (AIRE) Study Investigators. Effect of ramipril on mortality and morbidity of survivors of acute

myocardial infarction with clinical evidence of heart failure. *Lancet* 1993;**342**:821–828.

96 Swedberg K, Held P, Kjekshus J, Rasmussen K, Ryden L, Wedel H. Effects of the early administration of enalapril on mortality in patients with acute myocardial infarction. Results of the Cooperative New Scandanavian Enalapril Survival Study 2 (CONSENSUS 2). *N Engl J Med* 1992;**327**:678–684.

97 Gruppo Italiano per lo Studio della Sopravvivenza nell'infarto Miocardio. GISSI-3: effects of lisinopril and transdermal glyceryl trinitrate singly and together on 6-week mortality and ventricular function after acute myocardial infarction. *Lancet* 1994;**343**:1115–1122.

98 Luchi RJ, Taffet GE, Teasdale TA. Congestive heart failure in the elderly. *J Am Geriatr Soc* 1991;**39**:810–825.

99 Cody RJ, Torre S, Clark M, Pondolfino K. Age-related hemodynamic, renal and hormonal differences among patients with congestive heart failure. *Arch Intern Med* 1989;**149**:1023–1028.

100 Creasey WA, Funke PT, McKinstry DN. Pharmacokinetics of captopril in elderly healthy male volunteers. *J Clin Pharmacol* 1986; **26**:264–269.

101 Hockings N, Ajayi AA, Reid JL. Age and the pharmacodynamics of angiotensin converting enzyme inhibitors, enalapril and enalaprilat. *Br J Clin Pharmacol* 1986;**21**:341–345.

102 Gautam PC, Vargas E, Lye M. Pharmacokinetics of lisinopril (MK521) in healthy young and elderly subjects and in elderly patients with cardiac failure. *J Pharm Pharmacol* 1987;**39**:929–934.

103 Thomson AH, Kelly JG, Whiting B. Lisinopril population pharmacokinetics in elderly and renal disease patients with hypertension. *Br J Clin Pharmacol* 1989;**27**:157–160.

104 O'Neill CJ, Bowes SG, Sullens CM, et al. Evaluation of the safety of enalapril in the treatment of heart failure in the very old. *Eur J Clin Pharmacol* 1989;**35**:143–150.

105 Murphy PJ, Van der Cammen T, Malone-Lee J. Captopril in elderly patients with heart failure. *BMJ* 1986;**293**:239–240.

106 Jaeschke R, Oxman AD, Guyatt GH. To what extent do congestive heart failure patients in sinus rhythm benefit from digoxin therapy? A systematic overview and meta-analysis. *Am J Med* 1990;**88**:279–285.

107 Packer M, Gheorghiade M, Young JB, et al. Withdrawal of digoxin from patients with chronic heart failure treated with angiotensin-converting-enzyme inhibitors. *N Engl J Med* 1993;**329**:1–7.

108 Poole-Wilson PA, Robinson K. Digoxin: a redundant drug in the treatment of congestive heart failure. *Cardiovasc Drugs Ther* 1989; **2**:733–741.

109 Packer M, Carver JR, Rodeheffer RJ, et al. Effects of oral milrinone on mortality in severe chronic heart failure. *N Engl J Med* 1991; **325**:1468–1475.

110 Feldman AM, Bristow MR, Parmley WW, et al. Effects of vesnarinone on morbidity and mortality in patients with heart failure. *N Engl J Med* 1993;**329**:149–155.

111 Anonymous. Flosequinan withdrawn. *Lancet* 1993;**342**:235.

112 Aronow WS, Starling L, Etienne F. Lack of efficacy of digoxin in treatment of compensated congestive heart failure with third heart sound and sinus rhythm in elderly patients receiving diuretic therapy. *Am J Cardiol* 1986;**58**:168–169.

113 Krakauer R, Peterson B. The effects of discontinuing maintenance digoxin therapy: a study of elderly cardiac patients in sinus rhythm. *Dan Med Bull* 1979;**26**:10–13.

114 Ware JA, Snow E, Luchi JM, Luchi RJ. Effect of digoxin on ejection fraction in elderly patients with congestive heart failure. *J Am Geriatr Soc* 1984;**32**:631–635

115 Smith LH. Digitalis toxicity – turning over a new leaf? *West J Med* 1986;**145**:74–82.

116 McDonnell Cooke D. The use of central nervous system manifestations in the early detection of digitalis toxicity. *Heart Lung* 1993; **22**:477–481.

117 Rubinow A, Skinner M, Cohen AS. Digoxin sensitivity in amyloid cardiomyopathy. *Circulation* 1981;**63**:1285–1288.

118 Pritchett ELC. Management of atrial fibrillation. *N Engl J Med* 1992;**326**:1263–1271.

119 Lipkin DPP, Frenneaux M, Stewart R, Joshi J, Lowe T, McKenna WJ. Delayed improvement in exercise capacity after cardioversion of atrial

fibrillation to sinus rhythm. *Br Heart J* 1988; **59**:572–577.
120 Dittrich HC, Erickson JS, Schneiderman T, Blacky AR, Savides T, Nicol PH. Echocardiographic and clinical predictors for outcome of elective cardioversion of atrial fibrillation. *Am J Cardiol* 1989;**63**:193–197.
121 Henry WL, Morrganroth J, Pearlman AS, et al. Relation between echocardiographically left atrial size and atrial fibrillation. *Circulation* 1976;**53**:273–279.
122 Middlekauff HR, Wiener I, Saxon LA, Stevenson WG. Low-dose amiodarone for atrial fibrillation: time for a prospective study? *Ann Intern Med* 1992;**116**:1017–1020.
123 Repique LJ, Shah SN, Marais GE. Atrial fibrillation 1992. Management strategies in flux. *Chest* 1992;**101**:1091–1103.
124 Martin A, Benbow LJ, Leach C, Bailey RJ. Comparison of amiodarone and disopyramide in the control of paroxysmal atrial fibrillation and flutter (interim report). *Br J Clin Pract* 1986;**44(suppl)**:52–60.
125 Disch DL, Greenberg ML, Holzberger PT, Malenka DJ, Birkmeyer JD. Managing chronic atrial fibrillation: a Markov decision analysis comparing warfarin, quinidine and low-dose amiodarone. *Ann Intern Med* 1994;**120**:449–457.
126 Doval HC, Nul DR, Grancelli HO, Perrone SV, Bortman GR, Curiel R. Randomised trial of low-dose amiodarone in severe congestive heart failure. *Lancet* 1994;**344**:493–498.
127 Payne GE, Skehan JD. Issues in cardiac pacing: can agism be justified? *Br Heart J* 1994; **72**:102–103.
128 Bush DE, Finucane TE. Permanent cardiac pacemakers in the elderly. *J Am Geriatr Soc* 1994;**42**:326–334.
129 Santini M, Alexidou G, Ansalone G, Cacciatore G, Cini R, Turitto G. Relation of prognosis in sick sinus syndrome to age, conduction defects and modes of permanent cardiac pacing. *Am J Cardiol* 1990;**65**:729–735.
130 Rosenqvist M, Brandt J, Schuller H. Atrial versus ventricular spacing in sinus node disease: a treatment comparison study. *Am Heart J* 1986; **111**:292–297.
131 Heselson AB, Parsonnet V, Bernstein AD, Bonavita GJ. Deleterious effects of long-term single-chamber ventricular pacing in patients with sick sinus syndrome: the hidden benefits of dual-chamber pacing. *J Am Coll Cardiol* 1992;**19**:1542–1549.
132 Alpert MA, Curtis JJ, Sanfelippo JF, et al. Comparative survival after permanent ventricular and dual chamber pacing for patients with chronic high degree atrio-ventricular block with and without preexistent congestive heart failure. *J Am Coll Cardiol* 1986;**7**:925–932.
133 Saxon LA, Stevenson WG, Middlekauff HR, Stevenson LW. Increased risk of progressive hemodynamic deterioration in advanced heart failure patients requiring permanent pacemakers. *Am Heart J* 1993;**125**:1306–1310.
134 Amery A, Birkenhager W, Brixho P, et al. Mortality and morbidity results from the European Working Party of High Blood Pressure in the Elderly trial. *Lancet* 1985;**i**:1349–1354.
135 Dalhöf B, Hansson L, Lindholm L, Schersten B, Wester P. Morbidity and mortality in the Swedish Trial in Old People with Hypertension (STOP-Hypertension). *Lancet* 1991;**338**:1281–1285.
136 Gaasch WH. Diagnosis and treatment of heart failure based on left ventricular systolic or diastolic dysfunction. *JAMA* 1994;**271**:1276–1280.
137 Dahlöf B, Pennert K, Hansson L. Reversal of left ventricular hypertrophy in hypertensive patients: a meta-analysis of 109 treatment studies. *Am J Hypertens* 1992;**5**:95–110.
138 Cruichshank JM, Lewis J, Moore V, Dodd C. Reversal of left ventricular hypertrophy by differing types of antihypertensive therapy. *J Hum Hypertens* 1992;**6**:85–90.
139 Frishman WH, Glasser SP, Strom JA, Schoenberger JA, Liebson P, Poland MP. Effect of dilevalol, metoprolol and atenolol on left ventricular mass in elderly patients. *Am J Cardiol* 1989;**63**:691–701.
140 Schulman SP, Weiss JL, Becker LC, et al. The effects of antihypertensive therapy on left ventricular mass in elderly patients. *N Engl J Med* 1990;**322**:1350–1356.
141 Nagano N, Nagano M, Iwatsubo H, Hata T, Mikami H, Ogihara T. Regression of left ventricular hypertrophy in elderly hypertensive

patients treated with antihypertensive drugs. *Cardiol Elderly* 1994;**2**:219–225.
142 Grandi MA, Venco A, Barizizza F, Casadei B, Marchesi E, Finardi G. Effect of enalapril on left ventricular mass and performance in essential hypertension. *Am J Cardiol* 1989;**63**:1093–1097.
143 White W, Schulman P. Karimeddini M, Smith V. Regression of ventricular mass is accompanied by improvement in rapid left ventricular filling following antihypertensive therapy with metoprolol. *Am Heart J* 1989;**117**:145–150.
144 Timarco B, Deluca N, Rosiello, G. et al. Improvement of diastolic function after reversal of left ventricular hypertrophy induced by long term antihypertensive treatment with tertatol. *Am J Cardiol* 1989;**64**:45–51.
145 Granier P, Douste-Blazy MY, Tredez P, Coute D, Galinier F. Improvement in left ventricular hypertrophy and left ventricular diastolic function following verapamil therapy in mild to moderate hypertension. *Eur J Clin Pharm* 1990; **39(suppl 1)**:S45–S46.
146 Smith VE, White WB, Meeran MK, Karimeddini MK. Improved left ventricular filling accompanies reduced left ventricular mass during therapy of essential hypertension. *J Am Coll Cardiol* 1986;**8**:1449–1454.
147 Shahi M, Thom S, Poulter N, Sever PS, Foale RA. Regression of left ventricular hypertrophy and left ventricular diastolic function. *Lancet* 1990;**336**:458–461.
148 Inouye IK, Massie BM, Loge D, Simpson P, Tubau J. Failure of antihypertensive therapy with diuretic, beta blocking and calcium channel blocking drugs to consistantly reverse left ventricular diastolic filling abnormalities. *Am J Cardiol* 1984;**53**:1583–1587.
149 Frohlich ED. Cardiac hypertrophy in hypertension. *N Engl J Med* 1987;**317**:831–833.
150 Wilson JR, Reichek N, Dunkman WB, Goldberg S. Effect of diuresis on the performance of the failing ventricle. *Am J Med* 1981;**70**:234–239.
151 Kessler KM. Heart failure with normal systolic function. *Arch Intern Med* 1988;**148**:2109–2111.
152 Shunkert H, Dzau VJ, Tang SS, Hirsch AT, Apstein CS, Lorell BH. Increased rat cardiac angiotensin converting enzyme activity and mRNA expression in pressure overload hypertrophy: Effects on coronary resistance, contractility and relaxation. *J Clin Invest* 1990; **86**:1913–1929.
153 Friedrich SP, Lorell BH, Rousseau MF, et al. Intracardiac ACE inhibition improves diastolic distensibility in patients with left ventricular hypertrophy due to aortic stenosis. *Circulation* 1994;**90**:2761–71.
154 Aronow WS, Kronzon I. Effect of enalapril on congestive heart failure treated with diuretics in elderly patients with prior myocardial infarction and normal left ventricular ejection fraction. *Am J Cardiol* 1993;**71**:602–604.
155 Lorell BH, Isajama S, Grice WN, Weinberg EO, Apstein CS. Effects of oubain and isoproterenol on left ventricular diastolic function during low flow ischaemia in isolated blood perfused rabbit hearts. *Circ Res* 1988;**63**:457–467.
156 Lee DCS, Johnson RA, Bingham JB, et al. Heart failure in outpatients. A randomized trial of digoxin versus placebo. *N Engl J Med* 1982; **306**:699–705.
157 Hanrath P, Schluter M, Sonntag F, Diemart J, Bleifeld W. Influence of verapamil therapy on left ventricular performance at rest and during exercise in hypertrophic cardiomyopathy. *Am J Cardiol* 1983;**52**:544–548.
158 Bonow RO, Dilsizian V, Rosing DR, Maron BJ, Bacharach SL, Green MV. Verapamil-induced improvement in left ventricular diastolic filling and increased exercise tolerance in patients with hypertrophic cardiomyopathy: short- and long-term results. *Circulation* 1985;**72**:853–864.
159 Given BD, Lee TH, Stone PH, Dzau VJ. Nifedipine in severely hypertensive patients with congestive heart failure and preserved ventricular systolic function. *Arch Intern Med* 1985;**145**:281–285.
160 Lorell BH, Paulus WJ, Grossman W, Wynne J, Cohn PF. Modification of abnormal left ventricular diastolic properties by nifedipine in patients with hypertrophic cardiomyopathy. *Circulation* 1982;**65**:499–507.
161 Elkayam U, Amin J, Mehra A, Vasquez J, Weber L, Rahimtoola SH. A prospective, randomized, double-blind, crossover study to compare the efficacy and safety of chronic

nifedipine therapy with that of isosorbide dinitrate and their combination in the treatment of chronic congestive heart failure. *Circulation* 1990;**82**:1954–1961.
162 Gertz MA, Falk RH, Skinner M, Cohen AS, Kyle RA. Worsening of congestive heart failure in amyloid heart disease treated by calcium channel blocking agents. *Am J Cardiol* 1985; **55**:55–60.
163 Packer M. Calcium channel blockers in chronic heart failure. The risks of 'physiologically rational' therapy. *Circulation* 1990;**82**:2254–2256.
164 Eichorn EJ, Bedetto MB, Malloy CR, et al. Effect of beta-adrenergic blockade on myocardial function and energetics in congestive heart failure. *Circulation* 1990;**82**:473–483.
165 Bashir Y, McKenna WJ, Camm AJ. β blockers and the failing heart: is it time for a U-turn? *Br Heart J* 1993;**70**:8–12.
166 Waagstein F, Bristow MR, Swedberg K, et al. Beneficial effects of metoprolol in idiopathic dilated cardiomyopathy. *Lancet* 1993;**342**: 1441–1446.
167 The Norwegian Multicenter Study Group. Timolol-induced reduction in mortality and reinfarction in patients surviving acute myocardial infarction. *N Engl J Med* 1981;**304**:801–807.
168 Radack K, Deck C. Beta-adrenergic blocker therapy does not worsen intermittent claudication in subjects with peripheral vascular disease: a meta-analysis of randomized controlled trials. *Arch Intern Med* 1991;**151**:1769–1776.
169 Bright RA, Everitt DE. Beta-blockers and depression: evidence against an association. *JAMA* 1992;**267**:1783–1787.
170 Kjekshus J, Gilpin E, Cali G, Blackey AR, Henning H, Ross J. Diabetic patients and beta blockers after acute myocardial infarction. *Eur Heart J* 1990;**11**:43–50.
171 Kelly J, O'Malley K. Adrenoceptor function and ageing. *Clin Sci* 1984;**66**:509–515.
172 Gundersen T, Abrahamsen AM, Kjekshus J, Rønnevik PK. Timolol-related reduction in mortality and reinfarction in patients aged 65–75 years surviving acute myocardial infarction. *Circulation* 1982;**66**:1179–1184.
173 Forman DE, Bernal JLG, Wei JY. Management of acute myocardial infarction in the very elderly. *Am J Med* 1992; **93:315–326.**
174 Morey MC, Cowper PA, Feussner JR, et al. Two-year trends in physical performance following supervised exercise among community-dwelling older veterans. *J Am Geriatr Soc* 1991;**39**:986–992.
175 Fiatarone MA, Marks C, Ryan ND, Meredith CN, Lipsitz LA, Evans WJ. High-intensity strength training in nonagenerians: effect on skeletal muscle. *J Am Med Assoc* 1990; **262**:3029–3034.
176 Sullivan MJ, Higginbotham MB, Cobb FR. Exercise training in patients with severe left ventricular dysfunction: haemodynamic and metabolic effects. *Circulation* 1988;**78**:506–515.
177 Forman DE, Manning WJ, Hauser R, Gervino EV, Evans WJ, Wei JY. Enhanced left ventricular diastolic filling associated with long-term endurance training. *J Gerontol* 1992;**47**:M56–M58.
178 Monane M, Bohn RL, Gurwitz JH, Glynn RJ, Avorn J. Noncompliance with congestive heart failure therapy in the elderly. *Arch Intern Med* 1994;**154**:433–437.
179 Burch GE, Phillips J, Ansari A. The cachectic heart: a clinico-pathological, electrocardiographic and roentgenographic entity. *Chest* 1968;**54**:5–11.
180 King D. Cardiac cachexia in the elderly. *Cardiol Elderly* 1994;**2**:102–106.
181 Keys A, Haenschel A, Taylor HL. Size and function of the human heart at rest in semistarvation and in subsequent rehabilitation. *Am J Physiol* 1947;**50**:153–158.
182 Anon. Cardiovascular beriberi. *Lancet* 1982;**i**:1287.
183 Seligmann H, Halkin H, Rauchfleisch S, et al. Thiamine deficiency in patients with congestive heart failure receiving long-term furosemide therapy: a pilot study. *Am J Med* 1991; **91**:151–155.

5

What are we trying to achieve when we treat heart failure?

Philip A Poole-Wilson

Introduction

Heart failure is a common condition with a poor prognosis. The diagnosis can be made without undue use of high technology and at a reasonable cost. Effective treatment is available which both relieves symptoms and prolongs life. In the past decade major advances in management and treatment have been made as a consequence of the introduction of new therapies, improvements in the understanding of the pathophysiology of heart failure, and the availability of transplantation. A key consequence of these advances and of the epidemiological features of heart failure is that heart failure fulfils the criteria for being regarded as an important health problem worthy of specific action. Heart failure should receive the attention not only of the medical profession but of those concerned with the financing and delivery of health care to the community.

Recognition and definition of heart failure

Heart failure is a generic phrase used to describe a clinical condition with many different modes of presentation for which there are a variety of appropriate but different treatments. Heart failure is a clinical syndrome (readily diagnosed by doctors) caused by an abnormality of the heart and recognized by a characteristic pattern of haemodynamic, renal, neural, and hormonal responses.[1,2] The phrase is of great value in transmitting an impression of the expected condition of a patient from one doctor to another.

Many definitions conflict with common usage where the phrase 'heart failure' describes a clinical syndrome. A simple definition is that heart failure is cardiac dysfunction with symptoms. Most definitions require the demonstration of an abnormality of the heart and that this abnormality should have clinically relevant consequences. These definitions are difficult to apply in epidemiological studies. An alternative approach which has been advocated recently[3] is that heart failure should be diagnosed when there is an abnormality of ventricular function, symptoms of a type that can be attributed to heart failure, and improvement of symptoms and other features of the condition by treatment (see Chapter 1). This definition may exclude a few patients who have the syndrome but is more reliable than symptoms or signs alone.[4–6]

Heart failure is more common in the elderly and the symptoms and signs and even the results of investigations in those over the age of 75 may differ from younger persons. Most drug studies have been undertaken in selected patients usually presenting to hospitals. The average age of these patients is commonly around 60 years, with the prevalence of females around 20%. Studies in the community[7] suggest that, in reality, the average age of those with heart failure is 73 years and about 40% of cases are in females. The second and possibly more important consideration is that, although the syndrome of clinical heart failure begins with an abnormality of the heart, most of the manifestations result from changes in the peripheral circulation, which are the long-term consequence of heart failure.[8–11] Two key organs are the kidney and skeletal muscle. Underperfusion of the kidney combined with a raised venous pressure contributes to the failure of the kidney to excrete sodium and water, and this leads to the most obvious clinical manifestations of heart failure, namely oedema, raised venous pressure and liver enlargement. Recent work has shown that the function of skeletal muscle deteriorates in patients with heart failure and that this is not attributable to lack of fitness but to a fall in blood flow, reduction in muscle strength, and atrophy of skeletal muscle cells. These peripheral changes are the reason why, although some features of heart failure may respond quickly to treatment, full benefit is not observed until treatment has been continued for a period of weeks or months. A dramatic example of this delayed response is the time taken for an improvement of blood flow to the arm and relief of symptoms after heart transplantation.[12] If the symptoms were entirely related to central haemodynamics (which they are not), then immediate total benefit would be expected. Some contributory factors to symptoms are shown in Table 5.1.

Syndromes of heart failure

Numerous phrases are used by doctors to convey particular patterns of symptoms and signs in patients with heart failure. The commonest is the use of the phrases 'right-sided' and 'left-sided' heart failure. Right-sided heart failure usually refers to the major manifestations of sodium and water retention, such as a raised venous pressure, peripheral oedema and an enlarged liver. The commonest cause of these changes is an abnormality of the left ventricle, so the use of this phrase is not entirely logical. Left-sided heart failure usually means pulmonary congestion or pulmonary oedema and is generally due to an abnormality of the left ventricle. Other phrases which have been used are 'forward and backward failure', 'high and low

Lungs	Increased stiffness due to raised venous pressure and lymphatic distension Increased left atrial pressure Increased physiological dead space Increased respiratory rate Weakness of diaphragm Increased bronchial reactivity
Circulation	Reduced blood flow to skeletal muscle Increased production of metabolites Altered response to metabolites
Skeletal muscle	Rest atrophy Ischaemic atrophy Specific abnormality

Table 5.1
Origin of symptoms on exercise in chronic heart failure.

output failure', 'overt', 'treated', and 'compensated' heart failure. This is the jargon of cardiology.

Diastolic and systolic heart failure

A further common distinction is between systolic and diastolic heart failure[13,14]. This distinction has been the subject of recent controversy. Systolic heart failure is a phrase used when the ventricle enlarges (as it usually does in heart failure) and the major abnormality is an inability of the heart to generate a stroke volume during each beat. Diastolic heart failure is a phrase used to convey the idea that the abnormality of the heart is not due to the failure of the muscle to be able to contract and generate a stroke volume, but rather is due to a failure of the ventricle to fill during diastole (Table 5.2). A simple example would be mitral stenosis. Diastolic heart failure commonly occurs in the elderly, in the presence of hypertrophy and as a result of myocardial ischaemia. Diastolic heart failure is almost synonymous with heart failure in the presence of a small ventricular chamber. In theory, the true diagnosis of diastolic heart failure would depend on demonstrating failure of the ventricle to fill at peak exercise and that the abnormality of filling caused the symptoms of the patient. That is rarely the case in any patient. In the absence of such evidence, patients with heart failure and small hearts may have some degree of diastolic heart failure but can also have a failure of systolic ejection. Since at peak exercise there is a limitation to generating a cardiac output even in these patients, that limitation may well be the consequence of a systolic abnormality. Thus, most cases of diastolic heart failure are associated with an abnormality of systolic contraction. Diastolic heart failure has been claimed to be common in patients presenting to clinics with cardiac symptoms,[15–17] but is less common among patients admitted to hospital. In one study over a period of 68 months, 14% died, 45% developed new symptoms, and 27% were hospitalised. Those figures indicate a better outcome than in systolic heart failure.[18]

The natural history and origins of heart failure

The natural history of heart failure is not one of continuous deterioration of the patient. The heart failure may be treated so that the

- Heart failure with a near normal-sized heart and normal ejection fraction at rest
- Failure of the ventricle to fill at end-diastole
- Common in community not hospital practice
- Common in the elderly, hypertensives and those with coronary heart disease
- Often presents with breathlessness and fatigue
- Difficult to treat

Table 5.2
Diastolic heart failure.

symptoms and signs are obscured or become undulating. The phrases ‘undulating heart failure’, ‘treated heart failure’, and ‘overt heart failure’ are often used. Undulating heart failure is a useful phrase to describe the common observation that patients with heart failure may accumulate fluid and deteriorate for no apparent reason. Presumably such episodes are related to subtle disturbances of hormonal and fluid balance in the body.

A major and unresolved issue is how the syndrome of heart failure is initiated. One unifying scenario is that heart failure is a consequence of an attempt by the body to maintain the blood pressure.[19,20] The initial abnormality of the heart initially results in a fall in blood pressure. The body responds by activating many neurohormonal systems. Blood flow is distributed away from skin and skeletal muscle and is preferentially preserved to the brain and heart. The sympathetic system and the release of atrial natriuretic peptide are early responses. Activation of the renin–angiotensin system occurs later. These reflexes are those which are more commonly used to avoid fainting on standing and are similar to the response to exercise. Thus, heart failure may be considered as a syndrome which occurs in middle aged to elderly humans when the heart is damaged, and causes the activation of reflexes which emerged during evolution in order to promote survival of the species to be activated.

Objectives of treatment

The objectives of treating heart failure are no different from those for any other medical condition, which are to:

- prevent the occurrence of the condition;
- relieve symptoms and;
- prolong life.

In the context of heart failure, however, these three simple objectives become more complicated.

By far the commonest cause of heart failure is coronary heart disease.[7,21–23] Preventing coronary heart disease would lead to a substantial reduction in the occurrence of heart failure. Myocardial infarction is also common. Approximately half of those patients who sustain a myocardial infarct go on to suffer heart failure. Much interest has arisen in recent years with regard to the prevention of subsequent heart failure and to the preservation of myocardial function. This could be achieved in two ways. The first is to prevent the occurrence of further myocardial events, which are a common cause of the progression of heart failure. The second is to prevent the enlargement of the ventricle which may occur in the weeks and months following a myocardial infarction concurrent with the development of the symptoms of heart failure. This process has been called ‘remodelling’, a term that is slightly confusing. For many years physicians have known that the heart enlarges when heart failure develops and that this enlargement can often be reversed. It is not helpful to call that process remodelling. Remodelling refers to enlargement of the heart associated with specific biochemical and pathological changes, often in the context of myocardial infarction where these changes can be reversed by specific treatment.[24] For example, the reduction of ventricular size after myocardial infarction associated with the early use of angiotensin converting enzyme inhibitors could be partly due to the improved treatment of heart failure and partly due to modification of the inflammatory and healing processes occurring in the days and weeks following infarction.

Symptoms or mortality

Conventional wisdom is that drugs are given in heart failure in order to minimize symptoms. In addition, the drug should be shown to be safe, that is, it should not increase mortality. A reduction in mortality, as has been shown with ACE inhibitors, is an additional but not essential advantage.

Until recently, mortality studies were almost synonymous with safety studies. Efficacy was shown by an effect on symptoms, quality of life or mortality. This view has been challenged for two reasons. The first reason is that the surrogate efficacy end-points (e.g., exercise capacity) may not relate well to changes in mortality. In the SOLVD study quality of life was not greatly influenced by ACE inhibitors. In the VHeFT study, although enalapril had a greater effect on mortality than the combination of hydralazine and nitrates, the reverse was true for the ejection fraction. Thus drugs may have differing and at least unequal effects on the relief of symptoms and mortality.

The second reason for not equating surrogate end-points with mortality raises ethical and philosophical issues. The mortality studies have shown that many positive inotropic drugs increase mortality. These drugs include milrinone, xamoterol, flosequinan, vesarinone, ibopamine and pimobendan. However, some of these drugs, flosequinan for example, increase exercise capacity and quality of life in a group of patients with moderate to severe heart failure who are otherwise difficult to treat. Calculations suggest that the improved quality of life may be offset by a decrease in longevity of about two months in persons who may live for two to four years. Regulatory authorities, physicians, cardiologists, the public, and the patient, have not yet decided how such choices should be made. There is certainly a case for saying that the patient should be offered a choice and have input to the decision. The final decision should not be imposed by regulatory authorities.

In making such decisions many matters need to be taken into consideration. The severity of heart failure is one. In mild heart failure the objectives are directed more at preventing the worsening of heart failure and to increasing longevity, rather than to the relief of symptoms. Examples are the prevention of coronary heart disease and the avoidance of alcoholic intake in those with alcoholic dilated cardiomyopathy. In severe heart failure the reverse may be true; the patient seeks alleviation of symptoms as the prime objective.

Causes of heart failure

The clinical causes of heart failure are congenital heart disease and abnormalities of rhythm, the pericardium, valves, or the myocardium. The causes of myocardial failure are many. The simplest classification at present is to group patients into those with heart failure due to coronary heart disease and those with normal coronary arteries who have other causes of heart failure. This latter group are referred to as cardiomyopathies (Table 5.3). On clinical grounds these are subdivided into hypertrophic (usually characterized by a thickened septum), restrictive cardiomyopathy (limited late filling of the ventricle), and dilated cardiomyopathy (enlarged ventricle).

The commonest cause of an abnormality of the myocardium is coronary artery disease. This, in its various manifestations, probably accounts for 80% of heart failure. Hypertension was found to be a frequent cause of heart failure in the Framingham study. More recent studies suggest that it may be the major cause in 15% of cases and a contributory factor in 40%. The cardiomyopathies are a rare cause

Hypertrophic cardiomyopathy (HCM)		
Restrictive cardiomyopathy		
Dilated cardiomyopathy (DCM)	Identified cause Idiopathic dilated cardiomyopathy (IDCM)*	
*Putative causes of idiopathic dilated cardiomyopathy are: viral infection; immunological disorders; genetic abnormalities; familial		

Table 5.3
Clinical classification of cardiomyopathies.

of heart failure. Dilated cardiomyopathy is by far the commonest cardiomyopathy.

Epidemiology

The general epidemiology of heart failure is simply stated. Approximately 1–2% of the population have heart failure. Between 0.1 and 0.5% of patients admitted to hospital each year have heart failure. In a general district hospital at any particular moment, 5% of persons will be in that hospital with heart failure as a major cause for their admission. Of those admitted to hospital with heart failure, 40% will die in the following year. Approximately 60% of heart failure cases are men and 40% are women. The average age in the population of patients with heart failure is 73 years, and 10% of patients will be over 80 years old. The prognosis is poor, varying from 50% mortality in one year for severe heart failure to 50% at 4 years for all patients in a community. The cost of managing heart failure in a health service is 1–2% of the total health budget; 60% of this cost is spent on hospital admissions.

Heart failure is believed to be becoming more common because of the improved survival following myocardial infarction[25,26] and because heart failure is a disease of the elderly and the population is aging. The entity may also be being diagnosed more readily with an increase in awareness of therapeutic possibilities.

The epidemiology of heart failure[25,27–29] is not as well studied as that of coronary heart disease. There have been four population-based studies,[7,21–23,30] and further studies are currently being undertaken.

Cardiomyopathy has an incidence of between 5 and 10 per 100 000 per year.[30–36] The prevalence in the United States is claimed to be 36.5 per 100 000.[35] The incidence is commoner in men and 2.5 times more common in blacks after taking account of known confounding factors such as alcohol consumption, body size and poverty. A simple calculation would suggest that this form of heart disease accounts for about 2% of heart failure.

Though these data are probably reasonably correct, differences between countries and in subgroups of the population have not been fully evaluated. The sources of data are:

- population-based studies
- physician records
- hospital records for admissions and discharges
- controlled trials.

These global figures conceal much information which is important to doctors and health workers for the delivery of medical care. Some patients with heart failure live for a long time. In the Framingham study[23,37] 15% of patients were alive at 20 years. Some causes of heart failure, such as those where a single non-recurring event has damaged the heart, have an excellent prognosis. In other patients severe heart failure can persist for many months leading to incapacity and a wretched quality of life. The treatment of these patients requires detailed attention to optimize the use of drugs.

Readmission rates for heart failure vary from 35% to 78% in one year.[21,26,38] The causes of readmission are numerous (Table 5.4). Most (57%) are due to a reoccurrence of heart failure, but non-cardiac illness is also common (32%). Half the readmissions are preventable and attributable to non-compliance with drug or diet regimens, inadequate medical support, failed social support, or a failure to seek help (Table 5.5).[38]

Prognosis

The prognosis is variable (Fig. 5.1).[23,25,39–42] The data have been obtained largely from clinical trials and a limited number of population-based studies. Heart failure is progressive but there is considerable uncertainty as to whether the major determinant of progression is recurrence of the initial cause such a coronary event, an opportunistic arrhythmia, or progression of the syndrome of heart failure itself (Fig. 5.2). Knowing the cause of progression in a particular patient would allow more focused therapy to be initiated. There are several forms of information on prognosis (Table 5.6). The traditional prognostic factors are many. In general any factor which is more common in severe

• Ischaemic event, hibernation or stunning	
• Exposure to toxic agent:	alcohol viruses drugs
• Cell morphology and orientation – hypertrophy	
• Altered haemodynamics:	hypertension valve function
• Apoptosis	

Table 5.4
Causes of worsening myocardial function.

• Myocardial infarction or ischaemic episode	• Exposure to toxic agent
• Arrhythmia	• Stroke
• Pulmonary or systemic oedema	• Synergistic medical problem
• Dietary indiscretion	• Non-cardiovascular event
• Non-compliance with medicines	• Social circumstances
• Adverse drug related event	• Reassessment of medicines

Table 5.5
Causes of readmission or deterioration in patients with heart failure.

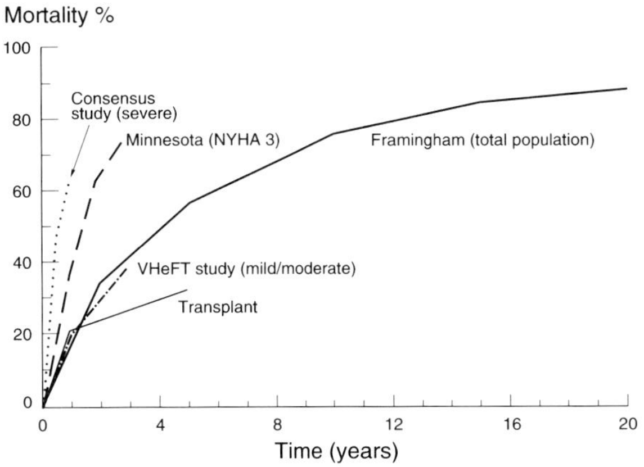

Fig. 5.1
Prognosis of heart failure.

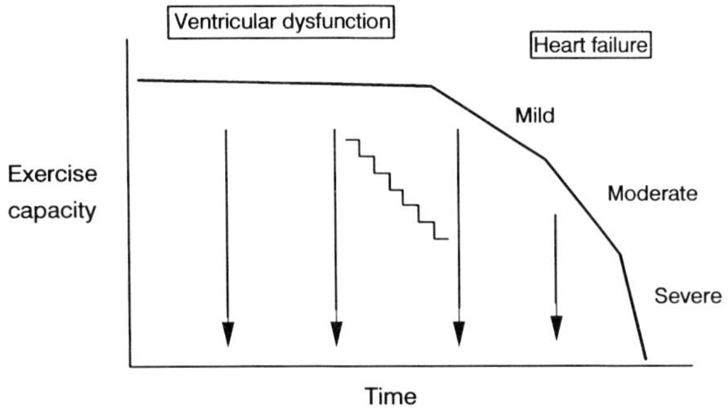

Fig. 5.2
Progression of heart failure.

heart failure predicts prognosis. Heart failure predicts worsening heart failure and severe heart failure predicts death from heart failure. Other variables to consider are risk factors for coronary events and acute recurrent causes of heart failure such as repeated exposure to noxious substances or viruses.

Conclusion

Heart failure is common, identifiable and treatable. Many patients are not being detected and treated appropriately.[43] Public and medical education programmes are required to alter not what is widely believed to be the correct course of action, but what is actually happening in clinical practice at the present time (Table 5.7).

Public education
- Campaigns to increase public awareness
- Inform and involve health authorities

Medical education
- Disseminate recent advances to doctors and health workers
- Educational programmes for the medical profession
- Guidelines for treatment

Table 5.7
Policies for detection and treatment of heart failure.

• Risk factors	Similar to those for coronary heart disease	
• Prognostic factors	Heart size Ventricular function Metabolic markers	Ejection fraction Peak $MV0_2$ Plasma sodium, atrial natriuretic factor, noradrenaline
• Acute causes		

Table 5.6
Types of data on progression of heart failure.

References

1 Poole-Wilson PA. Heart failure. *Medicine International* 1985;**2**:866–871.

2 Poole-Wilson PA. Chronic heart failure: cause, pathophysiology, prognosis, clinical manifestations, investigations. In: Julian DG, Camm AJ, Fox KF, Hall RJC, Poole-Wilson PA, eds. *Diseases of the Heart*. London: Baillière-Tindall, 1989:24–36.

3 The Task Force on Heart Failure of the European Society of Cardiology. Guidelines for the diagnosis of heart failure. *Eur Heart J* 1995;**16**:741–751.

4 Remes J, Miettinen H, Reunanen A, Pyorala K. Validity of clinical diagnosis of heart failure in primary health care. *Eur Heart J* 1991;**12**:315–321.

5 Dunselman PH, Kuntze CE, van-Bruggen A, et al. Value of New York Heart Association classification, radionuclide ventriculography, and cardiopulmonary exercise tests for selection of patients for congestive heart failure studies. *Am Heart J* 1988;**116**:1475–1482.

6 Marantz PR, Tobin JN, Wassertheil-Smoller S, et al. The relationship between left ventricular systolic function and congestive heart failure diagnosed by clinical criteria. *Circulation* 1988;**77**:607–612.

7 Parameshwar J, Shackell MM, Richardson A, Poole-Wilson PA, Sutton GC. Prevalence of heart failure in three general practices in north west London. *Br J Gen Prac 1992;***42**:287–289.

8 Poole-Wilson PA, Buller NP, Lipkin DP. Regional blood flow, muscle strength and skeletal muscle histology in severe congestive heart failure. *Am J Cardiol* 1988;**62**:49E–52E.

9 Poole-Wilson PA, Buller NP. Causes of symptoms in chronic congestive heart failure and implications for treatment. *Am J Cardiol* 1988;**62**:31A–34A.

10 Poole-Wilson PA. The origin of symptoms in patients with chronic heart failure. *Eur Heart J* 1988;**9** (**suppl H**):49–53.

11 Poole-Wilson PA. Relation of pathophysiologic mechanisms to outcome in heart failure. *J Am Coll Cardiol* 1993;**22** (**suppl 4**):22–29.

12 Sinoway LI, Minotti JR, Davis D, et al. Delayed reversal of impaired vasodilation in congestive heart failure after heart transplantation. *Am J Cardiol* 1988;**61**:1076–1079.

13 Brutsaert DL, Sys SU. Relaxation and diastole of the heart. *Physiol Rev* 1989;**69**:1228–1315.

14 Brutsaert DL, Sys SU, Gillebert TC. Diastolic failure: pathophysiology and therapeutic implications. *J Am Coll Cardiol* 1993;**22**:318–325.

15 Setaro JF, Soufer R, Remetz MS, Perlmutter RA, Zaret BL. Long-term outcome in patients with congestive heart failure and intact systolic left ventricular performance. *Am J Cardiol* 1992;**69**:1212-1216.

16 Dougherty AH, Naccarelli GV, Gray EL, Hicks CH, Goldstein RA. Congestive heart failure with normal systolic function. *Am J Cardiol* 1984;**54**:778–782.

17 Soufer R, Wohlgelernter D, Vita NA, et al. Intact systolic left ventricular function in clinical congestive heart failure. *Am J Cardiol* 1985;**55**:1032–1036.

18 Brogan WC, Hillis LD, Flores ED, Lange RA. The natural history of isolated left ventricular diastolic dysfunction. *Am J Med* 1992;**92**:627–630.

19 Harris P. Congestive cardiac failure: central role of the arterial blood pressure. *Br Heart J* 1987;**58**:190–203.

20 Harris P. Evolution and the cardiac patient. *Cardiovasc Res* 1983;**17**:313–319; 373–378; 437–445.

21 Parameshwar J, Poole-Wilson PA, Sutton GC. Heart failure in a district hospital. *J Roy Coll Phys* 1992;**26**:139–142.

22 Eriksson H, Svardsudd K, Larsson B, et al. Risk factors for heart failure in the general population: the study of men born in 1913. *Eur Heart J* 1989;**10**:647–656.

23 Kannel WB, Belanger JA. Epidemiology of heart failure. *Am Heart J* 1991;**121**:951–956.
24 Weber KT, Armstrong PW, Brilla CG, et al. Remodeling and reparation of the cardiovascular system. *J Am Coll Cardiol* 1992;**20**:3–16.
25 Ho KKL, Anderson KM, Kannel WB, Grossman W, Levy D. Survival after the onset of congestive heart failure in Framingham heart study subjects. *Circulation* 1993;**88**:107–115.
26 McMurray J, McDonagh T, Morrison CE, Dargie HJ. Trends in hospitalization for heart failure in Scotland 1980-1990. *Eur Heart J* 1993;**14**:1158–1162.
27 McFate-Smith W. Epidemiology of congestive heart failure. *Am J Cardiol* 1985;**55**:3A–8A.
28 Yusuf S, Thom T, Abbott RD. Changes in hypertension treatment and in congestive heart failure mortality in the United States. *Hypertension* 1989;**13 (suppl 1)**:74–79.
29 Sutton GC. Epidemiologic aspects of heart failure. *Am Heart J* 1990;**120**:1538–1540.
30 Remes J, Reunanen A, Aromaa A, Pyorala K. Incidence of heart failure in eastern Finland: a population-based surveillance study. *Eur Heart J* 1992;**13**:588–593.
31 Bagger JP, Baandrup U, Rasmussen K, Moller M, Vesterland T. Cardiomyopathy in western Denmark. *Br Heart J* 1984;**52**:327–331.
32 Williams DG, Olsen EGJ. Prevalence of overt dilated cardiomyopathy in two regions of England. *Br Heart J* 1985;**54**:153–155.
33 Gillum RF. Idiopathic cardiomyopathy in the United States. *Am Heart J* 1986;**111**:752–755.
34 Sugrue DD, Rodeheffer RJ, Codd MB, Ballard DJ, Fuster V, Gersh BJ. The clinical course of idiopathic dilated cardiomyopathy: a population-based study. *Ann Intern Med* 1992;**117**:117–123.
35 Codd MB, Sugrue DD, Gersh BJ, Melton LJ. Epidemiology of idiopathic dilated and hypertrophic cardiomyopathy. A population-based study in Olmsted County, Minnesota, 1975–1984. *Circulation* 1989;**80**:564–572.
36 Coughlin SS, Szklo M, Baughman K, Pearson TA. The epidemiology of idiopathic dilated cardiomyopathy in a biracial community. *Am J Epidemiol* 1990;**131**:48–56.
37 Kannel WB, Savage D, Castelli WP. Cardiac failure in the Framingham Study: twenty-year follow up. In: Braunwald E, Mock MB, Watson JT, eds. *Congestive Heart Failure. Current Research and Clinical Applications.* New York: Grune and Stratton, 1982:15–30.
38 Vinson JM, Rich MW, Sperry JC, Shah AS, McNamara T. Early readmission of elderly patients with congestive heart failure. *J Am Ger Soc* 1992;**38**:1290–1295.
39 The CONSENSUS Trial Study Group. Effects of enalapril on mortality in severe congestive heart failure. Results of the Cooperative North Scandinavian Enalapril Survival Study (CONSENSUS). *N Engl J Med* 1987;**316**: 1429–1435.
40 Cohn JN, Johnson G, Ziesche S, et al. A comparison of enalapril with hydralazine-isosorbide dinitrate in the treatment of chronic congestive heart failure. *N Engl J Med* 1991;**325**:302–310.
41 Cohn JN, Archibald DG, Ziesche S, et al. Effect of vasodilator therapy on mortality in chronic congestive heart failure. Results of a Veterans Administration Cooperative Study. *N Engl J Med* 1986;**314**:1547–1552.
42 Franciosa JA. Epidemiologic patterns, clinical evaluation, and long-term prognosis in chronic congestive heart failure. *Am J Med* 1986;**80**:14–21.
43 Clarke KW, Gray D, Hampton JR. Evidence of inadequate investigation and treatment of patients with heart failure. *Br Heart J* 1994;**71**:584–587.

SECTION II

AETIOLOGY

6

Human immunodeficiency virus infection and the heart

Peter F Currie, Nicholas A Boon

Epidemiology of HIV infection

The clinical entity now known as the acquired immunodeficiency syndrome (AIDS) was first recognized in 1981 when *Pneumocystis carinii* pneumonia and Kaposi's sarcoma were observed in homosexual men in the USA who were found to be immunodeficient.[1,2] It later became apparent that other groups are also at risk of infection from the human immunodeficiency virus (HIV), which is the accepted cause of AIDS. These other groups are injecting drug users,[3,4] blood product recipients,[5,6] heterosexual partners of HIV-positive subjects,[6] and the offspring of HIV-infected mothers.[7] Homosexual men constitute the largest group of HIV positive subjects in the developed world,[8] although heterosexual and vertical transmission has become an increasingly common route of infection.[9,10] The majority of new AIDS cases reported in Europe in the first half of 1994 were exposed to HIV as a result of injecting drug use.[11]

The World Health Organization has estimated that 18 million adults and $1\frac{1}{2}$ million children have been infected with HIV.[12] Over 128 000 AIDS cases have been reported in Europe[12] with the highest incidence, 6.6–8.7 cases per 100 000 people, occurring in France, Spain and Italy.[13] In the UK, 9865 cases had been notified by the end of 1994.[12]

The mortality associated with opportunistic infection is falling, possibly because of improved clinical surveillance, better diagnostic techniques and the advent of new antimicrobial agents. Although fewer HIV patients are dying of infections, more are surviving to the end stages of the disease only to succumb to malignancy[14] or end-organ failure such as cardiac dysfunction.[15]

Current predictions suggest that between 30 million and 40 million people worldwide will be HIV positive by the turn of the century,[12] and it has been speculated that 50% of these will develop AIDS within 10 years of the initial infection.[16] If only a small proportion of these patients survive to develop significant left ventricular dysfunction,[17] AIDS will become a major cause of heart failure.

Immunopathology of HIV infection

The retrovirus responsible for AIDS was isolated from patients in 1983 and 1984[18,19] and was initially named human T lymphotropic virus type III (HTLV III). The human immunodeficiency virus (HIV), as it is now known, gains entry into cells following high-affinity binding between its envelope glycoprotein group 120 and CD4 receptors which are found on T4 (helper) lymphocytes and some other cell types. The CD4 receptor is the normal ligand for major histocompatibility complex (MHC) class II molecules on antigen-presenting cells, allowing recognition of processed antigen and is therefore an integral part of the immune system.

After entering the cell, viral RNA begins the process of reverse transcription, producing circularized DNA which is incorporated in the host cell genome. The virus can remain latent for a prolonged period, so there is often a delay between the initial infection and clinical disease.

The events surrounding viral reactivation are not fully understood, but they lead to active intracellular RNA production. At this stage of the infection, the viral antigens group 40 and group 120, and p24 protein are expressed on the cell surface. Ultimately, cytolysis occurs, with resultant widespread dissemination of HIV.[20,21]

HIV infection therefore causes profound immunodeficiency by depleting helper cells and inducing functional abnormalities of other components of the immune system. When the body is no longer able to mount an effective immune response, the victim becomes susceptible to opportunistic infections, malignancy, and end-organ failure.

HIV has an affinity for helper lymphocytes, but the virus is also capable of infecting other cell types, including glial cells,[22] corneal epithelial cells,[23] peripheral nerve cells,[24] Kupfer cells of the liver,[25] and testicular Sertoli cells.[26] Many of these cell types do not possess the CD4 receptor and it is therefore possible that other unidentified mechanisms may promote viral entry into the cell.[15,20]

Although HIV can infect myocardial interstitial cells, the evidence that the virus can enter human cardiac myocytes, which do not possess CD4 receptors, is less clear. Immunohistochemistry studies have shown no evidence of p24 antigen expression in the heart,[27] and it is difficult to interpret polymerase chain reaction (PCR) or cell culture investigations because sample contamination with the subject's own HIV-infected blood cells may complicate the results.[28] In-situ hybridization studies have shown weak HIV DNA signals within myocytes[29–31] but these studies are also open to criticism.

Clinical presentation of cardiac disease related to HIV

The cardiac manifestations of HIV infection are listed in Table 6.1 and can present in several ways.

Incidental finding

Heart disease in HIV-positive patients is often overlooked, since symptoms of breathlessness or fatigue are frequently ascribed to other conditions such as anaemia or bronchopulmonary infection. Cardiac dysfunction is therefore sometimes revealed when chest radiographs or echocardiograms are requested for some other reason.

Sudden death

Although many unexpected deaths are clearly due to other causes such as trauma or drug overdose, sudden death and abnormalities of rhythm are responsible for many of the cardiac-related deaths in patients with AIDS.[32]

Tamponade

This is particularly common in Africa, where mycobacterial pericarditis is commonly the index condition for the diagnosis of AIDS.

Heart failure

This is increasingly important and is becoming better recognized in the developed world, where up to 6% of patients develop features.

Heart muscle disease	Myocarditis
	Primary HIV myocarditis
	Secondary myocarditis
	Opportunistic infections
	Mycobacterium tuberculosis
	Mycobacterium avium-intracellulare
	Cryptococcus neoformans
	Aspergillus fumigatus
	Toxoplasma gondii
	Histoplasma capsulatum
	Cytomegalovirus
	Pneumocystis carinii
	Candida species
	Dilated cardiomyopathy
	Left and biventricular dysfunction
	Isolated right ventricular dilatation
Endocarditis	Non-bacterial thrombotic (Marantic) endocarditis
	Infective endocarditis
Pericardial disease	Infectious pericarditis
	Non-infectious pericarditis
	Asymptomatic pericardial effusion
	Cardiac tamponade
Malignancy	Kaposi's sarcoma
	Lymphoma
Cardiac arrhythmia	Drug-induced
	Secondary to other pathology

Table 6.1
Cardiac pathology associated with HIV infection.

Non-bacterial thrombotic endocarditis

Marantic or non-bacterial thrombotic endocarditis (NBTE) is a condition in which friable clumps of platelets and red cells adhere to the cardiac valves. Unlike bacterial endocarditis, these lesions are not infective[33] and show no evidence of an inflammatory reaction.[34] NBTE was found in a homosexual male receiving chemotherapy for Kaposi's sarcoma in 1982,[35] and it had been reported in approximately 10% of adult AIDS patients at autopsy up to 1989 (Table 6.2).

The pathogenesis of NBTE is not fully understood, but hypercoagulability,[42] endothelial damage, or immune complex deposition may be important.[33] Intracardiac catheters or particulate matter from injecting drug use may cause endothelial damage in the right heart, predisposing to the development of thrombotic vegetations. Malnutrition and specific vitamin deficiencies are common in AIDS,[43] and these may also be implicated since the endothelium underlying the lesions often contains abnormal collagen and elastic fibres[44] similar to those seen in vitamin C deficiency.[45]

Systemic thromboembolism is a common sequel, contributing to or causing death in six of the 20 reported *post mortem* cases (see Table 6.2). However, in our experience, NBTE is rare, with only one case identified from a series of 118 *post mortem* examinations in Edinburgh, UK. Moreover, Lewis and Grody[46] have suggested that the incidence of NBTE in AIDS patients is falling in the USA. This is surprising given the growing interest in the cardiac manifestations of AIDS and the continuing echocardiological surveillance of these patients. It is possible, therefore, that the prevalence of NBTE was previously overestimated.

Infective endocarditis

The immunological abnormalities associated with HIV render patients susceptible to bacterial infections,[47] yet there are relatively few reports of infective endocarditis as a complication of AIDS outwith the setting of injecting drug use (Table 6.3). However, there are case reports of *Salmonella typhimurium* endocarditis[48,53] and *Streptococcus viridans* endocarditis[46] in AIDS patients who were not injecting drug users.

The clinical presentation of bacterial endocarditis is the same for both HIV-positive and HIV-negative patients, but it runs a more fulminant course in the late stages of AIDS.[54] Asymptomatic HIV infection, on the other hand, appears to have little effect on the susceptibility to or the mortality from the condition.[54,61] *Staphylococcus aureus* and *Streptococcus viridans* are the most frequently identified bacterial organisms in HIV-positive drug users with endocarditis.[54] *Aspergillus fumigatus*,[49] *Pseudallescheria boydii*,[55] and other forms of fungal endocarditis can occur in end-stage AIDS.[56]

The incidence of endocarditis in injecting drug users in general appears to be falling while hospitalization for HIV infection and AIDS has increased.[61,62] This may reflect a secondary benefit of needle exchange schemes and the continuing education of injecting drug users,

Reference	Year	Number of cases	Valve(s) involved	Symptoms
Garcia et al[35]	1983	1	mitral and aortic	systemic emboli
Snider et al[36]	1983	2	nr	systemic emboli
Fink et al[37]	1984	1	tricuspid and pulmonary	nil
Guarda et al[38]	1984	2	aortic, tricuspid, and mitral	disseminated intravascular coagulation systemic emboli
Cammarosano and Lewis[39]	1985	3	all	systemic emboli
Roldan et al[40]	1987	4	tricuspid and mitral	nil
Klatt and Meyer[41]	1988	7	nr	nr

Table 6.2
Non-bacterial thrombotic endocarditis in HIV infection. (nr – not reported.)

Reference	Year	Prevalence	Risk factor for HIV	Organism
Pitchenik et al[48]	1983	single case report	Haitian	*Salmonella* species
Henochowicz et al[49]	1985	single case report	injecting drug user	*Aspergillus fumigatus*
Roldan et al[40]	1987	1 of 54 autopsies	injecting drug user	healed infective endocarditis
Baroldi et al[50]	1988	1 of 26 autopsies	nr	myocardial abscess
Corallo et al[51]	1988	4 of 102 echocardiograms	injecting drug user	nr
Flomenbaum et al[52]	1989	1 of 4 autopsies	injecting drug user	*Staphylococcus aureus*
Kinney et al[53]	1989	1 of 18 patients	blood-product recipient	*Salmonella typhimurium*
Nahass et al[54]	1990	40 episodes of infective endocarditis	injecting drug user	*Staphylococcus aureus* 75% *Streptococcus viridans* 20% *Streptococcus pneumoniae* 2.5% enterococcus 2.5% *Haemophilus parainfluenzae* 2.5% *Staphylococcus epidermidis* 2.5%
Raffanti et al[55]	1990	single case report	homosexual	*Pseudallescheria boydii*
Cox et al[56]	1990	single case report	heterosexual	*Aspergillus fumigatus*
Bestetti et al[57]	1991	single case report	injecting drug user	*Salmonella* species
Eisenberg et al[58]	1992	2 of 14 patients	injecting drug user homosexual	nr nr
Lewis and Grody[46]	1992	single case report	homosexual	*Streptococcus viridans*
De Castro et al[59]	1992	5 of 72 patients	nr	*Staphylococcus aureus* (3); negative cultures (2)
Vazquez et al[60]	1993	single case report	injecting drug user	*Staphylococcus aureus*

Table 6.3
Infective endocarditis in HIV infection. (nr – not reported.)

although it has also been suggested that infective endocarditis is less common in HIV-positive addicts than in their HIV-negative counterparts.[63]

Cardiac malignancy

There is a well-recognized association between immune deficiency and the development of neoplasia, particularly Kaposi's sarcoma, B cell lymphoma, and other tumours of the lymphoid system.[64] These malignancies are commoner in patients with AIDS than in others, and they often occur in body sites that would be unusual in immunocompetent people.

Kaposi's sarcoma

Kaposi's sarcoma (KS) is the commonest AIDS-related neoplasia, affecting 25–35% of AIDS patients.[65] Male homosexuals appear to be most at risk[66] and, in contrast to the classical dermatological form of the disease, there is often disseminated and potentially fatal visceral involvement in these patients.

Although solitary cardiac involvement has been described,[67] myocardial KS usually occurs as part of a disseminated process. The tumour is an endothelial cell neoplasia and shows a predilection for the subpericardial fat around coronary arteries.[39] It may infiltrate these vessels,[50,68] the parietal pericardium, or the myocardium.

KS is seldom associated with symptoms of cardiac dysfunction; however, there are two reported cases of fatal tamponade associated with the tumour[69,70] and heart failure without ventricular dilatation may occur in cases with extensive myocardial infiltration.[71,72] Cutaneous KS is sensitive to radiotherapy and anthracyclines,[70] although there are no reports of these treatments being used for cardiac involvement.

Lymphoma

Primary cardiac lymphoma is extremely rare in HIV-negative people, accounting for less than 10% of all primary malignant cardiac tumours.[73] Disseminated lymphoma may involve the myocardium more frequently but usually only as part of widespread tumour involvement.[74] However, both patterns of malignant cardiac involvement are commoner in AIDS patients.

Non-Hodgkin's lymphoma can involve the pericardium or the myocardium, and intracavity masses and concomitant periocardial effusions are readily visible on echocardiography. Radionuclide[75] and MRI scans are occasionally useful for detecting more diffuse cardiac involvement.[76] In contrast to KS, cardiac lymphoma commonly gives rise to clinical symptoms of tamponade, heart failure, and conduction abnormalities.

Pericardial disease

Pericardial effusion is found in 10–38% of patients with HIV,[77] particularly when there is generalized fluid retention or advanced disease, but it is often idiopathic.[41,58] Small effusions are found in patients with heart failure or malignant infiltration, but cardiac tamponade occurs only rarely.[70] Pericardial effusion is common in Africa, where it is possibly secondary to mycobacterial pericarditis, which can occur early in the course of HIV infection and may be considered an index condition of AIDS in that continent.[78,79]

The presentation of pericarditis is often classical, though chest pain may be absent.[77] Friction rubs, diminished heart sounds, and ECG changes are found frequently,[80] whilst haemodynamic collapse and pulsus paradoxus should alert the clinician to the possibility of tamponade. Pericardiocentesis should be carried out on patients with tamponade as this can bring about long-term relief of symptoms.[81] Culture of pericardial biopsy or fluid from symptomatic effusions can help to identify treatable opportunitistic infections or malignancy.[82]

Heart muscle disease

Myocarditis

The Dallas criteria for the histological diagnosis of myocarditis requires the presence of an inflammatory infiltrate of the myocardium with adjacent myocyte necrosis or degeneration that is not typical of ischaemia.[83] However, the use of this strict definition may be inappropriate in the context of an impaired immune response.

Three histological patterns of myocarditis have been described in patients with AIDS:

- lymphocytic infiltration with myocyte necrosis,[40,50,84–86] which meets the Dallas criteria;
- lymphocytic infiltration without inflammation;[46,87] and
- myocyte damage in the absence of inflammatory infiltrate.[71,88,89]

The prevalence of myocarditis has therefore been difficult to establish, with estimates ranging from 12.5%[90] to 53%.[91]

Furthermore, immunohistochemical studies on histologically normal endomyocardial biopsies from HIV-positive patients with cardiac failure have revealed significant numbers of infiltrating CD8 and CD45 lymphocytes in association with increased MHC class I antigen expression.[92] These findings were indistinguishable from those in other HIV-positive heart failure patients who had histological evidence of myocarditis, and they suggest that a subgroup of AIDS patients may have immune-mediated heart disease despite seemingly normal biopsies.[92]

Left ventricular dysfunction and dilated cardiomyopathy

Cohen et al[90] were the first group to describe cardiac failure due to a dilated cardiomyopathy in three AIDS patients. *Post mortem* examinations in two of the patients revealed global dilation of the cardiac chambers and histological evidence of focal lymphocytic myocarditis but normal coronary arteries.

A number of subsequent, cross-sectional echocardiographic[15,37,51,88,90,91,93–99] and retrospective *post mortem* analyses[84,100,101] have confirmed the existence of left and biventricular failure in association with AIDS.

Cardiac dysfunction occurs in all the major risk groups for HIV infection, including homosexual men[94,96] and injecting drug users,[51,97,98] and in HIV-positive children.[93,95,101] The reported prevalence of left ventricular dysfunction in HIV infection varies from 2%[100] to over 40%,[51] with symptomatic heart failure developing in approximately 6% of patients,[15] most of whom have end-stage AIDS.[15,91,96,102]

The differential diagnosis of HIV-related heart muscle disease includes:

- left ventricular dysfunction secondary to ischaemic heart disease, diabetes or hypertension;
- hypersensitivity reactions to drugs or foreign injected material; and
- coronary spasm secondary to cocaine use.[103]

Left ventricular dysfunction was found to be common in hospitalized AIDS patients compared to a control group made up of 20 patients with acute leukaemia closely matched for body habitus and nutritional status, in whom there was no evidence of heart muscle disease.[96] Cardiac abnormalities were rare in an echocardiographic study of HIV-negative injecting drug users in contrast to an age-matched cohort of HIV-positive users,[104] suggesting that myocardial dysfunction in AIDS is not merely the result of lifestyle or a non-specific manifestation of a chronic and debilitating illness.

Dilated cardiomyopathy (DCM) has emerged as the most clinically significant cardiac complication of HIV infection in the western world.[17,105] A careful history should therefore always be taken to date the onset of symptoms such as fatigue, breathlessness, or palpitation along with a physical examination paying particular attention to the signs of heart failure including resting tachycardia with a third sound, elevated jugular venous pressure, basal crepitations, and peripheral oedema. Non-specific changes in the ECG are common and are often unhelpful. Chest X-ray may reveal cardiomegaly or pulmonary oedema. However, echocardiography remains the most useful diagnostic tool.

Echocardiographic studies involving a total of 816 patients with HIV infection show that between 3% and 41% (mean 15.6%) had ventricular dysfunction, and, although less commonly reported, around 6% had symptoms of cardiac failure (Table 6.4). Despite this, cardiac dysfunction is still often overlooked as a possible cause of breathlessness in AIDS patients.[95]

Anecdotal reports indicating that dilated cardiomyopathy is associated with a poor prognosis,[90,96,100] even in those patients with an apparent improvement in cardiac function after treatment,[94,107] have been confirmed by a large prospective study in Edinburgh.[17]

Over a 4-year period, 296 HIV-positive patients from all the major risk groups for HIV infection in the UK (203 injecting drug users, 52 homosexuals, 28 heterosexuals, seven bisexuals, three blood-product recipients, and three with multiple risk factors) underwent serial echocardiographic assessment in Edinburgh. A total of 100 patients had AIDS according to criteria from the Centers for Disease Control and Prevention in Atlanta, USA. A further 89 had advanced HIV infection without AIDS.

Thirteen of these patients had DCM (biventricular dysfunction) and their natural history was an early death from an AIDS-related condition. The median survival from the diagnostic echocardiogram was 101 days for the cardiomyopathy group compared to 713 days for those with structurally normal hearts despite evidence of advanced infection[17]

		Percentage			
Reference	No. of subjects	AIDS	Injecting drug users	Symptoms of heart failure	Ventricular dysfunction
Blanchard et al[94]	70	71	0	7	11
Corallo et al[51]	102	100	70	17	41
Herskowitz et al[15]	69	79	56	6	14
Himelman et al[96]	70	73	4	6	11
Currie et al[17]	296	34	69	5	15
Kinney et al[106]	63	30	93	nr	3
Levy et al[91]	60	58	0	nr	23
Monsuez et al[102]	86	50	34	nr	7

Table 6.4
Left ventricular dysfunction in HIV infection. (nr – not reported.)

(Fig. 6.1). Appropriate treatment remains worthwhile despite the seemingly hopeless prognosis and the opportunity for palliative therapy with diuretics, digoxin, and inotropes should not be overlooked.[95,99] However, in our experience, many end-stage AIDS patients have low systemic vascular resistance and tolerate ACE inhibition poorly.

Isolated right ventricular dysfunction

Right ventricular hypertrophy is one of the most common cardiac abnormalities found at *post mortem*,[100] and right ventricular functional abnormalities have been noted frequently in echocardiographic[94,98,108] and blood pool nucleotide studies of HIV-positive patients.[97] This may be part of the global process that leads to biventricular dysfunction and four-chamber dilatation,[88,90,95] but it can also occur in isolation.

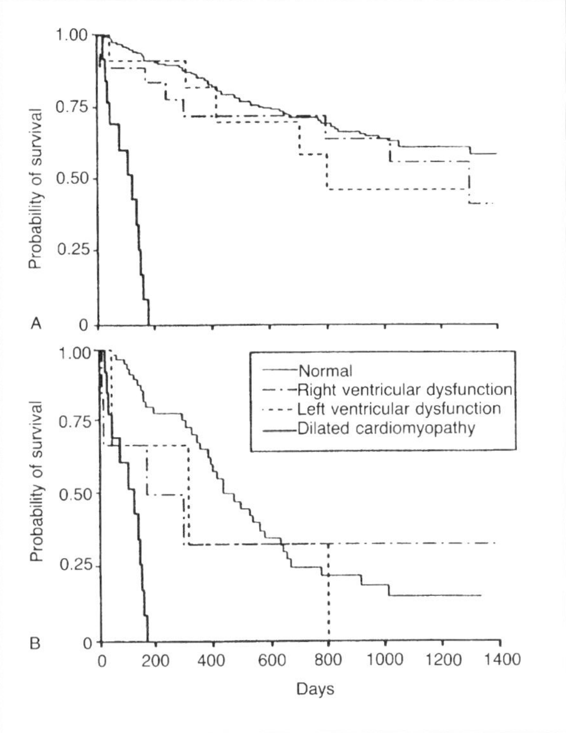

Fig. 6.1
(A) Survival curves for 296 HIV-positive patients with structurally normal hearts or with evidence of cardiac dysfunction. (B) Time to death related to AIDS in 81 patients with CD4 counts less than 20×10^6 *cells/litre.*

Most cases of isolated right ventricular dysfunction are probably secondary to changes in the pulmonary circulation rather than primary myocardial disease. They include pulmonary hypertension associated with multiple microvascular pulmonary emboli following drug injection,[108] HIV-induced pulmonary arteritis,[109] and the recurrent bronchopulmonary infections which are a hallmark of HIV infection.[108] Triscuspid incompetence may also result in volume overload and was a specific cause of right ventricular dysfunction in a man with non-bacterial thrombotic endocarditis and end-stage AIDS.[37]

Right ventricular hypertrophy may be evident on the ECG, but echocardiography remains the most useful method of assessing right ventricular function (Fig. 6.2). Doppler studies are also useful in determining right ventricular systolic pressure.[108]

Pathogenesis of HIV-related heart muscle disease

There may be an association between cardiac dysfunction and the lymphocytic myocarditis reported in some AIDS *post mortem* series. This is analogous to our current thinking on the pathogenesis of idiopathic dilated cardiomyopathy. The observation that isolated left ventricular dysfunction in HIV-positive patients may resolve spontaneously[94] suggests that a potentially self-limiting myocarditis could serve as a substrate for this. However, there seems to be only a loose correlation between clinical evidence of left ventricular dysfunction and histological evidence of myocarditis.

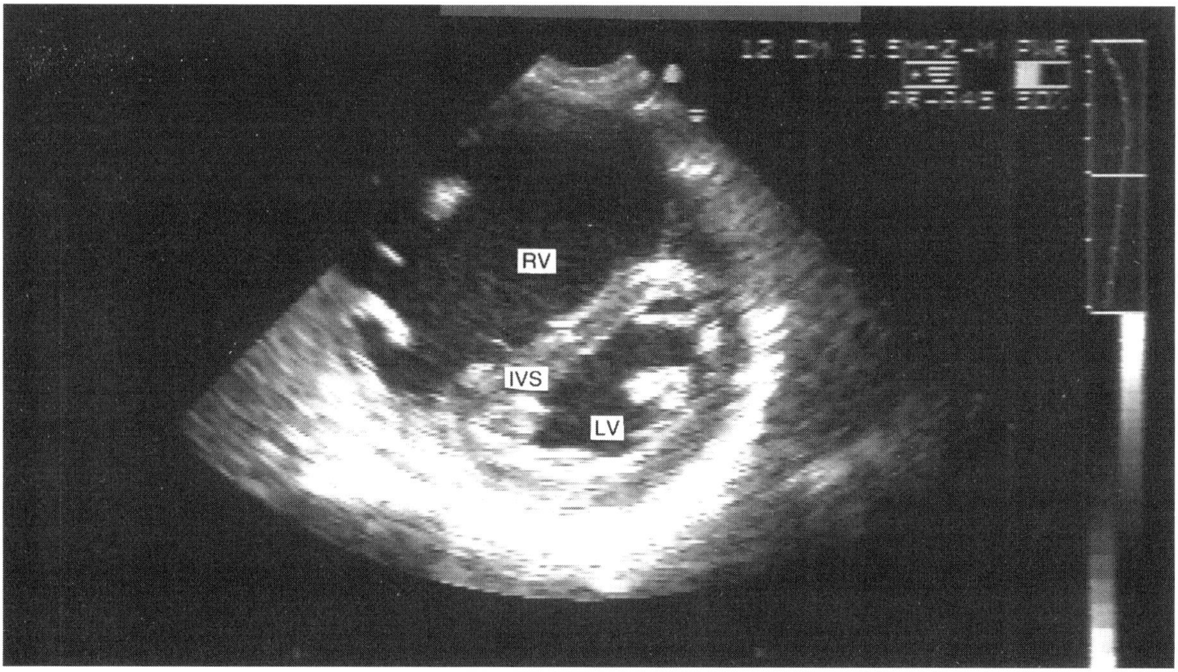

Fig. 6.2
Echocardiograph demonstrating right ventricular dysfunction in an HIV positive drug user. (RV – right ventricle; IVS – intraventricular septum; LV – left ventricle.)

In an autopsy study, Baroldi et al[50] reported on eight patients who had undergone echocardiographic assessment before death. Abnormal left ventricular shortening fractions were found in six of these patients; of these, three had ventricular dilatation, and five had diffuse hypokinesia. The two patients with structurally normal hearts had no evidence of myocarditis, but abnormal histology was found in the others. The Dallas criteria were met in four of these six patients, and lymphocytic infiltration alone was found in the remaining two. Five other patients with myocarditis had no macroscopic evidence of heart muscle disease.

Biventricular dilation was present in seven cases reported by Anderson et al.[84] Four of these died of heart failure and the three without cardiac symptoms succumbed to overwhelming sepsis. Evidence of myocarditis was found in all these cases but not in 12 other patients with isolated right ventricular enlargement. A further 30 patients also had myocarditis, and nine of these had evidence of myocardial infection by opportunistic pathogens.

Reilly et al[110] found histological evidence of myocarditis at *post mortem* in 26 AIDS patients, 15 of whom had clinical evidence of cardiac abnormalities including cardiac failure, pericarditis, and ventricular tachycardia, or a left ventricular ejection fraction of less than 44% using radionuclide ventriculography. Serious cardiac abnormalities were more common in patients with myocarditis than in those with normal histology.

Despite the marked variation in the prevalence of myocarditis found in other pathological studies, a preceding inflammatory process is undoubtedly important as a potential substrate for the development of cardiac dysfunction in HIV-positive patients. There are several hypotheses concerning the aetiology of HIV-related myocarditis; these include:

- primary HIV myocarditis – direct infection with HIV;
- secondary HIV myocarditis – an indirect effect of HIV infection;
- opportunistic infection; and
- toxic myocarditis – nutritional deficiencies, drug induced (zidovudine), or autonomic dysfunction.

Primary HIV myocarditis
Although it is clear that HIV can infect interstitial cells within the myocardium,[30] there is only scanty evidence to suggest the virus can enter the cardiac myocyte. The results of cell culture studies and PCR are summarized in Table 6.5. Contamination with the patient's own infected blood cells can make interpretation of PCR and culture investigations difficult,[111] and immunohistochemical studies have shown no evidence of group 120 or p24 antigen expression in the heart.[27,52]

Despite this, Rodriguez et al[112] demonstrated at least one HIV-1 gene sequence using PCR on microdissected endomyocardial biopsies from 15 HIV-positive patients, five of whom had cardiac symptoms. Although this finding did not correlate well with clinical or histological evidence of cardiac involvement, these authors found increased numbers of interstitial 'dendritic' cells in those patients with heart failure.

Weak HIV signals have been detected by in-situ hybridization in the myocytes of adults[31,92] and in a child with cardiac dysfunction.[29] However, the presence and extent of HIV hybridization often does not correlate well with histological evidence of myocarditis, and most of the positive signals appeared in relatively normal myocardium. Precise identification of cells targeted by *in situ* hybridization is difficult as the cells are often obscured by the positive reaction that occurs as part of the technique. It is possible, therefore, that some of these signals could emanate from infiltrating lymphocytes or endothelial cells. Other *in situ* hybridization studies have failed to demonstrate HIV within myocardium[111] despite microscopic evidence of myocarditis.[30,85]

Although *in vitro* studies on muscle cell lines have shown that HIV is unable to enter skeletal myocytes,[113] recent work on a newly developed human fetal cardiac myocyte cell line has suggested that, despite the absence of CD4 receptors on myocytes, HIV-1 may be ingested through a specific Fc receptor.[114] Therefore, it is still possible that HIV could play a direct role in the pathogenesis of HIV-related heart muscle disease.

Secondary HIV myocarditis
Many autoimmune processes have been described in HIV-positive patients; these include idiopathic thrombocytopenic purpura,[115,116] Sjögren's syndrome,[117] and bullous skin disease.[118] In addition, hypergammaglobulinaemia, elevated circulating immune complexes, and autoantibodies are well described,[119,120] and it seems plausible that myocyte damage could occur indirectly through autoimmune mechanisms.

It has been suggested that cardiotropic viruses such as Coxsackie B3, could modify existing surface antigens or expose other hidden epitopes on the cell surface. For example, MHC class I antigen is not normally expressed by myocytes but it is found in HIV-negative patients with myocarditis, in whom it possibly facilitates the removal of infected cells.[121] Such viral-induced myocyte antigen presentation could be responsible for the ongoing inflammation and cardiac injury seen in many cases of

Reference	Year	Microscopic findings	Evidence for direct HIV infection	Clinical details	Sample type (total no.)
Calabrese et al[28]	1987	no inflammatory infiltrate	cell culture positive for HIV	pericardial effusion, heart failure	single biopsy
Dittrich et al[111]	1988	no inflammatory infiltrate	cell culture positive for HIV, ISH study negative	dilated cardiomyopathy, heart failure	single biopsy
Flomenbaum et al[52]	1989	no inflammatory infiltrate, proliferative membranopathy	PCR positive for HIV in 3 cases, ISH study positive in 1 case	nil	autopsy myocardium (4)
Grody et al[31]	1990	nr	ISH study positive for HIV in 6 cases	nr	autopsy myocardium (22)
Lipshultz et al[29]	1990	lymphocytic infiltration, myocarditis	PCR and ISH study both positive for HIV	hyperdynamic left ventricle	autopsy myocardium (1 child)
Rodriguez et al[112]	1991	no inflammatory infiltrate	PCR positive for HIV	heart failure (4), chest pain (1)	biopsy and autopsy myocardium (15)
Herskowitz et al[92]	1994	21 cases myocarditis: active (4) or borderline (17)	ISH study positive for HIV in 5 cases	NYHA III or IV heart failure	biopsy (37)

Table 6.5
Evidence for primary HIV myocarditis. (PCR – polymerase chain reaction; ISH – in situ hybridization; nr – not reported.)

myocarditis,[121] although the precise mechanism behind this remains poorly understood.

A specific CD8 lymphocyte response targeting myocytes that are expressing viral peptides in association with MHC class I antigens has also been demonstrated in HIV-positive patients.[92] This could be the cause of cellular destruction and myocarditis through an aberrant autoimmune response against endogenous autoantigenic peptides associated with the MHC molecules.

Experimental evidence for these theories has been found in studies on cytomegalovirus (CMV) and Coxsackie B3 myocarditis;[122,123] in addition, high levels of autoantibodies against myosin and cardiac mitochondrial adenosine nucleotide translocator have been found in association with MHC class I antigen expression in a small group of HIV-positive patients with active myocarditis.[124]

HIV might also damage myocytes through 'innocent bystander destruction', a theory first proposed by Ho et al[125] to explain neuroglial cell damage in AIDS-related encephalitis. This hypothesis suggests that specific cells are damaged by proteolytic enzymes and cytokines released through HIV replication in the interstitium and it may be particularly relevant to the myocardium, since increased numbers of infected interstitial cells have been found in HIV-positive subjects with active myocarditis.[112]

Specific opportunistic infections and AIDS myocarditis

A variety of organisms have been identified in the myocardium of AIDS patients, including fungi, protozoa, bacteria, and viruses (Table 6.6). The majority of these have been part of a disseminated infection are are infrequently associated with localized myocarditis.

In an autopsy series of 71 patients, Anderson et al[84] discovered opportunistic infection in the myocardium of nine patients, all of whom had systemic infection with the corresponding organisms. These included CMV, acid-fast bacilli (AFB), *Toxoplasma gondii*, *Candida* species, *Histoplasma capsulatum*, and *Staphylococcus aureus*. Although evidence of myocarditis was found in all of these cases, myocyte necrosis and inflammatory infiltrate was found adjacent to the organism in only two instances (*Staphylococcus aureus* and AFB) and was found in separate sections in the others.

This finding has been confirmed by other workers,[46,50,71] and isolated infection with adjacent myocarditis has rarely been described.[129,130] A clear aetiological link between opportunistic infection and AIDS myocarditis has yet to be established, mirroring our experience in non-AIDS myocarditis where an infectious aetiology often remains obscure.

CMV infection is one of the most common opportunistic infections in AIDS patients. Despite this, it has been described only infrequently as a cause of myocarditis in these patients,[86,102,127] and always against a background of disseminated infection. The finding of CMV without an associated inflammatory infiltrate or the classical intranuclear inclusion bodies within myocytes may cast doubt on the role of the organism in the pathogenesis of myocarditis.[71,82,84] However, CMV can be present in tissue without histological confirmation,[132] and *in situ* hybridization has recently identified transcripts of DNA that are specific to the CMV genome within the the myocytes of HIV-positive patients with myocarditis and cardiomyopathy in whom typical inclusion bodies were not found.[86]

Herskowitz et al[92] studied 37 endomyocardial biopsies taken from HIV-positive patients with moderate to severe left ventricular dysfunction. Two patients had histological evidence of a CMV or cryptococcal myocarditis and two had changes secondary to drug hyper-

Reference	Year	Infective agent (No. of cases)	Isolated or disseminated infection	Incidence of infection
126	1983	variably acid fast organisms	disseminated	single case report
38	1984	cytomegalovirus	disseminated	1 of 13 patients
71	1984	cytomegalovirus	disseminated	1 of 36 patients
65	1985	*Toxoplasma*	nr	1 of 54 patients
127	1985	cytomegalovirus (4), *Candida* (1)	disseminated	5 of 56 patients
128	1987	*Pneumocystis carinii*	disseminated	single case report
40	1987	*Toxoplasma*	disseminated	6 of 54 patients
84	1988	alcohol acid-fast bacilli (2) cytomegalovirus (2) *Toxoplasma gondii* (2) *Histoplasma capsulatum* (1) *Candida* species (1) *Staphylococcus aureus* (1)	disseminated	9 of 71 patients
50	1988	*Toxoplasma* (1) *Sarcosporidium* (1) *Cryptococcus* (1)	nr	3 of 26 patients
89	1988	cytomegalovirus cultured	isolated	1 of 4 patients
41	1988	*Candida* species (5) cytomegalovirus (2) *Mycobacterium avium-intracellulare* (2) *Cryptococcus neoformans* (2) *Toxoplasma gondii* (2) *Histoplasma capsulatum* (1) *Mycobacterium tuberculosis* (1) *Coccidioides immitis* (2)	disseminated	17 of 216 patients
102	1988	*Cryptococcus* (2) *Toxoplasma gondii* (1)	nr	3 of 86 patients
129	1988	*Toxoplasma*	isolated	1 of 14 patients
130	1989	*Toxoplasma*	isolated	single case report
131	1989	*Toxoplasma gondii*	disseminated	single case report
56	1990	cardiac aspergilloma	disseminated	single case report
46	1992	*Cryptococcus* (2) *Candida* species (2) *Microsporidium* (1) *Pneumocystis carinii* (1)	disseminated	6 of 128 patients
86	1992	cytomegalovirus (6)	disseminated (2), isolated (4)	6 of 12 patients
92	1994	cytomegalovirus (16)	disseminated (6)	16 of 37 patients

Table 6.6
Specific cardiac opportunistic infections in HIV infection. (nr – not reported.)

sensitivity. Nine biopsies showed active myocarditis according to the Dallas criteria and a further eight samples showed histological evidence of borderline myocarditis. *In situ* hybridization for HIV-1 was positive in isolated myocytes from only five samples, but CMV DNA was discovered in 16 biopsies using the CMV IE-2 probe, suggesting latent viral infection.

Toxoplasma gondii has also been reported frequently as a possible cause of AIDS-related myocarditis, either as a part of disseminated infection or in cases where the organism has been isolated solely in the myocardium with adjacent myocyte necrosis and inflammation.[129,130] Both tachyzoites and *Toxoplasma* cysts have been reported as evidence of infection,[40] although cases without adjacent myocarditis have also been described.[50]

Myocardial disease secondary to *Histoplasma*, *Candida*, or *Mycobacteria* infection is rare and occurs almost exclusively in end-stage AIDS patients who have disseminated infection. This intramyocardial colonization is probably the result of severe immunodeficiency rather than primary myocardial infection.

Nutritional deficiencies

Nutritional deficiency is common in HIV infection as a result of reduced intake and malabsorption.[133,134] In particular, abnormally low levels of serum selenium have been discovered in paediatric AIDS patients[135,136] and in autopsy tissue samples of adult myocardium.[137] Selenium deficiency is responsible for Keshan disease, a form of dilated cardiomyopathy in China[138] and therefore may also be an important cofactor in the development of HIV-related heart muscle disease.[139]

Other specific nutritional deficiencies include B-group vitamins, folates and zinc,[140–143] some of which may be mediated by increased levels of circulating tumour necrosis factor.[144] These deficiencies could worsen immune function or contribute to cardiac dysfunction.[140,141]

Zidovudine

Zidovudine (azidothymidine), the first antiretroviral agent commonly used in the treatment of HIV infection, is a nucleoside analogue that acts as competitive inhibitor of HIV reverse transcriptase. The drug is phosphorylated in both infected and uninfected cells to the active triphosphate, which is incorporated into proviral DNA with subsequent chain termination.[145] Zidovudine triphosphate also inhibits gamma-DNA polymerase,[146] which is found specifically in the matrix of mitochondria where it disrupts mitochondrial replication. This is the cause of a specific, dose-dependent, reversible skeletal myopathy.[147] Specific histological changes have been noted in zidovudine skeletal myopathy, including focal necrosis, cytoplasmic bodies and sarcoplasmic, and mitochondrial abnormalities.[145] These are similar to those discovered in the myocardium of rats fed with the drug.[148]

The role of zidovudine in the pathogenesis of HIV-related heart muscle disease in humans remains unclear. Herskowitz et al[107] studied 26 HIV-infected patients with cardiac failure, 13 of whom had been treated with zidovudine. Three individuals developed cardiac dysfunction during treatment which resolved following its discontinuation. However, zidovudine did not appear to ameliorate or worsen the cardiac abnormalities in a prospective study of 24 children,[149] and in our experience the drug does not appear to be an important factor for the development of cardiac dysfunction.[98]

The autonomic nervous system

Patients with AIDS are subject to long-term exposure to high levels of endogenous circulating catecholamines. This may in turn lead to intermittent microvascular spasm and focal or widespread ischaemia,[150] resulting in cardiac damage as seen in some cases of phaeochromocytoma.[151] Autonomic imbalance may also be related to HIV-induced neural pathway damage[152] or it may be a result of direct beta-receptor stimulation by the group 120 protein.[153] These theories have yet to be explored, but they do offer a possible explanation for the presence of myocardial necrosis without accompanying inflammation.

Treatment of heart muscle disease

Grange et al[154] reported a patient with heart failure and dilated cardiomyopathy in whom *Toxoplasma* myocarditis was suspected on the basis of clinical findings and a positive bronchoalveolar lavage result. Although myocardial biopsy was normal, treatment with pyrimethamine and clindamycin was commenced. His general condition improved after this, and a repeat echocardiogram confirmed a complete recovery of ventricular function. Similarly, immunosuppressive therapy has been used to treat two patients with myocarditis that was presumed to be secondary to HIV itself.[87]

It is unclear whether the improvement in cardiac function noted in these cases is due to specific treatment or to the possibly self-limiting nature of the condition. However, the fact that some forms of myocarditis associated with HIV are potentially curable suggests that endomyocardial biopsy should be considered. Right ventricular dysfunction secondary to pulmonary infection may respond to treatment and is potentially reversible with antibiotic therapy.[94,102]

Although the outlook for patients with dilated cardiomyopathy is poor, the opportunity for appropriate palliative therapy should not be missed. Clinical trials evaluating the efficacy of conventional heart failure treatment would be worthwhile. However, there are anecdotal reports that vasodilators are poorly tolerated in advanced HIV infection, since these patients often have low systemic vascular resistance.

Disorders of rhythm associated with HIV infection

Sudden death and rhythm abnormalities are well recognized in HIV infection, and they account for more than 20% of cardiac-related deaths.[32,87,110] These may be secondary to other cardiac pathology or they may be a consequence of some forms of treatment.

Ventricular arrhythmias are associated with some drugs commonly used in the treatment of opportunistic infections. Pentamidine, used in the treatment and prophylaxis of *Pneumocystis carinii* infection, is structurally similar to procainamide and can cause torsade de pointes ventricular tachycardia when used intravenously or intramuscularly.[155–159] Concomitant electrolyte disturbance may be an important arrhythmogenic substrate and careful evaluation of the QT interval and magnesium concentration should be used as a guide to cardiac toxicity.[155] Gancyclovir, an acyclic nucleoside used in the treatment of severe cytomegalovirus infection, may also be arrhythmogenic.[160]

ECG abnormalities and rhythm disturbances are not uncommon findings in HIV-positive patients with myocarditis or heart muscle disease. Atrial and ventricular ectopics,[93] ventricular tachycardia[91] and sudden death[87,110] have all been reported.

Autonomic dysfunction is common in patients with HIV infection,[152] and this may predispose to syncopal events and even death.[161] Dysrhythmias due to excessive sympathetic tone are also recognized.[162] Conduction abnormalities and arrhythmias have been demonstrated in HIV-positive children with

ECG abnormalities; these are possibly related to small vessel vasculitis, neural tissue fibrosis, or myocarditis.[163,164]

Conclusion

Cardiac involvement can occur at any stage of HIV infection and it can present in diverse ways. Some conditions are seen early whereas others, such as the clinically important forms of heart muscle disease, are more commonly encountered in end-stage AIDS. Some of these cardiac manifestations can cause significant mortality and morbidity, and if they are not considered by the clinician are likely to remain undiagnosed, possibly to the detriment of the patient.

The pathogenesis of HIV-related heart muscle disease is probably multifactorial, but its similarity to idiopathic DCM cannot be ignored. It has been difficult to study the pathogenesis of DCM in HIV-negative people because the condition usually presents late when any putative autoimmune insult has largely subsided. HIV cardiomyopathy, on the other hand, occurs in a well-defined group of patients who can be studied prospectively and therefore offers a golden opportunity to learn more about the pathology of all forms of heart muscle disease.

Acknowledgements

The authors of this chapter wish to thank Mrs Jean Cunningham for her expert assistance in preparing the manuscript. Peter Currie is funded by the British Heart Foundation.

References

1 Centers for Disease Control and Prevention. *Pneumocystis carinii* pneumonia – Los Angeles. *MMWR* 1981;**30**:250.
2 Hymes KB, Cheung TL, Green JB, et al. Kaposi's sarcoma in homosexual men: a report of eight cases. *Lancet* 1981;**ii**:598–600.
3 Des Jarlais DC, Friedman SR, Novick M, et al. HIV-1 infection among intravenous drug users in Manhattan, New York City, from 1977 through 1987. *JAMA* 1989;**261**:1008–1012.
4 Chaisson RE, Moss AR, Oniski R, et al. Human immunodeficiency virus infection in heterosexual intravenous drug users in San Francisco. *Am J Public Health* 1987;**77**:169.
5 Evatt BL, Ramsey RB, Lawrence DN, et al. The acquired immunodeficiency syndrome in patients with haemophilia. *Ann Intern Med* 1984;**100**:499–504.
6 Curran JW, Lawrence DN, Jaffee H, et al. Acquired immunodeficiency syndrome (AIDS) associated with transfusions. *N Engl J Med* 1984;**310**:9–75.
7 Friedland GH, Klein RS. Transmission of the human immunodeficiency virus. *N Engl J Med* 1987;**317**:1125–1135.
8 Statistics from the World Health Organization and the Centers for Disease Control and Prevention. *AIDS* 1991;**5**:785–790.
9 Holmes KK, Karon JM, Kreiss JK. The increasing frequency of heterosexually acquired AIDS in the United States 1983–1988. *Am J Public Health* 1990;**80**:858–862.
10 European Collaborative Study: mother to child transmission of HIV infection. *Lancet* 1988; **332**:1039–1042.
11 European Centre for the Epidemiological Monitoring of AIDS. *AIDS Surveillance in Europe Quarterly Report* No 42, 1994.
12 World Health Organization. AIDS – data as at 31 December 1994. *Wkly Epidemiol Rec* 1995;**70**:5–12.
13 World Health Organization Global Statistics, July 1993. *AIDS* 1993;**7**:1287–1291.
14 Peters BS, Beck EJ, Coleman DG, et al. Changing disease patterns in patients with AIDS in a referral centre in the United Kingdom: the changing face of AIDS. *BMJ* 1991;**302**:203–207.
15 Herskowitz A, Vlahov D, Willoughby S, et al. Prevalence and incidence of left ventricular dysfunction in patients with human immunodeficiency virus infection. *Am J Cardiol* 1993;**71**:955–958.
16 Rutherford GW. Long term survival in HIV 1 infection. *BMJ* 1994;**309**:283–284.
17 Currie PF, Jacob AJ, Foreman AR, et al. HIV related heart muscle disease: prognostic implications. *BMJ* 1994;**309**:1605–1607.
18 Barre-Sinousie F, Chermann JC, Rey F, et al. Isolation of a T-lymphocyte retrovirus from a patient at risk for acquired immune deficiency syndrome (AIDS). *Science* 1983;**220**:868–870.
19 Gallo RC, Salahuddin SZ, Popovic M, et al. Frequent detection and isolation of cytopathic retroviruses (HTLV-III) from patients with AIDS and at risk for AIDS. *Science* 1984;**224**:500–504.
20 Levy JA. Changing concepts in HIV infection: challenges for the 1990s. *AIDS* 1991;**4**:1051–1058.
21 Yarchoan R, Broder S. Immunology of HIV infection. In: Paul WE, ed. *Fundamental Immunology*, 2nd edition. Raven Press, New York, 1989:1059–1079.
22 Wiley CA, Schrier RD, Nelson JA, Lampert PW, Oldstone MBA. Cellular localization of human immunodeficiency virus infection within the brains of acquired immune deficiency syndrome patients. *Proc Natl Acad Sci (USA)* 1986;**83**:7089–7093.
23 Salahuddin SZ, Palestine AG, Heck E, et al. Isolation of the human T-cell leukaemia/lymphotropic virus type III from the cornea. *Am J Ophthalmol* 1986;**101**:149–152.
24 Bailey RO, Baltch AL, Venkatesh R, Singh JK, Bishop MB. Sensor motor neuropathy associated with AIDS. *Neurology* 1988:**38**:886–891.
25 Hoda SA, Gerber MA. Immunohistochemical studies of human immunodeficiency virus type

1 (HIV 1) in liver tissues of patients with AIDS [abstract]. *Clin Pathol* 1990;**93**:452.

26 Da Silva M, Shevchuk MM, Cronin WJ, et al. Detection of HIV-related protein in testes and prostates of patients with AIDS. *Am J Clin Pathol* 1990;**93**:196–201.

27 Jacob AJ, Rebus S, Bird AG, Bell JE, Peutherer JF. Can HIV infect the heart? [abstract]. *Eur Heart J* 1992;**13**:P370.

28 Calabrese LH, Proffitt MR, Yen-Lieberman B, et al. Congestive cardiomyopathy and illness related to the acquired immunodeficiency syndrome (AIDS) associated with isolation of retrovirus from myocardium. *Ann Intern Med* 1987;**107**:691–692.

29 Lipshultz SE, Fox CH, Perez-Atayde AR, et al. Identification of human immunodeficiency virus-1 RNA and DNA in the heart of a child with cardiovascular abnormalities and congenital acquired immune deficiency syndrome. *Am J Cardiol* 1990;**66**:240–250.

30 Wu AY, Forouhar F, Cartun RW, et al. Identification of human immunodeficiency virus in the heart of a patient with acquired immunodeficiency syndrome. *Mod Pathol* 1990;**3**:625–630.

31 Grody WW, Cheng L, Lewis W. Infection of the heart by the human immunodeficiency virus. *Am J Cardiol* 1990;**66**:203–206.

32 Anderson DW, Virmani R. Emerging patterns of heart disease in human immunodeficiency virus infection. *Hum Pathol* 1990;**21**:253–259.

33 Freedman LR. *Current Topics in Infectious Diseases: Infective Endocarditis and Other Intravascular Infections.* Plenum, New York, 1982.

34 Angrist A, Marquiss J. The changing morphologic picture of endocarditis since the advent of chemotherapy and antibiotic agents. *Am J Pathol* 1954;**30**:39–63.

35 Garcia I, Fainstein V, Rios A, et al. Non bacterial thrombotic endocarditis in a male homosexual with Kaposi's sarcoma. *Arch Intern Med* 1983;**143**:1243–1244.

36 Snider WD, Simpson DM, Neilsen S, Gold JWM, Metroka CE, Posner JB. Neurological complications of acquired immune deficiency syndrome: analysis of 50 patients. *Ann Neurol* 1983;**14**:403–418.

37 Fink L, Reichek N, St John Sutton MG. Cardiac abnormalities in acquired immune deficiency syndrome. *Am J Cardiol* 1984;**54**:1161–1163.

38 Guarda LA, Luna MA, Smith JL, Mansell PWA, Gyorkey F, Roca AN. Acquired immune deficiency syndrome: *post mortem* findings. *Am J Clin Pathol* 1984;**81**:549–557.

39 Cammarosano C, Lewis W. Cardiac lesions in acquired immune deficiency syndrome (AIDS). *J Am Coll Cardiol* 1985;**5**:703–706.

40 Roldan EO, Moskowitz L, Hensley GT. Pathology of the heart in acquired immunodeficiency syndrome. *Arch Pathol Lab Med* 1987;**111**:943–946.

41 Klatt EC, Meyer PR. Pathology of the heart in acquired immunodeficiency syndrome (AIDS). *Arch Pathol Lab Med* 1988;**122**:114.

42 MacDonald RA, Robbins SL. The significance of non bacterial thrombotic endocarditis: an autopsy and clinical study of 78 cases. *Ann Intern Med* 1957;**46**:255–273.

43 Beach RS, Mantero-Atienza E, Shor-Posner G, et al. Specific nutrient abnormalities in asymptomatic HIV-1 infection. *AIDS* 1992;**6**:701–708.

44 Lopez JA, Fishbein MC, Siegel RJ. Echocardiographic features of non bacterial thrombotic endocarditis. *Am J Cardiol* 1987;**59**:478–480.

45 Rinehart JF, Mettier SR. Heart valves and muscle in experimental scurvy with superimposed infection with notes on the similarity of lesions to rheumatic fever. *Am J Pathol* 1964;**19**:135–143.

46 Lewis W, Grody WN. AIDS and the heart: review and consideration of pathogenic mechanisms. *Cardiovasc Pathol* 1992;**1**:53–64.

47 Wit DJ, Craven DE, McCabe WR. Bacterial infection in adult patients with the acquired immunodeficiency syndrome (AIDS) and AIDS related complex. *Am J Med* 1987;**82**:900–906.

48 Pitchenik AE, Fishl MA, Dickinson GM, et al. Opportunistic infections and Kaposi's sarcoma among Haitians: evidence of a new acquired immunodeficiency state. *Ann Intern Med* 1983;**98**:277–284.

49 Henochowicz S, Mustafa M, Lawrinson WE, Pistole M, Lindsay J Jr. Cardiac aspergillosis in acquired immune deficiency syndrome. *Am J Cardiol* 1985;**55**:1239–1240.

50 Baroldi G, Corallo S, Moroni M, et al. Focal lymphocytic myocarditis in acquired immunodeficiency syndrome (AIDS): a correlative morphologic and clinical study in 26 consecutive fatal cases. *J Am Coll Cardiol* 1988;**12**:463–469.
51 Corallo S, Mutinelli MR, Moroni M, et al. Echocardiography detects myocardial damage in AIDS: prospective study in 102 patients. *Eur Heart J* 1988;**9**:887–892.
52 Flomenbaum M, Soeiro R, Udem SA, et al. Proliferative membranopathy and human immunodeficiency virus in AIDS hearts. *J AIDS* 1989;**2**:129–135.
53 Kinney EL, Monsuez JJ, Kitzis M, Vittecoq D. Treatment of AIDS-associated heart disease. *Angiology* 1989;**40**:970–976.
54 Nahass RG, Weinstein MP, Bartels J, Gocke DJ. Infective endocarditis in intravenous drug users: a comparison of human immunodeficiency virus type 1-negative and -positive patients. *J Infect Dis* 1990;**162**:967–970.
55 Raffanti SP, Fyfe B, Carreiro S, Sharp SE, Hyma BA, Ratzan KR. Native valve endocarditis due to Pseudallescheria boydii in a patient with AIDS: case report and review. *Rev Infect Dis* 1990;**12**:993–996.
56 Cox JN, di Dio F, Pizzolato GP, Lerch R, Pochon N. Aspergillus endocarditis and myocarditis in a patient with the acquired immunodeficiency syndrome (AIDS). *Virchows Archiv [A]* 1990;**417**:255–259.
57 Bestetti RB, Figueiredo JF De C, Da Costa JC. Salmonella tricuspid endocarditis in an intravenous drug abuser with human immunodeficiency virus infection. *Int J Cardiol* 1991;**30**:361–362.
58 Eisenberg MJ, Gordon AS, Schiller NB. HIV-associated pericardial effusions. *Chest* 1992;**102**:956–958.
59 De Castro S, Migliau G, Silvestri A, et al. Heart involvement in AIDS: a prospective study during various stages of the disease. *Eur Heart J* 1992;**13**:1452–1459.
60 Vazquez R, Gomez J, Jimenez P, Sainz I, Manzaneque L. Triscuspid and Ebstein's anomaly in an intravenous drug abuser. *Eur J Med* 1993;**2**:247–249.
61 Weisse AB, Heller DR, Schimenti RJ, Montgomery RL, Kapila R. The febrile parenteral drug user: a prospective study in 121 patients. *Am J Med* 1993;**94**:274–280.
62 Sande MA, Lee BL, Mills J, Chambers HF. Endocarditis in intravenous drug users. In: Kay D, ed. *Infective Endocarditis*, 2nd edition. Raven Press, New York, 1992:345–359.
63 Roberts J. Navarro C, Johnson A, Brown J, Francis CK. Cardiac involvement in intravenous drug abusers with and without acquired immunodeficiency syndrome [abstract]. *Circulation* 1989;**80** suppl II:1285.
64 Centers for Disease Control and Prevention. Kaposi's sarcoma and Pneumocystis pneumonia among homosexual men – New York City and California. *MMWR* 1981;**30**:305.
65 Moskowitz L, Hensley GT, Chan JC, et al. Immediate causes of death in acquired immunodeficiency syndrome. *Arch Pathol Lab Med* 1985;**109**:735–738.
66 Ambrose RA, Eun-Young L, Sharer LR, et al. The acquired immunodeficiency syndrome in intravenous drug abusers and patients with a sexual risk. *Hum Pathol* 1987; **18**:1109–1114.
67 Autran BR, Gorin I, Leibowitch M, et al. AIDS in a Haitian woman with cardiac Kaposi's sarcoma and Whipple's disease. *Lancet* 1983;**i**:767–768.
68 Silver MA, Macher AM, Reichert CM, et al. Cardiac involvement by Kaposi's sarcoma in acquired immune deficiency syndrome (AIDS). *Am J Cardiol* 1984;**53**:983–985.
69 Steigman CK, Anderson DW, Macher AM, et al. Fatal cardiac tamponade in acquired immunodeficiency syndrome with epicardial Kaposi's sarcoma. *Am Heart J* 1988;**116**:1105–1107.
70 Stotka JL, Good CB, Downer WR, Kapoor WN. Pericardial effusion and tamponade due to Kaposi's sarcoma in acquired immunodeficiency syndrome. *Chest* 1989;**95**:1359–1361.
71 Welch K, Finkbeiner W, Alpers CE, et al. Autopsy findings in the acquired immune deficiency syndrome. *JAMA* 1984;**252**:1152–1159.
72 Guarner J, Brynes RK, Chan WC, et al. Primary non Hodgkins's lymphoma of the heart in two patients with the acquired immunodeficiency syndrome. *Arch Pathol Lab Med* 1987; **111**:254–256.

73 McAllister HA, Fenoglio JJ Jr. Tumors of the cardiovascular system. In: McAllister HA, Fenoglio JJ, eds. *Atlas of Tumor Pathology*. Armed Forces Institute of Pathology, Washington DC, 1978:111–119.

74 Roberts WC, Glancy DL, DeVitta VT Jr. Heart in malignant lymphoma (Hodgkin's disease, lymphosarcoma, reticulum cell sarcoma, and mycosis fungoides): a study of 196 autopsy cases. *Am J Cardiol* 1968;**22**:85–107.

75 Constantino A, West TE, Gupta M, Loghmanee F. Primary cardiac lymphoma in a patient with acquired immune deficiency syndrome. *Cancer* 1987;**60**:2801–2805.

76 Goldfarb A, King CL, Rosenzweig BP, et al. Cardiac lymphoma in the acquired immunodeficiency syndrome. *Am Heart J* 1989; **118**:1340–1344.

77 Hsia J, Ross AM. Pericardial effusion and pericardiocentesis in human immunodeficiency virus infection. *Am J Cardiol* 1994;**74**:94–96.

78 Cegielski JP, Ramaiya K, Lallinger GJ, Mtulia IA, Mbaga IM. Pericardial disease and human immunodeficiency virus in Dar es Salaam, Tanzania. *Lancet* 1990;**335**:209–212.

79 Taelman G, Kagame A, Batungwanayo J, et al. Pericardial effusion and HIV infection [letter]. *Lancet* 1990;**335**:924.

80 Woods GL, Goldsmith JC. Fatal pericarditis due to *Mycobacterium avium-intracellulare* in acquired immunodeficiency syndrome. *Chest* 1989;**95**:1355–1357.

81 Currie PF, Wright RA, Campanella C, Gray J, Boon NA. Long term survival following pericardiectomy for *Staphylococcus aureus* pericarditis in an HIV positive drug user. *Eur Heart J* (in press).

82 Andress JD, Polish LB, Clark DM, Hossack KF. Transvenous biopsy diagnosis of cardiac lymphoma in an AIDS patient. *Am Heart J* 1989;**118**:421–423.

83 Aretz TH, Billingham ME, Edwards WD, et al. Myocarditis: a histopathologic definition and classification. *Am J Cardiovasc Pathol* 1987;**1**:3–14.

84 Anderson DW, Virmani R, Reilly JM, et al. Prevalent myocarditis at necropsy in the acquired immunodeficiency syndrome. *J Am Coll Cardiol* 1988;**11**:792–799.

85 Beschorner WE, Baughman K, Turnicky RP, et al. HIV associated myocarditis: pathology and immunopathology. *Am J Pathol* 1990; **137**:1365–1371.

86 Wu TC, Pizzorno MC, Hayward GS, et al. In situ detection of human cytomegalovirus immediate-early gene transcripts within cardiac monocytes of patients with HIV-associated cardiomyopathy. *AIDS* 1992;**6**:777–785.

87 Levy WS, Varghese PJ, Anderson DW, et al. Myocarditis diagnosed by endomyocardial biopsy in human immunodeficiency virus infection with cardiac dysfunction. *Am J Cardiol* 1988;**62**:658–659.

88 Corboy JR, Fink L, Miller WT. Congestive cardiomyopathy in association with AIDS. *Radiology* 1987;**165**:139–141.

89 Kaminski HJ, Katzman M, Wiest PM, et al. Cardiomyopathy associated with the acquired immune deficiency syndrome. *AIDS* 1988;**1**:105–110.

90 Cohen IS, Anderson DW, Virmani R, et al. Congestive cardiomyopathy in association with the acquired immunodeficiency syndrome. *N Engl J Med* 1986;**315**:628–630.

91 Levy WS, Simon GL, Riso JC, Ross AM. Prevalence of cardiac abnormalities in human immunodeficiency virus infection. *Am J Cardiol* 1989;**63**:86–89.

92 Herskowitz A, Wu TC, Willoughby S, et al. Myocarditis and cardiotropic viral infection associated with severe left ventricular dysfunction in late stage infection with human immunodeficiency virus. *J Am Coll Cardiol* 1994;**24**:1025–1032.

93 Lipshultz SE, Chanock S, Sanders SP, et al. Cardiovascular manifestations of human immunodeficiency virus infection in infants and children. *Am J Cardiol* 1989;**63**:1489–1497.

94 Blanchard DG, Hagenhoff C, Chow LC, et al. Reversibility of cardiac abnormalities in human immunodeficiency virus (HIV)-infected individuals; a serial echocardiographic study. *J Am Coll Cardiol* 1991;**17**:1270–1276.

95 Stewart JM, Kaul A, Gromische DS, et al. Symptomatic cardiac dysfunction in children with human immunodeficiency virus infection. *Am Heart J* 1989;**117**:140–144.

96 Himelman B, Chung WS, Chernoff DN, et al. Cardiac manifestations of human immunodeficiency virus infection: a two-dimensional echocardiographic study. *J Am Coll Cardiol* 1989;**13**:1030–1036.

97 Raffanti SR, Chiaramida AJ, Sen P, et al. Assessment of cardiac function in patients with the acquired immunodeficiency syndrome. *Chest* 1988;**93**:592–594.

98 Jacob AJ, Sutherland GR, Bird AG, et al. Myocardial dysfunction in patients infected with HIV: prevalence and risk factors. *Br Heart J* 1992;**68**:549–553.

99 Steinherz LJ, Brochstein JA, Robins J. Cardiac involvement in congenital acquired immunodeficiency syndrome. *Am J Dis Child* 1986;**140**:1241–1244.

100 Lewis W. AIDS: cardiac findings from 115 autopsies. *Prog Cardiovasc Dis* 1989;**32**:207–215.

101 Joshi VV, Gadol C, Connor E, et al. Dilated cardiomyopathy in children with acquired immunodeficiency syndrome: a pathologic study of five cases. *Hum Pathol* 1988;**19**:69–73.

102 Monsuez J, Kinney EL, Vittecoq D, et al. Comparison among acquired immune deficiency syndrome patients with and without clinical evidence of cardiac disease. *Am J Cardiol* 1988;**62**:1311–1313.

103 Zimmerman FH, Gustafson GM, Kemp HG. Recurrent myocardial infarction associated with cocaine abuse in a young man with normal coronary arteries: evidence for coronary artery spasm culminating in thrombosis. *J Am Coll Cardiol* 1987;**9**:964–968.

104 Willoughby SB, Vlahov D, Herskowitz A. Frequency of left ventricular dysfunction and other echocardiographic abnormalities in human immunodeficiency virus seronegative intravenous drug users. *Am J Cardiol* 1993;**71**:446–447.

105 De Castro S, D'Amati G, Gallo P, et al. Frequency of development of acute global left ventricular dysfunction in human immunodeficiency virus infection. *J Am Coll Cardiol* 1994;**24**:1018–1024.

106 Kinney EL, Brafman D, Wright RJ. Echocardiographic findings in patients with acquired immunodeficiency syndrome (AIDS) and AIDS related complex (ARC). *Cathet Cardiovasc Diag* 1989;**16**:182–185.

107 Herskowitz A, Willoughby S, Baughman KL, et al. Cardiomyopathy associated with antiretroviral therapy in patients with HIV infection: a report of six cases. *Ann Intern Med* 1992;**116**:311–313.

108 Himelman RB, Dohrmann M, Goodman P, et al. Severe pulmonary hypertension and cor pulmonale in the acquired immunodeficiency syndrome. *Am J Cardiol* 1989;**64**:1396–1399.

109 Coplan NL, Shimony RY, Ioachim HL, et al. Primary pulmonary hypertension associated with human immunodeficiency viral infection. *Am J Med* 1990;**89**:906–909.

110 Reilly JM, Cunnion RE, Anderson DW, et al. Frequency of myocarditis, left ventricular dysfunction and ventricular tachycardia in the acquired immune deficiency syndrome. *Am J Cardiol* 1988;**62**:789–793.

111 Dittrich H, Chow L, Denaro F, Spector S. Human immunodeficiency virus, Coxsackie virus, and cardiomyopathy [letter]. *Ann Intern Med* 1988;**108**:308.

112 Rodriguez ER, Nasim S, Hsia J, et al. Cardiac monocytes and dendritic cells harbor human immunodeficiency virus in infected patients with and without cardiac dysfunction: detection by multiplex, nested, polymerase chain reaction in individually microdissected cells from right ventricular endomyocardial biopsy tissue. *Am J Cardiol* 1991;**68**:1511–1520.

113 Clapham PR, Weber JN, Whitby D, et al. Soluble CD4 blocks the infectivity of diverse strains of HIV and SIV for T cells and monocytes but not for brain or muscle cells. *Nature* 1989;**337**:368–370.

114 Herskowitz A, Willoughby S, Wu TC, et al. Immunopathogenesis of HIV-1 associated cardiomyopathy. *Clin Immunol Immunopathol* 1993;**68**:234–241.

115 Sloand EM, Klein HG, Banks SM, Vareldzis B, Merritt S, Pierce P. Epidemiology of thrombocytopenia in HIV infection. *Eur J Haematol* 1992;**48**:168–172.

116 Bettaieb A, Fromont P. Louache F, et al. Presence of cross-reactive antibody between human immunodeficiency virus (HIV) and platelet glycoproteins in HIV-related immune

thrombocytopenic purpura. *Blood* 1992; **80**:162–169.
117 Procaccia S, Blasio R, Villa P, et al. Rheumatoid factors and circulating immune complexes in HIV-infected individuals. *AIDS* 1991;**5**:1441–1446.
118 Chou K, Kauh YC, Jacoby RA, Webster GF. Autoimmune bullous disease in a patient with HIV infection. *J Am Acad Dermatol* 1992;**24**:1022–1023.
119 Golding H, Robey FA, Gates FT, et al. Identification of homologous regions in human immunodeficiency virus I gp 41 and human MHC class II beta 1 domain I. Monoclonal antibodies against the gp 41-derived peptide and patients' sera react with native HLA class II antigens, suggesting a role for autoimmunity in the pathogenesis of acquired immune deficiency syndrome. *J Exp Med* 1988;**167**:914–923.
120 Klaassen RJLK, Vlekke ABJ, von dem Borne AEGK. Neutrophil-bound immunoglobulin in HIV infection is of autoantibody nature. *Br J Haematol* 1991;**77**:403–409.
121 Herskowitz A, Ahmed-Ansari A. Myocarditis. *Curr Opin Cardiol* 1992;**7**:469–475.
122 Price P, Eddy KS, Papadimitriou JM, Faulkner DL, Shellam GR. Genetic determination of cytomegalovirus-induced and age-related cardiomyopathy in inbred mice. Characterization of infiltrating cells. *Am J Pathol* 1991;**138**:59–67.
123 Lodge PA, Herzum M, Olszewski J, Huber SA. Coxsackie virus B-3 myocarditis. Acute and chronic forms of the disease caused by different immunopathogenic mechanisms. *Am J Pathol* 1987;**128**:455–463.
124 Herskowitz A, Ansari AA, Neumann DA, et al. Cardiomyopathy in acquired immunodeficiency syndrome: evidence for autoimmunity. *Circulation* 1989;**80**:II322.
125 Ho DD, Pomerantz RJ, Kaplan JC. Pathogenesis of infection with human immunodeficiency virus. *N Engl J Med* 1987;**317**:278–286.
126 Cantwell AR. Necroscopic findings of variably acid-fast bacteria in a fatal case of acquired immunodeficiency syndrome and Kaposi's sarcoma. *Growth* 1983;**47**:129–134.
127 Neidt GW, Schinella RA. Acquired immunodeficiency syndrome: Clinico-pathological study of 56 autopsies. *Arch Pathol Lab Med* 1987;**111**:943–946.
128 Grimes MM, LaPook JD, Bar MH, et al. Disseminated *Pneumocystis carinii* infection in a patient with acquired immunodeficiency syndrome. *Hum Pathol* 1987;**18**:307–308.
129 Tschirhart D, Klatt EC. Disseminated toxoplasmosis in acquired immunodeficiency syndrome. *Arch Pathol Lab Med* 1988;**122**:1237–1241.
130 Adair OV, Randive N, Krasnow N. Isolated toxoplasma myocarditis in acquired immune deficiency syndrome. *Am Heart J* 1989; **118**:856–857.
131 Tolat D, Kim HS. Toxoplasmosis of the brain and heart: autopsy report of a patient with AIDS. *Tex Med* 1989;**85**:40–42.
132 Meyerson D, Hackman RC, Nelson JA, et al. Widespread presence of histologically occult cytomegalovirus. *Hum Pathol* 1984;**15**:430–439.
133 Kotler DP. Nutritional effects and support in the patient with acquired immunodeficiency syndrome. *J Nutr* 1992;**122**:723–727.
134 Anon. Nutrition and HIV [editorial]. *Lancet* 1991;**338**:86–87.
135 Kavanaugh-McHugh AL, Ruff A, Perlman E. Selenium deficiency and cardiomyopathy in acquired immunodeficiency syndrome. *J Parenter Enter Nutr* 1991;**15**:347–349.
136 Jacob AJ, Fell GS, Boon NA. Is HIV cardiomyopathy related to deficiency of selenium? *Br Heart J* 1992;**68**:137.
137 Dworkin BM, Antonecchia PP, Smith F, et al. Reduced cardiac selenium content in the acquired immunodeficiency syndrome. *J Parenter Enter Nutr* 1989;**13**:644–647.
138 Keshan Disease Research Group. Observations on the effect of sodium selenite on prevention of Keshan Disease. *Chin Med J* 1979;**92**:471–476.
139 Zazzo JF, Chalas J, Lafont A, et al. Is non obstructive cardiomyopathy in AIDS a selenium deficiency-related disease? *J Parenter Enter Nutr* 1988;**12**:537–538.
140 Beach RS, Cabrejos C, Mantero-Atienza E, et al. Effect of zinc normalization on immunological function in early HIV-1 infection. Proceedings of the VIIth International Conference on AIDS. Florence, June 1991: Abstract MC 3128.

141 Baum MK, Mantero-Atienza EM, Shor-Posner G, et al. Association of vitamin B6 status with parameters of immune function in early HIV-1 infection. *J Acquir Immune Defic Syndr* 1991;**4**:1122–1132.
142 Mantero-Atienza E, Beach RS, Gavancho MC, Morgan R, Shor-Posner G, Fordyce-Baum MK. Selenium, status of HIV-1 infected individuals. *J Parenter Enter Nutr* 1991;**15**:693–694.
143 Dworkin BM, Rosenthal WS, Wormser GP, Weiss L. Selenium deficiency in the acquired immunodeficiency syndrome. *J Parenter Enter Nutr* 1986;**10**:405–407.
144 Beutler B. The presence of cachectin/tumor necrosis factor in human disease states. *Am J Med* 1988;**85**:287–288.
145 Fischl MA. State of antiretroviral therapy with zidovudine. *AIDS* 1989;3(**suppl 1**):S137–S142.
146 Simpson MV, Chin CD, Keilbaugh SA, Lin TS, Prusoff WH. Studies on inhibition of mitochondrial DNA replication of 3′-azido-3′-dioxythymidine and other dideoxynucleoside analogues which inhibit HIV-1 replication. *Biochem Pharmacol* 1989;**38**:1033–1036.
147 Peters BS, Winer J, Landon DN, Stotter A, Pinching AJ. Mitochondrial myopathy associated with chronic zidovudine therapy in AIDS. *Q J Med* 1993;**86**:5–15.
148 Dalakas MC, Illa I, Pezenshkpour GH, et al. Mitochondrial myopathy caused by long term zidovudine therapy. *N Engl J Med* 1990;**322**:1098–1105.
149 Lipshultz SE, Orav EJ, Sanders SP, et al. Cardiac structure and function in children with human immunodeficiency virus infection treated with zidovudine. *N Engl J Med* 1992;**327**:1260–1265.
150 Factor SM, Sonnenblick EH. The pathogenesis of clinical and experimental congestive cardiomyopathies: recent concepts. *Prog Cardiovasc Dis* 1985;**27**:395–420.
151 Sardesai SH, Mourant AJ, Sivathandon Y, et al. Phaeochromocytoma and catecholamine induced cardiomyopathy presenting as heart failure. *Br Heart J* 1990;**63**:234–237.
152 Freeman R, Roberts MS, Friedman LS, Broadbridge C. Autonomic function and human immunodeficiency virus infection. *Neurology* 1990;**40**:575–580.
153 Glulio L, Petrucci T, Patrizio M, Bernado A. HIV envelope glycoprotein gp 120 interacts with astroglial beta-adrenergic receptors. Proceedings of the VIIth International Conference on AIDS. Florence, June 1991: Abstract MA 1037.
154 Grange F, Kinney EL, Monsuez J, et al. Successful therapy for *Toxoplasma gondii* myocarditis in acquired immunodeficiency syndrome. *Am Heart J* 1990;**120**:443–444.
155 Wharton JHM, Demopulos PA, Goldschlager N. Torsades de pointes during administration of pentamidine isethionate. *Am J Med* 1987;**83**:571–576.
156 Pujol M, Carratala J, Mauri J, Viladrich PF. Ventricular tachycardia due to pentamidine isethionate [letter]. *Am J Med* 1988;**84**:980.
157 Mitchell P, Dodek P, Lawson L, et al. Torsades de pointes during intravenous pentamidine isethionate therapy. *Can Med Assoc J* 1989;**140**:173–174.
158 Loescher TH, Loeschke K, Niebel J. Severe ventricular arrhythmia during pentamidine treatment of AIDS-associated *Pneumocystis carinii* pneumonia [letter]. *Infection* 1987;**45**:455.
159 Stein KM, Haronian H, Mensah GA, et al. Ventricular tachycardia and torsades de pointes complicating pentamidine therapy of *Pneumocystis carinii* pneumonia in the acquired immunodeficiency syndrome. *Am J Cardiol* 1990;**66**:888–889.
160 Cohen AJ, Weiser B, Afzal Q, Fuhrer J. Ventricular tachycardia in two patients with AIDS receiving ganciclovir (DHPG). *AIDS* 1990;**4**:807–809.
161 Craddock C, Pasvol G, Bull R, et al. Cardiorespiratory arrest and autonomic neuropathy in AIDS. *Lancet* 1987;**i**:16–18.
162 Lipshultz SE, Luginbuhl L, McIntosh K. Dysrhythmias, unexpected arrest and sudden death in pediatric HIV infection. Proceedings of the VIIth International Conference on AIDS. Florence, June 1991: Abstract TU B 36.
163 Bharati S, Lev M. Pathology of the heart in AIDS. *Prog Cardiol* 989;**2/2**:261–272.
164 Bharati S, Joshi VV, Connor EM, et al. Conduction system in children with acquired immunodeficiency syndrome. *Chest* 1989; **96**:406–413.

7

ACE genotype, myocardial infarction, and heart failure

Frank Kee, Alun Evans

Introduction

The structure and function of angiotensin converting enzyme and its gene

Angiotensin converting enzyme (ACE) is a member of a family of zinc metallopeptidases. It acts primarily as a dipeptidyl carboxypeptidase in the metabolism of two major vasoactive peptides, angiotensin II and bradykinin. ACE generates the potent vasopressor hormone angiotensin II by cleaving the carboxy-terminal dipeptide from angiotensin I and inactivates the vasodepressor hormone bradykinin by the sequential removal of two carboxy-terminal dipeptides.[1] It is an extensively glycosylated protein that occurs predominantly as a singular molecular form of 170 kDa, although a distinct germinal isoform of 100 kDa is expressed in the testes after puberty. Other somatic forms, such as occur in various neuronal pathways, vary primarily in the degree of N-glycosylation.[2] Human ACE, a membrane-bound enzyme of 1306 amino acids that displays ubiquitous tissue distribution, is oriented so that the catalytic sites are exposed on the extracellular surface of the endothelial cells. The rates of hydrolysis of various substrates, bradykinin excepted, are markedly influenced by the presence of monovalent anions, especially chloride, probably through a change in the protein's tertiary structure.

Molecular cloning of endothelial ACE cDNA has revealed that the enzyme consists of two highly homologous domains (the *amino* and *carboxy*), indicating probable gene duplication in the course of evolution. The overall sequence similarity between the two domains is more than 60% at the nucleotide level, increasing to 89% at the amino acid level in the vicinity of the active site. The complete intron–exon structure of the human ACE gene was determined by restriction mapping of genomic clones and by sequencing of the intron–exon boundaries.[3] The ACE gene, located on chromosome 17q, contains 26 exons, and numbers 4–11 and 17–24 encode the two homologous domains.

The 5′ flanking region has several identifiable sequences for known promoters and regulatory elements, some of which contain motifs resembling glucocorticoid and cAMP responsive units. Although little is known about the regulation of ACE mRNA expression, ACE can be induced by corticosteroids in cultured endothelial cells, and protein-kinase-C- and cAMP-dependent mechanisms both appear to increase its activity.

The role of angiotensin II in vascular biology

Although proof of a functional local renin–angiotensin system is as yet lacking, the localization of the mRNA of angiotensinogen, renin, and converting enzyme[4–7] has provided definitive evidence of local angiotensin II synthesis in cardiac tissues, and it is very likely that its impact will extend beyond any central vasopressor effect. Angiotensin II also has direct inotropic and chronotropic effects on myocardial cells,[8] increases DNA turnover and protein synthesis in isolated atria and ventricles,[9] and increases connective tissue deposition.[10] The factors that regulate growth of vascular cells, or that are involved in remodelling, are beyond the scope of this chapter, but it seems clear that the interdependence of autocrine and paracrine promoters and inhibitors of vascular smooth muscle cell and fibroblast growth is complex. For instance, transforming growth factor-β1 (TGF-β1) may exert stimulating or inhibiting effects depending on the type of cell involved or on the local cellular milieu, while angiotensin II causes vascular smooth muscle growth by inducing autocrine factors TGF-β1 and platelet derived growth factor. Arguably some of the mitogenic effects of angiotensin II are mediated by transcriptional effects on *c-fos* and *c-myc* oncogene expression.[11] The biological significance of these effects is unclear but characterizing the changes at a DNA level should allow a sharper focus on genotypes and phenotypes that are associated with disease.

Following the cloning of human ACE cDNA, a polymorphism has been detected which depends on the presence or absence of a 287 bp fragment located in intron 16, corresponding to an *Alu* repetitive sequence.[12] The deletion (D) is codominantly associated with the immunoreactive level[13] and activity[14] of circulating ACE levels. Although plasma ACE concentration is stable within subjects, this polymorphism is probably a neutral marker for a functional variant explaining 25–44% of the interindividual variability of plasma ACE activity. In one study,[15] subjects who were homozygous for the D allele had a mean serum ACE activity nearly double that of subjects with the II genotype. Furthermore, it is probable that induction of ACE synthesis in subjects on ACE inhibitors may be modulated by the functional variant for which the insertion/deletion (I/D) genotype is a marker.[15]

Until recently it was unclear whether ACE genotype would have any real importance to human disease, but epidemiological research has now found a number of intriguing associations with myocardial infarction and heart failure. These are discussed in this chapter.

ACE genotype and myocardial infarction

The first report of an association between ACE genotype and myocardial infarction (MI) was by Cambien et al in 1992.[16] In a large case-control study (ECTIM – Etude Cas-Temoin de l'Infarctus Myocarde), in three French WHO MONICA Project centres and one centre in Northern Ireland, the prevalence of the DD genotype among 610 cases recruited within 9 months of MI was 1.34 times that in 733 randomly selected controls (Fig. 7.1).

Despite their varying baseline risk of infarction, there was no statistical heterogeneity of effect across the populations. Because the odds ratios were higher in subjects who were other-

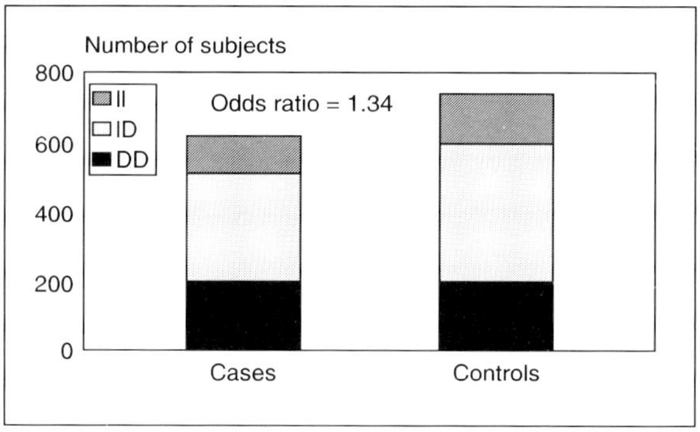

Fig. 7.1
Distribution of ACE genotypes in cases and controls of the ECTIM study.

wise at low risk by virtue of their low body mass index (BMI) and apolipoprotein B levels, it was postulated that selective mortality of DD subjects could have caused an underestimation of the true risk associated with the genotype.

This has been given some weight by several other observations. The same group subsequently studied the prevalence of DD genotype in the hearts of 213 autopsied subjects from Belfast who died suddenly after definite and possible MI. Compared to population controls, the odds ratio for DD versus II was 2.2 ($p < 0.02$), with a stronger relationship observed in older than in younger subjects (2.8 versus 1.9).[17] Furthermore, a parental history of fatal MI was strongly related to the ACE D allele in offspring, and this association was stronger (odds ratio 2.6) than would have been predicted by the differences between cases and controls.[18]

The ECTIM investigators have acknowledged that the reported associations are probably the result of linkage disequilibrium between the ACE I/D polymorphism and a nearby functional mutation, but they have subsequently confirmed that the case–control differences in genotype are associated with serum ACE levels.[15] However, higher ACE levels were found only in cases under 55 years (when compared to age-matched controls) and these younger cases had consistently higher mean ACE levels within all three ACE genotypes. It may be important to bear in mind this age variation when assessing the degree to which subsequent research has substantiated the findings of ECTIM.

The findings lend some support to the involvement of the renin–angiotensin system in myocardial infarction risk. Two well designed longitudinal studies have investigated this issue. One of these, a prospective study of 1717 mildly hypertensive subjects (the majority of whom were African Americans), found MI risk to be associated with a high renin–sodium profile.[19] In the other, which studied 803 normotensive and hypertensive men (predominantly white), there was no significant relationship between renin profile and risk.[20] The disparate findings may be related to differences in the racial composition of the samples or to the more extreme renin profile values investigated in the American study. Further work is clearly indicated.

In a relatively small Norwegian study, the DD genotype was less common in 185 male MI cases than it was in 172 controls (23% versus 35%, $p = 0.03$).[21] However, when categorized as low and high risk groups on the basis of apolipoprotein B level and BMI, the DD genotype was marginally more frequent in cases than it was in controls in low risk subjects (46% versus 33%, $p = 0.14$). No significant differences were found (in either direction) in women.

Although the authors speculated that the divergence from the earlier ECTIM findings could have reflected real differences in the interaction between genetic and environmental factors in Norway (compared to France or Ireland), there were important differences in their study's recruitment strategy. Male cases were eligible for inclusion if their MI occurred before their 56th birthday (there was a mean age of 47 years) and if they were examined up to 14 years (mean 2.8 years) after the event. Thus there may have been a selective loss of DD genotypes in the high risk group. Interestingly the same researchers corroborated the findings of Tiret et al,[18] showing an increased prevalence of a positive family history of premature MI in subjects carrying the DD genotype.[22]

Clearly, a range of genetic and environmental factors affecting atherosclerotic or thrombotic traits may mediate MI risk, and these may vary widely across populations.[23] Caution must therefore be exercised when assessing the impact of ACE genotype on intermediate phenotypes such as angina pectoris or angiographically proven coronary heart disease (CHD).

The evidence incriminating the DD genotype with other such traits is mixed. A small Finnish study[24] found virtually identical frequencies of the D allele in 82 patients with angina (mean age 41 years) to those in age-matched controls. On the other hand, in the prospective Caerphilly Study,[25] although there was no association shown between DD genotype and prevalent coronary heart disease (angina or MI) in the group as a whole ($n = 1225$), in those at otherwise low risk by virtue of a low apolipoprotein B or a high HDL level, the DD genotype was significantly more common in those who developed disease.

Two further studies from the USA have produced somewhat discrepant results. In the Physicians' Health Study,[26] 1250 men with angina or a history of MI or revascularization were compared with 1464 controls matched for age and smoking history. The presence of DD genotype was associated with a non-significant age-adjusted relative risk of 1.1 (0.93–1.29) for all endpoints. When the same group subsequently compared genotype frequencies between the 387 men with definite MI and controls, no association with risk was demonstrated between ACE genotype and MI risk.[27] Additional analyses of the same data set have been published subsequently[28] and no demonstrable effect on MI risk has been shown. Although the Physician's Health Study is one of the few prospective evaluations of the influence of ACE genotype on risk, it differs in other potentially important ways from the original ECTIM study. Firstly, it represents a highly selected subgroup of the population – of 261 248 invitations initially sent out, approximately 5% were eventually recruited and gave a blood sample. The highly selected nature of the sample may have explained the fact that the death rate was approximately 15% of what would have been expected for a population of white American males of the same age. Given the duration of the follow-up (10 years) and a mean age at baseline of all CHD cases of 59.4 years, it could be expected that the mean age of occurrence of MI was at least 65 years, at least 12 years later than for individuals in the ECTIM study. Given the steeply decreasing effect of genetic factors on MI risk with age and the fact that the distribution of fatal and non-fatal infarctions among the genotype groups in the Physician's Health Study is not known, these differences may have a bearing on the differences between their results and those of earlier studies.

In an angiographically defined series of patients from Utah, the frequency of the DD genotype was compared in 359 men and women who had over 60% stenosis in any major coronary vessel with that in 335 subjects who had 10% or less stenosis in any vessel.[29] There was no significant overall difference between the two groups but the frequency of DD genotype was significantly increased in a subset of 123 men with a past history of myocardial infarction ($p = 0.025$). Curiously, there was also a significant and independent association between the D allele and low BMI.

In one of the few other longitudinal studies, the Caerphilly Prospective Heart Disease Study, no association was found between DD genotype and the development of coronary artery disease among all 1226 subjects, but among those at low risk (by virtue of their cholesterol or blood pressure levels at baseline), the D allele was more frequent in those who developed disease.[25]

Several other European studies have now been published which tend to support the DD-risk association. In one, from Leeds, serum ACE levels were associated with the anatomical extent of coronary artery disease in a sample of 388 patients.[30] The DD genotype was more frequent in those with single vessel disease than in those with more extensive disease, leading the authors to conclude that it may be a more important risk factor for subjects at relatively low risk. In another study from Sweden the allele and genotype frequencies in 180 MI cases were compared with those in 430 controls. While the D allele frequency was significantly greater in cases ($p<0.05$) the odds ratio for DD genotype was 1.35 (95% confidence intervals 0.94–1.97).[31]

Two reports have recently emerged from Japan demonstrating an association between MI risk and DD genotype. In the first, by Zhao et al,[32] the frequency of the deletion allele was compared in 101 men with a history of MI before the age of 65 (mean age 53.6 years) and 102 age-matched controls attending the hospital outpatient department (but with no ECG evidence of coronary heart disease at rest or after a stress test). The overall odds ratio for DD versus ID or II was 3.8. The association was present both in low risk and in high risk groups (odds ratios 4.3 and 3.4 respectively) when categorized by the level of total cholesterol and BMI. In the second study, by Nakai et al,[33] 178 patients with CHD (70 angina patients and 108 with MI; mean age 59 years) were compared to 100 unmatched 'healthy subjects' (mean age 42 years). The frequency of the D allele in cases in the CHD group (0.58) was significantly greater than in the control group (0.42). Furthermore, among the patients the frequency seemed to depend on the severity of disease, with a prevalence of 0.71 in those with triple vessel disease and 0.54 for those with only one affected vessel.

Although the strength of the association in these Japanese studies seems to be greater than in many others, the details of control recruitment are not clear, nor were Hardy–Weinberg equilibrium proportions confirmed. (For a given pair of autosomal alleles with a frequency of p and q (where $p + q = 1$), in a large random mating population, the frequency of genotypes should attain the equilibrium proportions of p^2, $2pq$, and q^2, provided that the forces of selection, migration and mutation are not significant.)

Finally, a recent but smaller study from Quebec found the frequency of DD genotype to be 0.61 in young MI survivors (mean age 35 years) and 0.41 in young (but not age-matched) controls ($p < 0.02$).[34]

The association between DD genotype and risk has not, however, been confirmed in all studies. No differences in genotype frequencies were observed in a sample of 315 Austrian CHD cases when compared to 149 controls.[35] In a sample of 882 German patients undergoing angiography, the allele frequency in those with angiographically-significant disease (n=711) was similar to that in those without disease (n=128).[36]

Although some of the variation in the observed frequency of the D allele in different studies is potentially attributable to different genotyping methods,[37] because both case and controls samples in each study will have been performed by an identical method, the estimated odds ratios should not be biased.

While longitudinal studies of angiographically defined CHD may ultimately shed light on plausible biological mechanisms for genotype–phenotype associations, cross-sectional investigations like these can be subject to a number of well-recognized biases.[38] Alternatively, the not entirely consistent results from these studies may be a consequence of unmeasured factors, which, in differently defined populations, may modify the effect of the DD genotype on MI risk.

One such factor may be genetic variation at the angiotensin II receptor locus. Most of the known actions of angiotensin II are exerted through this 'AT_1' receptor. A polymorphism in the 3′ untranslated region of the gene, corresponding to an A to C transversion at nucleotide 1166 of the mRNA sequence, has recently been identified.[39] In ECTIM, the overall odds ratio for DD genotype was 1.05 in subjects homozygous for the common AT_1 allele ('AA') but 3.95 for those who were 'CC' at this locus. Indeed, among subjects at otherwise low risk (as defined previously) the synergism was even more apparent (odds ratios for DD genotype 1.64_{AA} versus 13.3_{CC}) (Fig. 7.2).[40]

Although the frequency of double homozygotes in the population is only 2.5%, the attributable risk for myocardial infarction is 6.9% overall but 27% in subjects at otherwise low risk. Even these data should not be perceived as offering support for a population screening programme, but there may clearly be some groups in the population for whom the risk–benefit ratio is justified.

The biological mechanism and thus the clinical relevance by which the ACE and AT_1 genes interact on the risk of myocardial infarction is

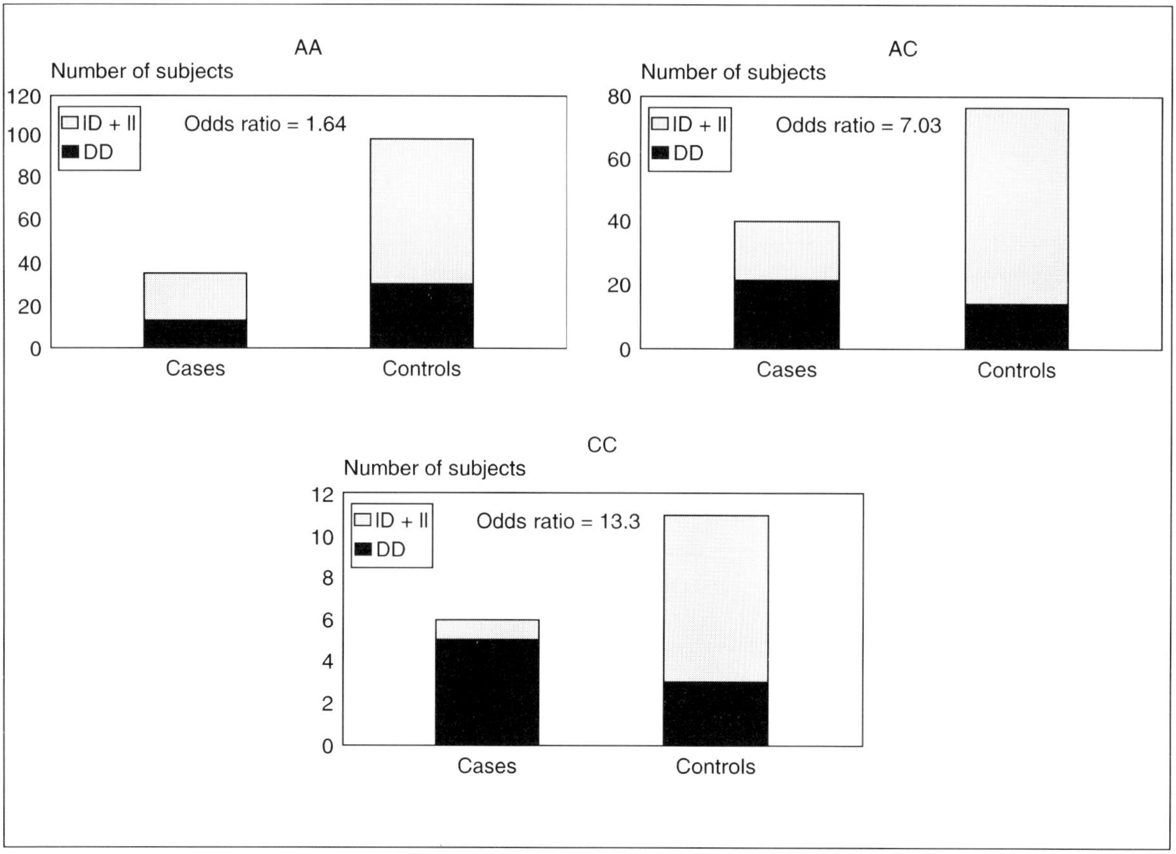

Fig. 7.2
Odds ratios for DD genotype in low risk subjects according to AGT_1R genotype class. (II, insertion/insertion; ID, insertion/deletion; DD, deletion/deletion.)

unknown, but an epistatic interaction would be consistent with this data. Whereas the association of the ACE D allele with increased expression of ACE is known, no intermediate phenotype associated with the AT_1 C allele has been identified. Since the AT_1 gene polymorphism does not seem to be independently and directly associated with MI, but rather modulates the relative risk conferred by the ACE D allele, it is possible that the AT_1 C allele is associated with a modified receptor response to angiotensin II. Several G-protein-coupled receptors, including the vascular AT_1 receptor, show desensitization after exposure to their agonists. One might speculate that the AT_1 C allele is in linkage disequilibrium with a functional variant that could alter the down regulation of the AT_1 gene in response to angiotensin II, the latter being present in increased concentrations in the presence of the D allele of the ACE gene. Alternatively, it is conceivable that increased activity of the AT_1 receptor, under genetic control, is associated with over-expression of the ACE gene, since in a rat model AT_1 receptor blockade induces decreased plasma and tissue ACE activities.[41] Local paracrine mechanisms of interaction may also be speculated, since it is clear that angiotensin II can alter the expression of renin, angiotensinogen, and ACE messenger RNA.[42] It is known that ACE inhibitors do not completely block ACE activity and so, apart from the variations in methodology and definitions of CHD, the ultimate impact of ACE I/D genotype on MI risk will only be defined when plausible biological mechanisms and the potential for other risk factor interactions have been clarified.

Although the underlying mechanism by which the ACE genotype may be linked to MI risk is not known, a recent study from Japan has suggested that subjects who restenose after angioplasty for MI are more likely to be of DD genotype.[43] The study was small and the authors could not account for potential confounders such as smoking, adverse diet, or other gene loci. Although it may suggest an association with neo-intimal proliferation, atherogenesis is clearly a much more complex process. Given the variety of biological effects of ACE inhibition, ranging from a reduction in sympathetic stimulation, a reduction in left ventricular preload and afterload, improvement in endothelial function, and activation of endogenous fibrinolysis, it would be wise not to compare too closely studies implicating the effect of ACE genotype on the risk of different conditions such as angina and myocardial infarction.[44] Whether a varying international frequency of the ACE gene could contribute to variation in CHD risk (the frequency of the I allele is much higher in the Chinese[45]) is unknown. Nor is the extent to which different environments might affect the penetrance of abnormal phenotypes. Although a recent study showed no association between ACE genotype and endothelium-dependent relaxation in young healthy life-long non-smokers (with no family history of heart disease), it is uncertain whether this might also hold in older subjects at greater risk.[46]

ACE genotype and heart failure

Heart failure may not be a single disease and, in fact, could be better regarded as a disorder of the circulation, and not merely a disease of the heart.[47] By far the commonest risk factors for heart failure are hypertension and ischaemic injury following MI, which together underlie 90% of all cases; both have multifactorial aetiologies.

A decrease in the ability of the ventricles to eject blood activates the sympathetic nervous system. At the same time, there is peripheral vasoconstriction due to circulating noradrenaline and angiotensin II, which ultimately leads to salt and water retention. As a consequence, either in response to the low output state itself or to predisposing causes such as infarction or hypertension, a variety of architectural changes develop in myocardial tissue, such as hypertrophy, abnormal interstitial collagen deposition, and the expression of 'slower' fetal isoforms of actin and tropomyosin. However the mechanism directly linking afterload with the transcriptional and mitogenic response is unclear.

At the population level, one of the most important risk factors for heart failure is essential hypertension. There is now fairly clear evidence linking polymorphisms of the angiotensinogen gene and the risk of essential hypertension.[48] Therefore, although it seems that the renin–aldosterone system is involved in defining risk,[49] there is only indirect evidence linking ACE genotype with heart failure and this is perhaps explained by its association with the major predisposing causes, MI (reviewed above), and hypertension. This evidence is discussed below.

One of the most intriguing predisposing causes of ventricular hypertrophy is hypertension, but there is relatively little evidence linking hypertension with the ACE genotype itself. Although one small Australian study found a lower prevalence of the D allele in 85 young hypertensives with a family history of early onset hypertension compared to 95 controls, most other association[50–52] and linkage[53] studies have found no relationship.

Perhaps the most notable report is that by Schunkert et al, who compared the ACE genotype of 290 men and women with electrocardiographically defined left ventricular hypertrophy, usually a precursor of heart failure, with 290 control subjects. Both groups were selected randomly from the Augsburg MONICA Project screening population.[54] For all men and women combined, the odds ratio for left ventricular hypertrophy associated with DD genotype was 1.76 (1.22–2.53). Interestingly, the relationship was stronger among men and normotensive subjects and remained after adjustment for BMI, cigarette consumption, and history of myocardial infarction.

In another study, the ACE genotype was determined in 102 subjects with ischaemic cardiomyopathy and 112 subjects with idiopathic cardiomyopathy (who were receiving transplantation for end-stage heart failure).[55] Compared to the DD frequency in a control population ($n = 79$) with normal ECGs or coronary angiograms, the frequency of the ACE DD genotype was 48% higher in the idiopathic group and 63% higher in the ischaemic cardiomyopathy group.

There are few prospective data to determine whether DD genotype may affect the prognosis in heart failure. However, Anderson et al recently described five-year survival data in a group of 185 patients with idiopathic congestive heart failure.[56] About 20% fewer patients possessing DD genotype (compared to ID and II) survived five years and it would be intriguing to speculate whether such a group might have benefited from treatment with ACE inhibitors.

Conclusion

In 1992, Arnold Katz predicted that by 2001 an improved understanding of heart failure as an abnormality of cardiac gene expression, particularly with regard to the variable effects of ACE inhibition, would underpin cardiac therapeutics.[57] Certainly it is clear that following MI, comparatively few patients (only a proportion of those with prognostically important left ventricular dysfunction) will benefit from an ACE inhibitor. While some variability in the results of ACE inhibitor trials may depend on differences in subject eligibility or on differences between the possible early and later actions of the drugs,[58,59] it is tempting to speculate that ACE genotype may also modulate the clinical effects of the drugs.[60] However, this is still in the realm of speculation and it should be remembered that even the epidemiological evidence linking ACE genotype and the risk of myocardial infarction and heart failure leaves several questions unanswered. To date the evidence has primarily been from cross-sectional and case–control studies, and it is important to replicate the findings in larger prospective investigations. Such studies are already underway.

So far, the majority of the research has concerned the risk in men and, while the number of women in previous studies has been small, the evidence relating adverse outcomes with DD genotype in women is much less compelling. Indeed the differences between the sexes could not be more apparent than in a recent study of French centenarians (85% female), in whom the frequency of the D allele was 0.62, much higher than in the younger control populations with which they were compared.[61] This apparent protective effect of the D allele flies in the face of the evidence from ECTIM[15] and elsewhere[46] that DD genotypes may be under-represented in older age groups, at least in men, through selective mortality. Previous studies have not been large enough to study interactions adequately but clearly, from what is known about the biology and distribution of ACE, a wide range of potentially important physiological actions are possible; whether these are deleterious or beneficial may well depend on age and the presence of other genetic and environmental risk factors.[62] An unanswered question is why, through the course of evolution, a potentially harmful allele of the ACE gene is relatively common and it could be speculated that for some (perhaps for women during the child-bearing years) the vasopressor effects of ACE (and perhaps the DD genotype) could confer an advantage.

References

1 Erdos EG. Angiotensin I converting enzyme and the changes in our concepts through the years: Lewis K Dahl Memorial Lecture. *Hypertension* 1990;**16**:363–370.

2 Hooper NM, Turner AJ. Isolation of two differentially glycosylated forms of peptidyl dipeptidase A (angiotensin converting enzyme) from pig brain: a re-evaluation of their role in neuropeptide metabolism. *Biochem J* 1987;**241**: 625–633.

3 Hubert C, Houot AM, Corvol P, Soubrier F. Structure of the angiotensin I converting enzyme gene: two alternate promoters correspond to evolutionary steps of a duplicated gene. *J Biol Chem* 1991;**266**:15377–15383.

4 Hellman W, Suzuki F, Ohkubo H, Nakanishi S, Ludwig G, Ganten D. Angiotensinogen gene expression in extrahepatic rat tissues: application of a solutions hybridisation assay. *Naunyn Schmiedesbergs Arch Pharmacol* 1988;**338**: 327–331.

5 Paul M, Wagner D, Metzger R, et al. Quantification of renin mRNA in various mouse tissues by a novel solution hybridization assay. *J Hypertens* 1988;**6**:247–252.

6 Rainer RS, Ellridge CS, Gilliland GK, Naftilan AJ. Antisense oligonucleotide to c-fos blocks the angiotensin induced stimulation of protein synthesis. *Hypertension* 1990;**16**:326 (abstract).

7 Schunkert H, Dzau V, Tang SS, Hirsch A, Apstein CS, Lorell BA. Increased rat cardiac angiotensin converting enzyme activity and mRNA expression in pressure overload left ventricular hypertrophy. *J Clin Invest* 1990;**86**: 1913–1920.

8 Lindpainter K, Ganten D. The cardiac renin–angiotensin system: a synopsis of current experimental and clinical data. *Acta Cardiol* 1991;**46**:385–397.

9 Khairallah PA, Robertson Al, Davila D. Effect of angiotensin II on DNA, RNA, and protein synthesis. In: Genest J, Krow E, eds, *Hypertension*. Springer Verlag, New York, 1972.

10 Tan LB, Brilla C, Weber KT. Prevention of structural changes in the heart in hypertension by ACE inhibition. *J Hypertens* 1992; **10(suppl)**: S31–S34.

11 Paul M, Ganten D. The molecular basis of cardiovascular hypertrophy: the role of the renin–angiotensin system. *J Cardiovasc Pharmacol* 1992;**19(suppl 5)**:S51–S58.

12 Rigat B, Hubert C, Corvol P, Soubrier F. PCR detection of the insertion/deletion polymorphism of the human angiotensin converting enzyme gene (DCPI). *Nucleic Acid Res* 1992; **20**:1433.

13 Rigat B, Hubert C, Alhenc-Gelas F, et al. An insertion/deletion polymorphism in the angiotensin I-converting enzyme gene accounting for half the variance of serum enzyme levels. *J Clin Invest* 1990;**86**:1343–1346.

14 Tiret L, Rigat B, Visvikis S, et al. Evidence from combined segregation and linkage analysis that a variant of the angiotensin I converting enzyme (ACE) gene controls plasma ACE. *Am J Hum Genet* 1992;**51**:197–205.

15 Cambien F, Costerousse O, Tiret L, et al. Plasma level and gene polymorphism of angiotensin converting enzyme in relation to myocardial infarction. *Circulation* 1994;**90**:669–676.

16 Cambien F, Poirier O, Lecerf L, et al. Deletion polymorphism in the gene for angiotensin converting enzyme is a potent risk factor for myocardial infarction. *Nature* 1992;359:641–644.

17 Evans A, Poirier O, Kee F, et al. Polymorphisms of the angiotensin converting enzyme gene in subjects who die from coronary heart disease. *Q J Med* 1994;**87**:211–215.

18 Tiret L, Kee F, Poirier O, et al. Deletion polymorphism in the angiotensin converting enzyme gene associated with parental history of myocardial infarction. *Lancet* 1993;**341**:991–992.

19 Alderman M, Madhavan S, Ooi W, Cohen H, Sealey J, Laragh J. Association of renin–sodium profile with the risk of myocardial infarction in

patients with hypertension. *N Engl J Med* 1991; **324**:1098–1104.
20 Meade T, Cooper J, Peart W. Plasma renin activity and ischaemic heart disease. *N Engl J Med* 1993;**329**:616–619.
21 Bohn M, Berge K, Bakken A, Frikssen J, Berg K. Insertion/deletion (I/D) polymorphism at the locus for angiotensin I converting enzyme and myocardial infarction. *Clin Genet* 1993; **44**:292–297.
22 Bohn M, Berge K, Bakken A, Frikssen J, Berg K. Insertion/deletion (I/D) polymorphism at the locus for angiotensin I converting enzyme and parental history of myocardial infarction. *Clin Genet* 1993;**44**:298–301.
23 Shephard J. Importance and interaction of genetic and environmental factors in development of atheroscelerosis. In: Vuylsteek K, Hallen M, eds, *Epidemiology*. Amsterdam: IOS Press, 1994.
24 Meittinen H, Korpela K, Hamalainen L, Kontula K. Polymorphisms of the apolipoprotein and angiotensin converting enzyme genes in young North Karelian patients with coronary heart disease. *Hum Genet* 1994;**94**:189–192.
25 Mattu RK, Needham EWA, Galton DJ, Frangos E, Clark AJ, Caulfield M. A DNA variant at the angiotensin converting enzyme gene locus associates with coronary artery disease in the Caerphilly Heart Study. *Circulation* 1995;**91**:270–274.
26 Kreutz R, Lindpainter K, Pfeffer MA, et al. Angiotensin converting enzyme genotype and risk for coronary heart disease. *Circulation* 1993;**88**:I510.
27 Lindpainter K, Kreutz R, Stampfer M, et al. A prospective case-control study of angiotensin-converting enzyme genotype and the risk of myocardial infarction. *Circulation* 1994; **90**:I472.
28 Lindpainter K, Pfeffer MA, Kreutz R, et al. Prospective evaluation of an angiotensin-converting enzyme gene polymorphism and the risk of ischaemic heart disease. *N Engl J Med* 1995;**332**:706–711.
29 Ludwig E, Cornell PS, Anderson JL, Marshall H, Lalouel JM, Ward RH. The ACE insertion/deletion polymorphism is independently associated with myocardial infarction and Body Mass Index but not with stenosis. *Circulation* 1993;**88**:I-364.
30 Ossei-Gerning N, Foy C, Wilson J, Grant P. Angiotensin converting enzyme gene polymorphism and plasma levels in relation to the extent of coronary artery disease. *Eur Heart J* 1995;**16(suppl)**:abstract P472.
31 Ahnve S, Eggersten G, Hot-Bjelak A, Flodin T, Gabriel A, Sylven C. Angiotensin converting enzyme gene polymorphism and acute myocardial infarction. *Eur Heart J* 1995;**16(suppl)**: abstract P468.
32 Zhao Y, Higashimori K, Higaki J, et al. Significance of the deletion polymorphism of the angiotensin converting enzyme gene as a risk factor for myocardial infarction. *Hypertens Res* 1994;**17**:55–57.
33 Nakai K, Itoh C, Miura Y, Hotta K, Musha T, Itoh T. Deletion polymorphism of the angiotensin I converting enzyme gene is associated with serum ACE concentration and increased risk for CAD in the Japanese. *Circulation* 1994; **90**:2199–2202.
34 Robitaille M, Bogarty P, Asselin MJ, et al. Genotype distribution of the angiotensin converting enzyme insertion/deletion polymorphism differs among young cardiac and young healthy Canadian subjects. *Circulation* 1994; **90**:I110.
35 Friedl W, Krempler F, Paulweber B, Pichler N, Sandhofer F. A deletion polymorphism in the angiotensin converting enzyme gene is not associated with coronary artery disease in an Austrian population. *Atherosclerosis* 1995;**112**:137–143.
36 Haberbosch W, Weiss T, Schwartz O, et al. Deletion polymorphism of the angiotensin converting enzyme gene is independently associated with coronary artery disease and myocardial infarction. *Eur Heart J* 1995;**16(suppl)**:abstract 230.
37 Fogarty D, Maxwell AP, Doherty K, Hughes A, Nevin N. Ace genotyping [letter]. *Lancet* 1994; **343**:851.
38 Pearson TA. Coronary arteriography in the study of the epidemiology of coronary heart disease. *Epidemiol Rev* 1984;**6**:140–166.
39 Bonnardeaux A, Davies E, Jeunemaitre X, et al. Angiotensin II type 1 receptor gene polymorph-

isms in human essential hypertension. *Hypertension* 1994;**24**:63–69.
40 Tiret L, Bonnardeaux A, Poirier O, et al. Synergistic effects of angiotensin-converting enzyme and angiotensin II type 1 receptor gene polymorphism on risk of myocardial infarction. *Lancet* 1994;**344**:910–913.
41 Schieffer B, Wirger A, Meybrunn M, et al. Comparative effects of chronic angiotensin converting enzyme inhibition and angiotensin II type 1 receptor blockade on cardiac remodelling after myocardial infarction in the rat. *Circulation* 1994;**89**:2273–2282.
42 Kohara K, Brosnihan B, Ferrario C, Milsted A. Peripheral and central angiotensin II regulates expression of genes of the renin–angiotensin system. *Am J Physiol* 1992;**262**:E651–E657.
43 Ohishi M, Fujii K, Minamino T, et al. A potent genetic risk factor for restenosis. *Nat Genet* 1993;**5**:324–325.
44 Lonn E, Yusuf S, Jha P, et al. Emerging role of angiotensin converting enzyme inhibitors in cardiac and vascular protection. *Circulation* 1994;**90**:2056–2069.
45 Lee E. Population genetics of the angiotensin converting enzyme in Chinese. *Br J Clin Pharmacol* 1994;**37**:212–214.
46 Celermajer D, Sorensen K, Barley J, Jeffrey S, Carter N, Deanfield J. Angiotensin converting enzyme genotype is not associated with endothelial dysfunction in subjects without other coronary risk factors. *Atherosclerosis* 1994;**111**:121–126.
47 Packer M. Pathophysiology of chronic heart failure. *Lancet* 1992;**340**:88–92.
48 Caulfield M, Lavender P, Farrall, et al. Linkage of the angiotensinogen gene to essential hypertension. *N Engl J Med* 1994;**330**:1629–1633.
49 Weber KT, Brilla CG. Pathological hypertrophy and cardiac interstitium. Fibrosis and renin–aldosterone system. *Circulation* 1991; **83**:1849–1865.
50 Schmidt S, van Hooft I, Grobbee D, Ganten D, Ritz E. Polymorphism of the angiotensin I converting enzyme gene is apparently not related to high blood presure: Dutch Hypertension and Offspring Study. *J Hypertens* 1993;**11**:345–348.
51 Harrap S, Davidson R, Connor M, et al. The angiotensin I converting enzyme gene and predisposition to high blood pressure. *Hypertension* 1993;**21**:455–460.
52 Morris B, Zee R, Schrader A. Different frequencies of angiotensin converting enzyme in older hypertensive individuals. *J Clin Invest* 1994; **94**:1085–1089.
53 Jeunemaitre X, Lifton RP, Hunt S, Williams RR, Lalouel M. Absence of linkage between the angiotensin converting enzyme locus and human essential hypertension. *Nat Genet* 1992;**1**:72–75.
54 Schunkert H, Hense HW, Holmer S, et al. Association between a deletion polymorphism of the angiotensin converting enzyme gene and left ventricular hypertrophy. *N Engl J Med* 1994;**330**:1634–1638.
55 Raynolds M, Bristow M, Bush E, et al. Angiotensin converting enzyme in patients with ischaemic or idiopathic dilated cardiomyopathy. *Lancet* 1993;**342**:1073–1075.
56 Anderson B, Sylven C. The DD genotype of the ACE gene is associated with increased mortality in idiopathic heart failure. *Eur Heart J* 1995;**16** (**suppl**):abstract 705.
57 Katz A. Heart failure in 2001: a prophecy. *Am J Cardiol* 1992;**70**:126C–131C.
58 Ertl G, Jugdutt B. ACE inhibition after myocardial infarction: can megatrials provide the answer? *Lancet* 1994;**344**:1068–1069.
59 Cody RJ. Comparing angiotensin converting enzyme inhibitor trial results in patients with acute myocardial infarction. *Arch Intern Med* 1994;**154**:2029–2036.
60 Morgan K. Diverse factors influencing angiotensin metabolism during ACE inhibition: insights from molecular biology and genetic studies. *Br Heart J* 1994;**72**(**suppl**):3–10.
61 Schachter F, Faure-Delanef L, Guenot F, et al. Genetic associations with human longevity at the APOE and the ACE loci. *Nat Genet* 1994;**6**:29–32.
62 Slud E, Byar D. How dependent causes of death can make risk factors appear protective. *Biometrics* 1988;**44**:265–269.

SECTION III

PATHOPHYSIOLOGY

8

The effects of chronic heart failure on pulmonary function

Sundeep Puri, John GF Cleland

Introduction

Cardiac and pulmonary function are intimately linked, both anatomically and functionally. It is therefore not surprising that dysfunction in one may lead to abnormalities in the other. Wright et al reported an incidence of abnormal pulmonary function tests of 67% in a series of 132 heart failure patients being evaluated for heart transplantation[1] that could not simply be accounted for by smoking history, differences in drug therapy, or aetiology of heart failure[1,2] (Table 8.1).

This chapter considers in turn the abnormalities of pulmonary function that have been described in chronic heart failure (CHF), their functional significance, and the possible mechanisms involved in these changes.

Airway function

Reductions in peak expiratory flow rate (PEFR), forced expiratory volume in 1 second (FEV_1), the ratio of FEV_1 to vital capacity (VC), and acute bronchospasm are well described in acute heart failure. Acute bronchospasm resolves with the resolution of pulmonary oedema, but other indices of airways resistance sometimes require weeks of diuretic therapy before they stabilize and they may never normalize.[3] Even in the absence of pulmonary oedema, reductions in FEV_1 and VC have been shown to mirror the increasing severity of symptoms as graded by the NYHA criteria.[4] In addition, not only does FEV_1 correlate significantly with the peak exercise oxygen uptake (VO_{2max}) in patients with CHF[5] (Fig. 8.1), but some investigators have found that inhaled bronchodilators such as ipratropium bromide and salbutamol acutely improve both FEV_1[6,7] and VO_{2max},[7] which suggests that airway calibre may be of some importance in the limitation of exercise performance in heart failure. However, an improvement in FEV_1 or exercise duration after a combination of salbutamol and ipratropium could not be demonstrated by Moore et al.[15]

The magnitude of the increase in airway resistance in CHF is approximately 25%, and is greatest in the supine position.[8] There is little evidence, however, for significant airways occlusion in CHF; nitrogen washout, a sensitive index of airways occlusion and ventilatory inhomogeneity, is normal.[9] Chronic changes in peripheral bronchovascular sheaths secondary to pulmonary venous hypertension and submucosal oedema have been proposed as possible mechanisms for the reduction in airway calibre seen in CHF.[10] More controversially, the presence or absence of bronchial hyper-reactivity has received much attention. Cabanes et al have demonstrated that the bronchoconstrictor response to inhaled methacholine in heart failure patients can be abolished by the action of the inhaled vasoconstrictor methoxamine,[11] and that treatment with methoxamine can acutely

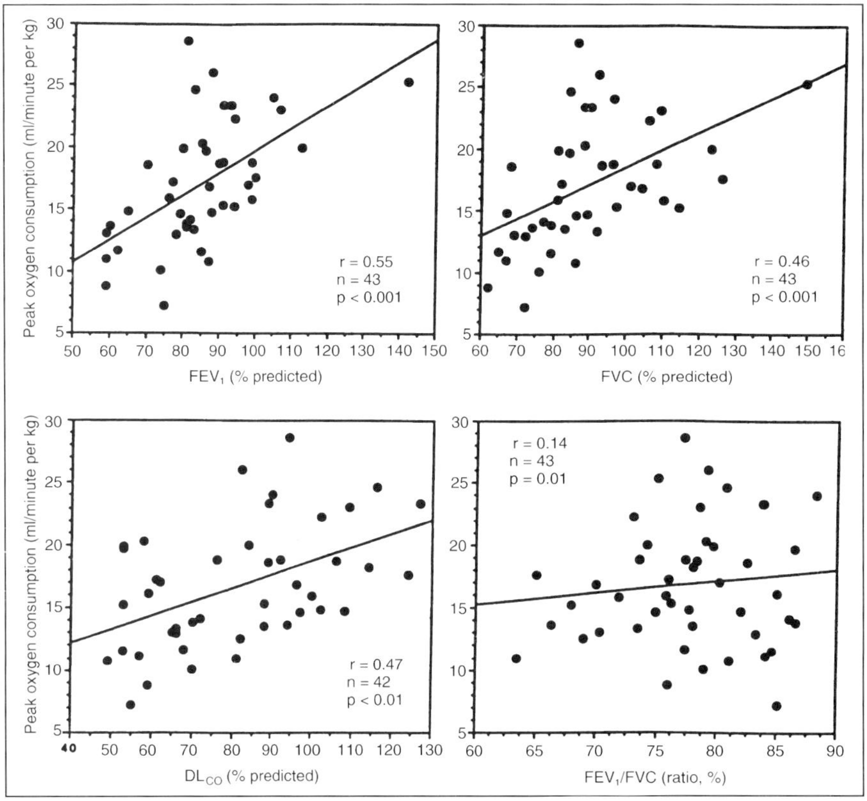

Fig. 8.1
Scatter plots of pulmonary function variables versus peak oxygen uptake. The relations between forced expiratory volume in 1 second (FEV_1), forced vital capacity (FVC), and diffusing capacity for carbon monoxide (DL_{CO}) versus oxygen uptake were all significant. The ratio of FEV_1/FVC was not correlated with peak oxygen uptake. (From reference 5, with permission.)

cause a significant increase in both VO_{2max} and exercise duration at a constant workload[12] (mean VO_{2max} increasing from 18.5 to 20.0 ml/minute per kg, $p < 0.05$; and mean constant workload exercise duration increasing from 293 to 612 seconds, $p < 0.001$). Cabanes et al propose that elevation of left ventricular filling pressures in CHF causes vasodilatation of bronchial wall vessels leading to transudation of plasma into the interstitium and hence to bronchial hyper-responsiveness and functional limitation. Although the evidence is persuasive, and although pulmonary venous hypertension has been shown to be associated with bronchial hyperreactivity,[13,14] bronchial hyper-responsiveness in patients with heart failure could not be demonstrated by other workers.[15,16]

Pulmonary diffusion

Reduction in the pulmonary diffusing capacity for carbon monoxide (DL_{CO}) is well documented in CHF.[1,2,17] It had previously been assumed that a reduction in lung volumes secondary to cardiomegaly and intrathoracic venous congestion was the main mechanism responsible for the reduction in DL_{CO}. Reduction in DL_{CO} can however occur in the absence of any reduction in lung volumes in a significant proportion of heart failure patients[1] (see Table 8.1), suggesting that this may not be the case. More recently, DL_{CO} has been partitioned into its two subcomponents in CHF patients,[4,18] using the classic Roughton and Forster method:[19,20] D_M (the molecular diffusion of carbon monoxide across the alveolar–

		SMOKING STATUS		
	All (n = 132)	Never (n = 22)	Former (n = 96)	Current (n = 14)
Diffusion impairment (D) only	31.1	36.4	28.1	42.9
Restriction (R) only	8.3	4.5	10.4	0.0
Obstruction (O) only	3.8	0.0	3.1	14.3
Restriction and diffusion impairment	20.5	27.3	21.9	0.0
Obstruction and diffusion impairment	11.4	0.0	12.5	21.4
Restriction and obstruction	0.8	0.0	1.0	0.0
Restriction, obstruction, and diffusion impairment	3.8	0.0	4.2	7.1
Normal	20.5	31.8	18.8	14.3

Table 8.1
Frequency of pulmonary function abnormality by smoking status (%). (From reference 1, with permission.)

capillary membrane) and $\theta.Vc$ (the chemical reaction [θ] of carbon monoxide with pulmonary capillary blood [Vc] (Fig. 8.2). The reduction of DL_{CO} in CHF has been shown to be predominantly due to a reduction in D_M (Fig. 8.2), the alveolar–capillary membrane forming

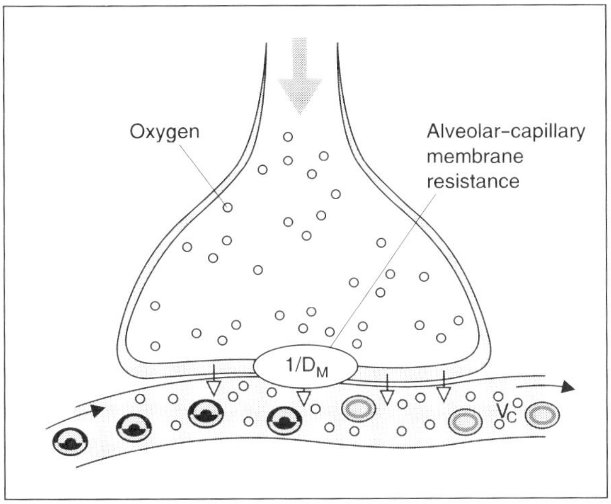

Fig. 8.2
Diagram to illustrate the relationship between D_M and $\theta.V_C$, the two sub-components of DL_{CO}. Total pulmonary diffusive resistance = $\frac{1}{DL_{CO}} = \frac{1}{D_M} + \frac{1}{\theta V_C}$, where $\frac{1}{D_M}$ = alveolar–capillary membrane resistance, θ = rate of reaction of carbon monoxide with haemoglobin, and V_C = pulmonary capillary blood volume.

a larger proportion of the total pulmonary diffusive resistance than in normal subjects (Fig. 8.3). This reduction in D_M cannot be accounted by a reduction in lung volumes (see Fig. 8.3),[18] which implies that there are causes other than reduced lung volumes that must be important in impairing pulmonary diffusing capacity. Further evidence to support this hypothesis comes from the results of pulmonary function studies in heart transplant recipients.[21–23] The effect of heart transplantation on FEV_1, VC, TLC and DL_{CO} from three studies is summarized in Table 8.2. In brief, these studies demonstrate that, despite normalization of cardiopulmonary haemodynamics and lung volumes, pulmonary diffusing capacity fails to improve and may actually fall after cardiac transplantation.[21–23]

Pulmonary diffusion limitation, however, has not been thought to be of great functional significance in CHF because exertional arterial oxygen desaturation is not prominent.[24,25] In addition, it has been proposed that the relatively reduced cardiac output on exercise and prolonged pulmonary capillary transit time would allow increased time for gas exchange, thereby limiting the importance of any impairment of diffusion that might be present at the

	Pre-transplant	1 year post-transplant
FEV1 (% predicted)	75	88
VC (% predicted)	77	90
FEV1/VC (%)	77	77
TLC (% predicted)	86	94
DL_{CO} (% predicted)	75	69
KCO (% predicted)	102	86

Table 8.2
The effects of heart transplantation on pulmonary function tests in patients with chronic heart failure. (Pooled data from three studies with a total of 94 patients.[21–23] FEV1 – forced expiratory volume in 1 second; VC – vital capacity; TLC – total lung capacity; DL_{CO} – the pulmonary diffusing capacity for carbon monoxide; KCO – the diffusion coefficient for carbon monoxide.)

alveolar–capillary membrane.[26] There is, however, evidence that patients with CHF are at increased risk of arterial oxygen desaturation,[27] especially if they have a greater impairment of alveolar–capillary membrane function.[28]

DL_{CO} is an independent predictor of VO_{2max} in heart failure[5] (see Fig. 8.1), and its alveolar–capillary membrane component, D_M, shows an even stronger correlation, both with VO_{2max} ($R = 0.72$, $p < 0.001$) and NYHA functional class[18] (see Fig. 8.2). In addition, increasing the inspired oxygen concentration has been shown to improve both arterial oxygen saturation and exercise performance in heart failure,[29] which suggests that impairment of pulmonary gas exchange may play a role in the limitation of exercise capacity in CHF. Indeed, alveolar–arterial gradients of oxygen ($AaPO_2$) up to 32 mmHg have been reported on exercise in heart failure,[24] implying that either singly, or in combination, some degree of oxygen diffusion limitation or ventilation–perfusion mismatch exists. Although a reduction in D_M may contribute to the widening of $AaPO_2$ gradients in heart failure, gradients of the magnitude reported in the literature would not in themselves cause significant arterial hypoxaemia, and therefore alternative mechanisms may be responsible for the strong correlation of pulmonary diffusing capacity and its alveolar–capillary membrane component with VO_{2max}.

Recent studies have highlighted a possible mechanism leading to a reduction of DL_{CO} and D_M in CHF. In the rabbit lung model, raising lung capillary transmural pressures leads to disruption and fractures of the endothelial and epithelial layers,[30] which in the short term may be reversible. The stereotyped response to pressure-induced trauma in the pulmonary microvasculature is proliferation of alveolar type II cells, thickening of the alveolar–capillary interstitium, and some fibrotic change.[31] Such changes would increase alveolar–capillary membrane thickness and reduce D_M. Extensive studies of pulmonary function have been performed in patients with mitral stenosis,[9,32] including measurement of D_M and pulmonary capillary blood volume.[33] The reduction in DL_{CO} and D_M in this patient group with chronic venous hypertension correlates with NYHA functional class[33] and the severity of histological lung damage.[34] The structural

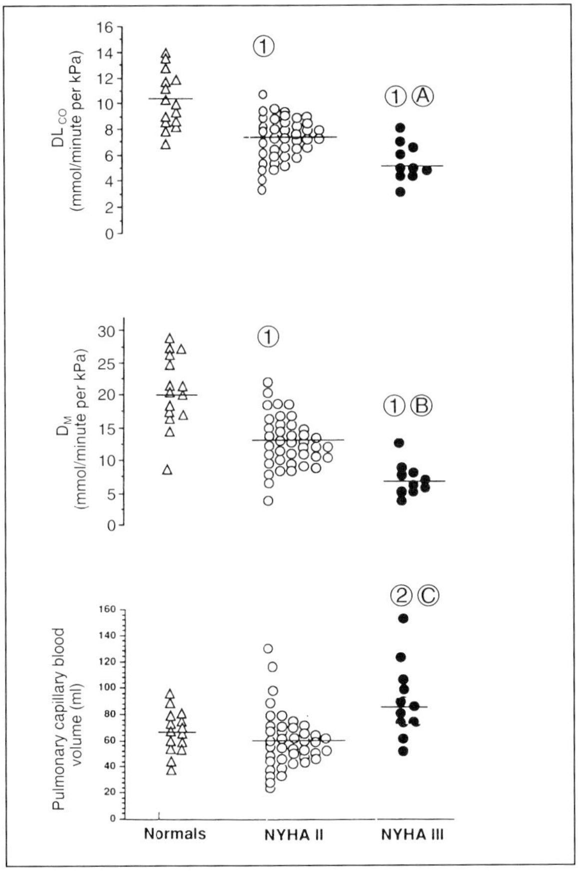

Fig. 8.3
Individual results and mean values of the pulmonary diffusing capacity for carbon monoxide (DL_{CO}), alveolar–capillary membrane diffusing capacity (D_M) and pulmonary capillary blood volume for all normal subjects and heart failure patients. Statistical analysis was performed using analysis of variance. (Compared to normal subjects: (1) $p < 0.0001$ (2) $p < 0.05$. Compared to NYHA II: (A) $p < 0.01$ (B) $p < 0.001$. (C) $p < 0.05$.) (From reference 18, with permission.)

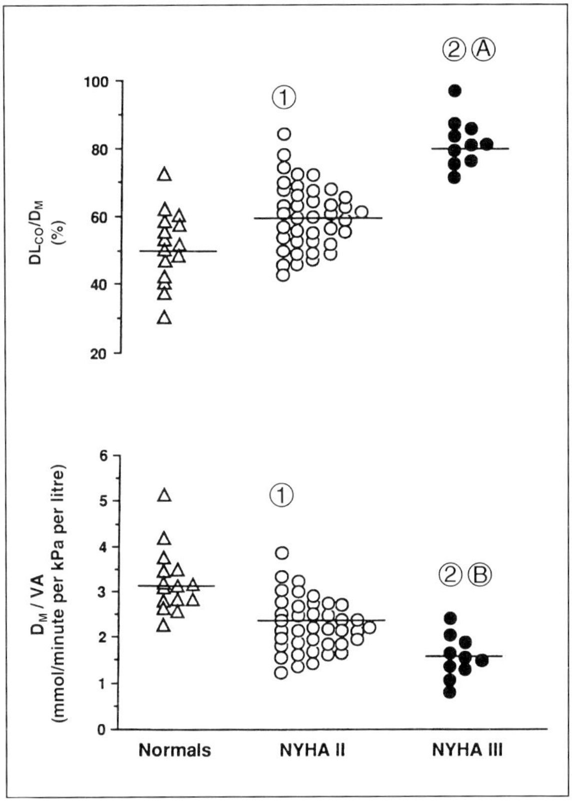

Fig. 8.4
Individual results and mean values of the proportion of total pulmonary diffusive resistance due to the alveolar–capillary membrane (DL_{CO}/D_M) and the alveolar–capillary membrane diffusing capacity per unit effective alveolar volume (D_M/VA) in all normal subjects and heart failure patients. Statistical analysis was performed using analysis of variance. (Compared to normal subjects: (1) $p < 0.05$ (2) $p < 0.001$. Compared to NYHA II: (A) $p < 0.001$ (B) $p < 0.01$.) (From reference 18, with permission.)

changes in the pulmonary vasculature in CHF are similar to those as a result of mitral valve disease,[35] and therefore it is likely that similar mechanisms of injury and remodelling apply to alveolar–capillary membrane injury in both conditions. A reduction in D_M may therefore reflect stress failure of the alveolar–capillary interface induced by pulmonary capillary hypertension. The inverse correlation of pulmonary vascular resistance with D_M that has been demonstrated in chronic heart failure provides further evidence in support of this hypothesis.[18]

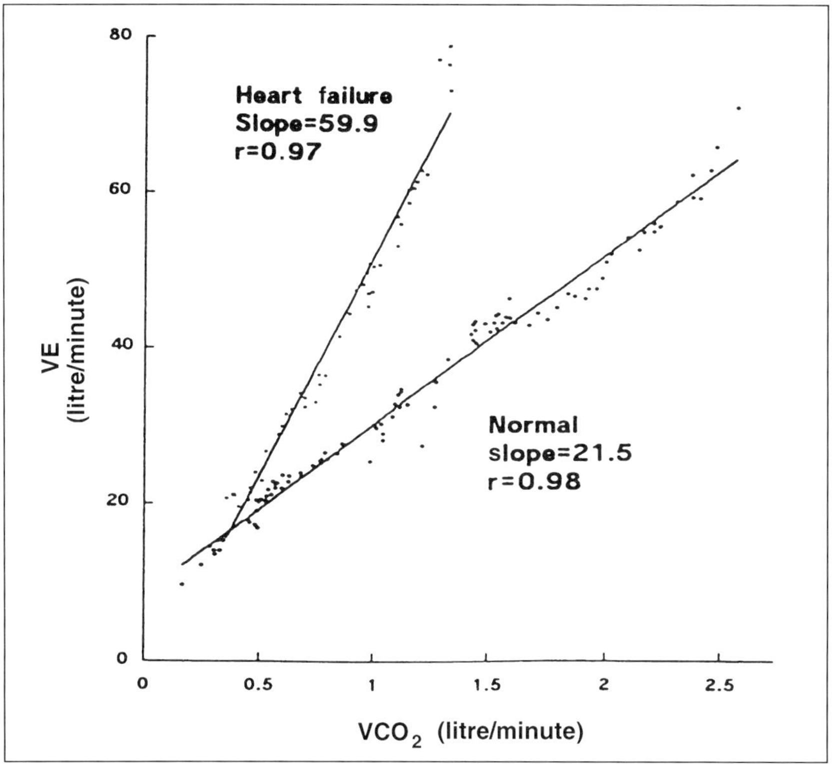

Fig. 8.5
Examples of calculation of the slope of the relation between minute ventilation (VE) and carbon dioxide production (VCO_2) in a normal subject and a patient with heart failure. (From reference 40, with permission.)

Ventilation

Exertional dyspnoea is a common symptom and cause of morbidity in CHF. It therefore comes as no surprise that an increased ventilatory response to exercise is one of the characteristic features of CHF, ventilatory levels being higher for any given workload or level of carbon dioxide production in heart failure patients than in normal subjects.[36,37] A high level of correlation between ventilation and carbon dioxide production exists in normal subjects, and this is retained in CHF patients,[38–40] but the slope of ventilation against carbon dioxide production (VE/VCO_2) is steeper than normal in heart failure (Fig. 8.4), and it has been shown to correlate with the reduction of VO_{2max}.[40–42] Despite extensive research, the pathophysiology of exertional hyperventilation in CHF remains controversial. Several mechanisms have been proposed as possible causes, and these are discussed below.

Increased pulmonary artery pressures

Undoubtedly, pulmonary hypertension is a significant prognostic factor in chronic heart failure,[43,44] and interventions that improve pulmonary haemodynamics also improve exercise capacity.[45–47] The inability to decrease pulmonary vascular resistance appropriately has also been implicated in the limitation of exercise capacity[48] and poor therapeutic response to ACE inhibition[47,49] in heart failure patients. Pulmonary vascular pressures may be elevated at rest in heart failure,[50] and then rise further on exercise.[36,51,52] There is little evidence, however, to support the hypothesis that a rise in pulmonary vascular pressures is a significant stimulus to ventilation, and several studies have failed to show a correlation between exercise pulmonary haemodynamic measurements and the ventilatory response to exercise in CHF.[36,53] It therefore seems unlikely that abnormal pulmonary haemodynamics are the sole cause of exertional hyperventilation in CHF.

Early metabolic acidosis

Patients with CHF have impairment of the cardiac output response to exercise, and therefore develop anaerobic metabolism at an earlier stage of exercise than normal,[37,54,55] leading to an accumulation of lactic acid. It has been proposed that buffering of this lactate accumulation causes carbon dioxide to be displaced, and therefore stimulates increased ventilation. Although there is no doubt that this does occur, the increased ventilatory response to exercise is present both above and below the anaerobic threshold in CHF, which suggests that other significant factors are important in the modulation of ventilatory drive.

Increased dead space ventilation

Several studies have proposed that an increase in physiological dead space is responsible for the exaggerated ventilatory response in chronic heart failure.[39,40,53] These studies have demonstrated a significant correlation between the ratio of dead space to tidal ventilation (VD/VT) and the values of VE/VCO_2 slopes in such patients. Examination of the modified alveolar equation:

$$VE = \frac{863 \times VCO_2}{PaCO_2 \times (1 - VD/VT)}$$

where VE is the total ventilation, VCO_2 the production of carbon dioxide, and PaCO_2 the partial pressure of arterial carbon dioxide, is in keeping with this hypothesis.

There are problems, however, when applying this equation to the aforementioned studies. First of all, these studies used progressive incremental exercise protocols and, strictly speaking, the modified alveolar equation relates to steady state conditions. Secondly, measurement of VD/VT is sensitive to the overall level of ventilation,[56] and therefore spurious positive correlations between VE/VCO_2 slopes and VD/VT ratios may be obtained. However, even with these reservations, it is likely that the pattern of dead space to tidal ventilation is abnormal in CHF. Traditionally, the explanation offered for the rise in physiological dead space in heart failure is an increase in ventilation–perfusion mismatch. By definition, if the ventilatory response to exercise is increased and the cardiac output response decreased, global ventilation–perfusion mismatching must be present in CHF.

The pathophysiological link between lung perfusion and ventilatory drive, however, remains controversial. Wada et al[57] examined the relationship between resting pulmonary blood distribution and the ventilatory response to exercise (VE/VCO_2 slope) in 23 patients with chronic heart failure using a radioisotope technique. They identified two groups of patients – a group with normal VE/VCO_2 slopes (eight patients), and a group with high VE/VCO_2 slopes (15 patients). The patients with increased VE/VCO_2 slopes had increased perfusion of the lung apices, suggesting that ventilation–perfusion matching at rest might actually be improved in these patients compared to normal, the relatively overventilated upper lobes now receiving increased blood flow, presumably secondary to elevated pulmonary vascular pressures. This is in keeping with the increase of pulmonary capillary volume reported in patients with NYHA class III heart failure as determined by the Roughton and Forster method.[4] Uren et al[58] examined both ventilation and perfusion at rest and on exercise in 10 patients with CHF using radionuclide techniques. They calculated a global ventilation–perfusion mismatch index, and demonstrated that overall this index decreased on exercise from baseline resting values. Although peak exercise values of this index did not correlate with VO_{2max}, the magnitude of its change did ($R = 0.88$, $p < 0.01$). From this it may be inferred that the ability to improve ventilation–perfusion matching on exercise may be impaired in CHF because resting ventilation–perfusion matching is already enhanced, leaving less reserve available to meet the increased requirements demanded by exercise.

Oscillatory ventilation

It has been proposed that patients with CHF may exhibit an abnormal pattern of ventilation characterized by alternating hyperpnoea and hypopnoea. This has been classically described as Cheyne–Stokes respiration in the moribund or severely decompensated patient. More recently, cyclical variations in ventilation have been described in patients with treated stable heart failure in the absence of pulmonary oedema, both during sleep[59,60] and during exercise,[61–64] as occurring in up to 25% of patients in NYHA class III.[62,64] Kremser et al[64] were able to show that oscillatory hyperventilation during exercise in patients with a diagnosis of idiopathic dilated cardiomyopathy was associated with cyclical fluctuations in arterial PO_2 and a lower VO_{2max} (11.7 *vs* 17.9 ml/minute per kg compared to non-oscillators), suggesting that such a pattern of ventilation might compound impaired oxygen delivery and thereby limit exercise performance. The pathogenesis of cyclical breathing patterns in CHF at present remains unresolved, but it would appear that oscillatory ventilation during exercise tends to occur more frequently in patients with severe systolic cardiac impairment,[62] and may be accompanied by cyclical fluctuations of pulmonary blood flow.[63]

Respiratory skeletal muscle function

Much interest has focused on abnormalities of skeletal muscle in CHF,[65–68] and similar changes are observed in respiratory muscles. Respiratory muscle strength is reduced, particularly in patients with severe symptoms[69,70] (NYHA classes III and IV), and has been shown to correlate with the sensation of dyspnoea[71] and VO_{2max}.[70] Respiratory muscle deoxygenation on exercise has been demonstrated in chronic heart failure,[72] even in the absence of arterial deoxygenation, suggesting that this may also be a mechanism causing dyspnoea and fatigue.

References

1 Wright RS, Levine MS, Bellamy PE, et al. Ventilatory and diffusion abnormalities in potential heart transplant recipients. *Chest* 1990;**98**:816–820.

2 Naum CC, Sciurba FC, Rogers RM. Pulmonary function abnormalities in chronic severe cardiomyopathy preceding cardiac transplantation. *Am Rev Respir Dis* 1992;**145**:1334–1338.

3 Light RW, George RB. Serial pulmonary function in patients with acute heart failure. *Arch Intern Med* 1983;**143**:429–433.

4 Puri S, Baker BL, Oakley CM, Hughes JMB, Cleland JGF. Increased alveolar–capillary membrane resistance to gas transfer in patients with chronic heart failure. *Br Heart J* 1994;**72**:140–144.

5 Kraemer MD, Kubo SH, Rector TS, Brunsvold N, Bank AJ. Pulmonary and peripheral vascular factors are important determinants of peak exercise oxygen uptake in patients with heart failure. *J Am Coll Cardiol* 1993;**21**:641–648.

6 Kindman LA, Vagelos RH, Willson K, Prikazky L, Fowler M. Abnormalities of pulmonary function in patients with congestive heart failure, and reversal with ipratropium bromide. *Am J Cardiol* 1994;**73**:258–262.

7 Uren NG, Davies SW, Jordan SL, Lipkin DP. Inhaled bronchodilators increase maximum oxygen consumption in chronic left ventricular failure. *Eur Heart J* 1993;**14**:744–750.

8 Yap JCH, Moore DP, Cleland JGF, et al. Mechanisms of the supine increase in airflow resistance in chronic left ventricular failure [abstract]. *Am Rev Respir Dis* 1991;**143**:A345.

9 Jebavy P, Widimsky J, Stanek V. Distribution of inspired gas and pulmonary diffusing capacity at rest and during graded exercise in patients with mitral stenosis. *Respiration* 1971;**28**:216–235.

10 Fishman AP. Cardiac asthma – a fresh look at on old wheeze. *N Engl J Med* 1989;**320**:1346–1348.

11 Cabanes LR, Weber SN, Matran R, et al. Bronchial hyperresponsiveness to methacholine in patients with impaired left ventricular function. *N Engl J Med* 1989;**320**:1317–1322.

12 Cabanes L, Costes F, Weber S, et al. Improvement in exercise performance by inhalation of methoxamine in patients with impaired left ventricular function. *N Engl J Med* 1992;**326**:1661–1665.

13 Brunnee T, Graf K, Kastens B, Fleck E, Kunkel G. Bronchial hyperreactivity in patients with moderate pulmonary circulation overload. *Chest* 1993;**103**:1477–1481.

14 Nishimura Y, Maeda H, Yokoyama M, Fukuzaki H. Bronchial hyperreactivity in patients with mitral valve disease. *Chest* 1990;**98**:1085–1090.

15 Moore DP, Weston A, Hughes JM, Oakley CM, Cleland JG. Bronchial hyperresponsiveness in heart failure. *N Engl J Med* 1993;**328**:1424–1425.

16 Snashall PD, Chung KF. Airway obstruction and bronchial hyperresponsiveness in left ventricular failure and mitral stenosis. *Am Rev Respir Dis* 1991;**144**:945–955.

17 Siegel JL, Miller A, Brown LK, DeLuca A, Teirstein AS. Pulmonary diffusing capacity in left ventricular dysfunction. *Chest* 1990; **98**:550–553.

18 Puri S, Baker BL, Dutka DP, Oakley CM, Hughes JMB, Cleland JGF. Reduced alveolar–capillary membrane diffusing capacity in chronic heart failure: its pathophysiological relevance and relationship to exercise performance. *Circulation* 1995;**91**:2769–2774.

19 Roughton FJW, Forster FE. Relative importance of diffusion and chemical reaction rates in determining rate of exchange of gases in human lung, with special reference to true diffusing capacity of pulmonary membrane and volume of blood in the lung capillaries. *J Appl Physiol* 1957;**11**:290–302.

20 Cotes JE, ed. *Lung Function*, 4th edition. Blackwell Scientific, Oxford, 1979:239–249.

21 Ohar J, Osterloh J, Ahmed A, Miller L. Diffusing capacity decreases after heart transplantation. *Chest* 1993;**103**:857–861.

22 Ravenscraft SA, Gross CR, Kubo SH, et al. Pulmonary function after successful heart transplantation. One year follow-up. *Chest* 1993;**103**:54–58.

23 Groen HJM, Bogaard JM, Balk AHMM, Kho SG, Hop WCJ, Hilvering C. Diffusion capacity in heart transplant recipients. *Chest* 1992;**102**:456–460.

24 Rubin SA, Brown HV, Swan HJ. Arterial oxygenation and arterial oxygen transport in chronic myocardial failure at rest, during exercise and after hydralazine treatment. *Circulation* 1982;**66**:143–148.

25 Clark AL, Coats AJS. Usefulness of arterial blood gas estimations during exercise in patients with chronic heart failure. *Br Heart J* 1994;**71**:528–530.

26 Burgess JH. Pulmonary diffusing capacity in disorders of the pulmonary circulation. *Circulation* 1974;**49**:541–550.

27 Munger MA, Stanek EJ, Nara AR, Kingman SP, Decker MJ, Nair RN. Arterial oxygen saturation in chronic congestive heart failure. *Am J Cardiol* 1994;**73**:180–185.

28 Puri S, Baker BL, Oakley CM, Hughes JMB, Cleland JGF. Raised alveolar–capillary membrane resistance to gas exchange is associated with arterial desaturation on exercise in chronic heart failure [abstract]. *Eur Heart J* 1994;**15**:523.

29 Moore DP, Weston AR, Hughes JM, Oakley CM, Cleland JG. Effects of increased inspired oxygen concentrations on exercise performance in chronic heart failure. *Lancet* 1992;**339**:850–853.

30 Costello ML, Mathieu Costello O, West JB. Stress failure of alveolar epithelial cells studied by scanning electron microscopy. *Am Rev Respir Dis* 1992;**145**:1446–1455.

31 Kay JM, Edwards FR. Ultra-structure of the alveolar-capillary wall in mitral stenosis. *J Pathol* 1973;**111**:239–245.

32 Rhodes KM, Evemy K, Nariman S, Gibson GJ. Relation between severity of mitral valve disease and results of routine lung function tests in non-smokers. *Thorax* 1982;**37**:751–755.

33 Gazioglu K, Yu PN. Pulmonary blood volume and pulmonary capillary blood volume in valvular heart disease. *Circulation* 1967;**35**:701–709.

34 Aber CP, Campbell JA. Significance of changes in the pulmonary diffusing capacity in mitral stenosis. *Thorax* 1965;**20**:135–145.

35 Smith RC, Howard MD, Burchell B, Edwards JE. Pathology of the pulmonary vascular tree IV. Structural changes in the pulmonary vessels in chronic left ventricular failure. *Circulation* 1954;**10**:801–809.

36 Fink LI, Wilson JR, Ferraro N. Exercise ventilation and pulmonary artery wedge pressure in chronic stable congestive heart failure. *Am J Cardiol* 1986;**57**:249–253.

37 Weber KT, Kinasewitz GT, Janicki JS, Fishman AP. Oxygen utilization and ventilation during exercise in patients with chronic cardiac failure. *Circulation* 1982;**65**:1213–1223.

38 Clark AL, Poole Wilson PA, Coats AJ. Relation between ventilation and carbon dioxide production in patients with chronic heart failure. *J Am Coll Cardiol* 1992;**20**:1326–1332.

39 Myers J, Salleh A, Buchanan N, et al. Ventilatory mechanisms of exercise intolerance in chronic heart failure. *Am Heart J* 1992;**124**:710–719.

40 Metra M, Dei Cas L, Panina G, Visioli O. Exercise hyperventilation in chronic congestive heart failure, and its relation to functional capacity and hemodynamics. *Am J Cardiol* 1992;**70**:622–628.

41 Davies SW, Emery TM, Watling MI, Wannamethee G, Lipkin DP. A critical threshold of exercise capacity in the ventilatory response to exercise in heart failure. *Br Heart J* 1991;**65**:179–183.

42 Buller NP, Poole Wilson PA. Mechanism of the increased ventilatory response to exercise in patients with chronic heart failure. *Br Heart J* 1990;**63**:281–283.

43 Jackle AC, Fowler MB. Influence of preoperative artery pressure on mortality after heart transplantation: testing of potential reversibility of pulmonary hypertension with nitroprusside is useful in defining a high risk group. *J Am Coll Cardiol* 1992;**19**:48–54.

44 Abramson SV, Burke JF, Kelly JJ, et al. Pulmonary hypertension predicts mortality

and morbidity in patients with dilated cardiomyopathy. *Ann Intern Med* 1992; **116**:888–895.

45 Leier CV, Huss P, Magorien RD, Unverferth DV. Improved exercise capacity and differing arterial and venous tolerance during chronic isosorbide dinitrate therapy for congestive heart failure. *Circulation* 1983;**67**:817–822.

46 A placebo-controlled trial of captopril in refractory chronic congestive heart failure. Captopril Multicenter Research Group. *J Am Coll Cardiol* 1983;**2**:755–763.

47 Pelliccia F, Borghi A, Ruggeri A, Cianfrocca C. Morgagni GL, Bugiardini R. Changes in pulmonary hemodynamics predict benefits in exercise capacity after ACE inhibition in patients with mild to moderate congestive heart failure. *Clin Cardiol* 1993;**16**:607–612.

48 Franciosa JA, Baker BJ, Seth L. Pulmonary versus systemic hemodynamics in determining exercise capacity of patients with chronic left ventricular failure. *Am Heart J* 1985;**110**: 807–813.

49 Packer M, Lee WH, Medina N, Yushak M. Hemodynamic and clinical significance of the pulmonary vascular response to long term captopril therapy in patients with severe chronic heart failure. *J Am Coll Cardiol* 1985;**6**:635–645.

50 Franciosa JA, Leddy CL, Wilen M, Schwartz DE. Relation between hemodynamic and ventilatory responses in determining exercise capacity in severe congestive heart failure. *Am J Cardiol* 1984;**53**:127–134.

51 Higginbotham MB, Morris KG, Conn EH, Coleman RE, Cobb FR. Determinants of variable exercise performance among patients with severe left ventricular dysfunction. *Am J Cardiol* 1983;**51**:52–60.

52 Lipkin DP, Canepa Anson R, Stephens MR, Poole-Wilson PA. Factors determining symptoms in heart failure: comparison of fast and slow exercise tests. *Br Heart J* 1986;**55**:439–445.

53 Sullivan MJ, Higginbotham MB, Cobb FR. Increased exercise ventilation in patients with chronic heart failure: intact ventilatory control despite hemodynamic and pulmonary abnormalities. *Circulation* 1988;**77**:552–559.

54 Sullivan MJ, Higginbotham MB, Cobb FR. Exercise training in patients with chronic heart failure delays ventilatory anaerobic threshold and improves submaximal exercise performance. *Circulation* 1989;**79**:324–329.

55 Roubin GS, Anderson SD, Shen WF, et al. Hemodynamic and metabolic basis of impaired exercise tolerance in patients with severe left ventricular dysfunction. *J Am Coll Cardiol* 1990;**15**:986–994.

56 West JB. State of the art: ventilation–perfusion relationships. *Am Rev Respir Dis* 1977;**116**: 919–943.

57 Wada O, Asanoi H, Miyagi K, et al. Importance of abnormal lung perfusion in excessive exercise ventilation in chronic heart failure. *Am Heart J* 1993;**125**:790–798.

58 Uren NG, Davies SW, Agnew JE, et al. Reduction of mismatch of global ventilation and perfusion on exercise is related to exercise capacity in chronic heart failure. *Br Heart J* 1993;**70**:241–246.

59 Hanly P, Suberi N, Gray R. Pathogenesis of Cheyne–Stokes respiration in patients with congestive heart failure. Relationship to arterial PCO_2. *Chest* 1993;**104**:1079–1084.

60 Naughton M, Benard D, Tam A, Rutherford R, Bradley TD. Role of hyperventilation in the pathogenesis of central sleep apneas in patients with congestive heart failure. *Am Rev Respir Dis* 1993;**148**:330–338.

61 Ben Dov I, Sietsema KE, Casaburi R, Wasserman K. Evidence that circulatory oscillations accompany ventilatory oscillations during exercise in patients with heart failure. *Am Rev Respir Dis* 1992;**145**:776–781.

62 Feld H, Priest S. A cyclic breathing pattern in patients with poor left ventricular function and compensated heart failure: a mild form of Cheyne–Stokes respiration? *J Am Coll Cardiol* 1993;**21**:971–974.

63 Yajima T, Koike A, Sugimoto K, Miyahara Y, Marumo F, Hiroe M. Mechanism of periodic breathing in patients with cardiovascular disease. *Chest* 1994;**106**:142–146.

64 Kremser CB, O'Toole MF, Leff AR. Oscillatory hyperventilation in severe congestive heart failure secondary to idiopathic dilated cardiomyopathy or to ischemic cardiomyopathy. *Am J Cardiol* 1987;**59**:900–905.

65 Mancini DM, Walter G, Reichek N, et al. Contribution of skeletal muscle atrophy to exercise intolerance and altered muscle metabolism in heart failure. *Circulation* 1992;85:1364–1373.
66 Wilson JR, Mancini DM, Dunkman WB. Exertional fatigue due to skeletal muscle dysfunction in patients with heart failure. *Circulation* 1993;**87**:470–475.
67 Minotti JR, Christoph I, Massie BM. Skeletal muscle function, morphology, and metabolism in patients with congestive heart failure. *Chest* 1992;**101**:333S–339S.
68 Minotti JR, Christoph I, Oka R, Weiner MW, Wells L, Massie BM. Impaired skeletal muscle function in patients with congestive heart failure. Relationship to systemic exercise performance. *J Clin Invest* 1991;88:2077–2082.
69 Ambrosino N, Opasich C, Crotti P, Cobelli F, Tavazzi L, Rampulla C. Breathing pattern, ventilatory drive and respiratory muscle strength in patients with chronic heart failure. *Eur Respir J* 1993;7:17–22.
70 Nishimura Y, Maeda H, Tanaka K, Nakamura H, Hashimoto Y, Yokoyama M. Respiratory muscle strength and hemodynamics in chronic heart failure. *Chest* 1994;**105**:355–359.
71 McParland C, Krishnan B, Wang Y, Gallagher CG. Inspiratory muscle weakness and dyspnea in chronic heart failure. *Am Rev Respir Dis* 1992;**146**:467–472.
72 Mancini DM, Ferraro N, Nazzaro D, Chance B, Wilson JR. Respiratory muscle deoxygenation during exercise in patients with heart failure demonstrated with near-infrared spectroscopy. *J Am Coll Cardiol* 1991;**18**: 492–498.

9

The ABC of natriuretic peptides: pathophysiology, diagnostic and therapeutic potential

Neil C Davidson, Allan D Struthers

Introduction

The natriuretic peptide system consists of three peptides with similar structures that circulate in plasma and share common receptors. These peptides cause a wide range of actions in the kidney, the vasculature, the heart, and the central nervous system. Atrial natriuretic peptide (ANP) was first sequenced in 1984[1] and has subsequently been the subject of extensive investigation. This peptide is secreted from the cardiac atria and has profound natriuretic and diuretic properties, as well as vasodilatory effects.[2] Brain natriuretic peptide (BNP) was subsequently discovered in porcine brain[3] – hence its name – but in humans this peptide is secreted almost exclusively from the heart, predominantly from the ventricles.[4] It has similar actions to those of ANP and has more recently been called B-type natriuretic peptide. The third member of the group, C-type natriuretic peptide (CNP), is present mainly in the central nervous system and the vascular endothelium, and it appears to have very limited natriuretic and vasodilatory properties.[5] Although the nomenclature of these peptides, especially BNP, is misleading, it is now well established in the scientific literature.

Pathophysiology

The structures of the natriuretic peptides are shown in Fig. 9.1. They share a common central ring structure with variable carboxy (C-) and amino (N-) terminal tails.[6] Each peptide also exists as a relatively high molecular weight storage form; this is cleaved prior to release into the circulation and these larger peptides are detectable in the peripheral blood, although their biological significance is uncertain. ANP and BNP are released from storage granules in the myocardium; animal studies have suggested that the main trigger for their secretion is stretching of the atrial and ventricular walls respectively,[7] and in patients with heart failure a recent study has demonstrated that the release of both ANP and BNP is regulated by the tension of the wall of the left ventricle.[8] The physiological factors that control the release of CNP have not been clearly defined. All three natriuretic peptides are detectable at picomolar concentrations in the venous blood of normal subjects.

In patients with heart failure, the plasma levels of ANP and BNP – but not CNP – are markedly elevated.[9] This is associated with increased expression of messenger RNA (mRNA) for ANP and BNP in all cardiac chambers, indicating increased synthetic activity. CNP mRNA has also recently been detected in relatively small quantities in failing myocardium. The plasma levels of ANP and especially of BNP show close negative correlations with indices of ventricular systolic function, including left ventricular ejection fraction and cardiac

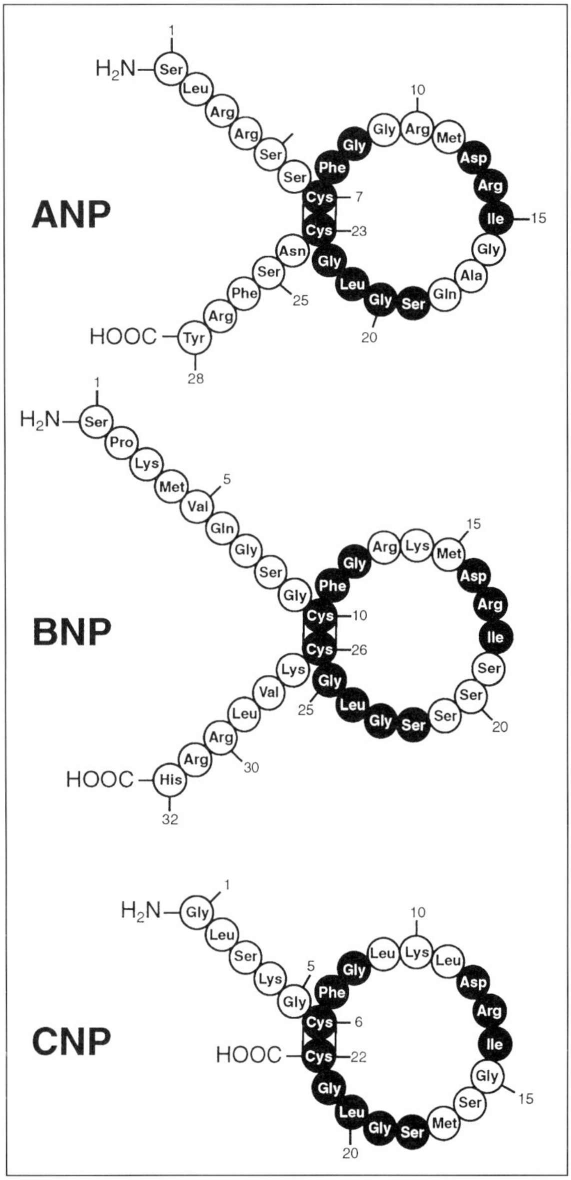

Fig. 9.1
Structure of predominant circulating forms of human atrial natriuretic peptide (ANP), B-type natriuretic peptide (BNP) and C-type natriuretic peptide (CNP).

output.[10,11] Despite this augmented production of natriuretic peptides in association with ventricular dysfunction, their release in response to fluid loading is diminished.[12] The release of ANP and BNP is also stimulated by conditions that are associated with ventricular pressure overload, such as hypertrophic cardiomyopathy[13] and hypertensive left ventricular hypertrophy.[14] Following myocardial infarction (MI), the plasma levels of ANP and BNP rise acutely, presumably due to release of stored peptide from the myocardium, and in some patients a second peak of BNP occurs several days after infarction;[15] this appears to signify the development of ventricular dysfunction.

Three different natriuretic peptide receptors have been identified and unfortunately, although these have been named A, B and C, the designations do not correspond to their relative affinities for ANP, BNP and CNP.[16] The A and B receptors are linked to guanylate cyclase and cause increased production of cyclic guanosine monophosphate (cGMP), which acts as a second messenger for most of the known biological effects of natriuretic peptides. The C receptor was originally described as a clearance receptor with no function other than the removal of natriuretic peptides from the circulation, but it is now recognized that this receptor may be linked with biological actions that are mediated by second messengers other than cGMP.[17] All three receptors are widely distributed and have been localized in the kidney, the heart, the vascular endothelium, the adrenals, and throughout the central nervous system.[18]

Clearance of natriuretic peptides from the circulation occurs via two mechanisms: firstly via receptor-mediated endocytosis and secondly via degradation by a zinc-containing enzyme, neutral endopeptidase 24.11 (NEP).[19] This is a non-specific enzyme that is present in the kidney and in vascular beds and that catalyses the degradation of many endogenous peptides including substance P and angiotensin II. The relative importance of these two mechanisms in the clearance of natriuretic peptides is controversial. The approximate plasma half-lives of natriuretic peptides in humans are: ANP 3 minutes;[20] BNP 22 minutes;[21] and CNP 2.6 minutes.[5] The stability of BNP reflects a relative resistance to degradation by NEP.[19]

An important feature of the actions of natriuretic peptides is their interaction with other neurohormonal mechanisms. ANP antagonises the renin–angiotensin–aldosterone system directly at three separate sites: it inhibits renin secretion from juxtaglomerular cells;[22] it reduces angiotensin-converting enzyme activity;[23] and it inhibits angiotensin II-mediated release of aldosterone from the adrenal cortex.[24] Both ANP and BNP inhibit the release of endothelins,[25] potent vasoconstrictors that originate in the vascular endothelium. Moreover, ANP has a modulatory effect on the activity of the sympathetic nervous system; it appears to inhibit baroreceptor-mediated tachycardia[26] and to reduce the levels of circulating catecholamines.[27]

In addition to modulating the effects of the renin–angiotensin–aldosterone system, ANP and BNP produce natriuresis and diuresis by numerous renal actions, the most prominent of which is probably a direct effect on the collecting duct, although they also act on glomerular and proximal tubular cells and inhibit the actions of antidiuretic hormone.[28] The effects of ANP and BNP within the heart are less well defined. ANP is a coronary vasodilator[29] and has been shown to reduce symptoms of angina in patients with coronary spasm.[30] In contrast with the other natriuretic peptides CNP is neither a potent vasodilator nor a diuretic agent. It is thought to act mainly as a neurotransmitter involved in central cardiovascular control mechanisms, and it may also have important paracrine effects on vascular growth.[31]

Clinical uses of natriuretic peptides

Diagnostic uses

There has been recent interest in the use of natriuretic peptides as indicators of left ventricular function (Table 9.1). This follows the results of trials such as SOLVD[32] and SAVE,[33] which have demonstrated benefits from the treatment of patients with symptomatic and asymptomatic ventricular dysfunction with ACE inhibitors. Most cardiologists agree that, ideally, all patients with suspected heart failure should be investigated with an echocardiogram, but this is incompatible with the current level of provision of echocardiography services in many countries. Plasma levels of N-terminal proatrial natriuretic peptide

- Assessment of patients with suspected chronic heart failure (to target further investigation)
- Assessment of the need for ACE inhibition after myocardial infarction
- Risk stratification in chronic heart failure
- Risk stratification after myocardial infarction

Table 9.1
Possible uses of natriuretic peptide assays.

(N-ANP), which is a prohormone for ANP that appears to be more stable than ANP, have been shown to be good indicators of asymptomatic ventricular dysfunction.[34] Another report has suggested that an elevated plasma level of BNP identifies post-MI patients with impaired ventricular function who will benefit from ACE inhibition.[35] Commercial kits for the measurement of N-ANP, ANP, and BNP are now available; such assays, which could be performed cheaply in a standard laboratory, may provide a useful screening test that could enable general practitioners to decide which patients require further investigation, especially since clinical methods of diagnosing systolic dysfunction are insensitive and lack specificity.[36] Therefore, the selection of patients for cardiac investigations by prescreening in this way could lead to large cost savings.

Natriuretic peptide levels may be useful not merely as markers of left ventricular function but also as independent prognostic indicators. A substudy of the SAVE trial has demonstrated that the plasma concentration of N-ANP is a powerful predictor of long-term mortality, independent of any of the other neurohormonal or haemodynamic parameters that were measured, including the left ventricular ejection fraction.[37] Moreover, a recent study has suggested that elevated plasma levels of BNP are an independent predictor of mortality in patients with chronic heart failure.[38] This may reflect additional risk factors, other than the degree of systolic dysfunction, which affect the release of natriuretic peptides and which are of prognostic significance, such as the presence of diastolic dysfunction, left ventricular asymmetry, or the level of neuroendocrine activation. For example the release of both ANP and BNP is stimulated in cultured cells by endothelins,[39] which circulate at increased concentrations in the plasma of patients with heart failure.[40] Further studies are required to determine the exact role of natriuretic peptide assays in the assessment and risk stratification of patients with suspected heart failure.

Therapeutic uses

The recognized natriuretic, diuretic and vasodilatory properties of natriuretic peptides make them very attractive as therapeutic agents in heart failure. In contrast with loop diuretics and many vasodilators, natriuretic peptides cause inhibition rather than stimulation of the renin–angiotensin–aldosterone system, which is now recognized as a key determinant of the long-term efficacy of such agents. ANP may also have important additional beneficial effects such as reducing cardiac ischaemia and modulating vascular growth.

The intravenous infusion of pharmacological doses of ANP in patients with heart failure produces a decrease in pulmonary capillary wedge pressure and an increased stroke index.[41] However, the renal effects of ANP are less prominent in heart failure patients than in normal subjects.[42] A recent study of the effects of intra-arterial infusions of natriuretic peptides on the forearm vasculature of patients with heart failure has shown that the vasodilatory effects of ANP, but not those of CNP, are attenuated.[43] In as yet unpublished work, the authors have found that intravenous BNP produces a more dramatic natriuresis than ANP in patients with heart failure. These findings, which may at first appear to be surprising, may be partly explained by a selective down-regulation of different natriuretic peptide receptors, which has been demonstrated but not yet clearly defined in heart failure.[44] It is also likely that the activation of the renin–angiotensin system will significantly reduce the effects of the natriuretic peptides.

Unfortunately, the peptide structure of ANP and BNP precludes their use as oral preparations. For reasons of cost and convenience, intravenous infusion of synthetic peptides is not a viable long-term therapeutic strategy and attention has therefore turned to alternative methods of increasing the effects of natriuretic peptides. Candoxatril is an orally-active prodrug that is metabolized to candoxatrilat, a specific inhibitor of the enzyme NEP responsible for natriuretic peptide degradation. There is conflicting evidence regarding the effects of treatment with oral candoxatril in normal volunteers, patients with essential hypertension, and patients with heart failure. Studies have demonstrated either no change[45] or an increase[46] in plasma levels of ANP, although urinary levels of ANP and the second messenger cGMP have consistently increased with candoxatril therapy. The plasma levels of BNP have been reported to increase on treatment with candoxatril in patients with heart failure[47] and to fall in patients with essential hypertension.[48] In the study by Richards et al,[48] the drug caused an increase in plasma ANP levels and had a hypotensive effect, which may have caused a secondary reduction in BNP release.

A study of candoxatril in patients with heart failure has demonstrated a natriuresis comparable to that produced by frusemide, but greater falls in pulmonary artery wedge pressure;[49] predictably, candoxatril produced a more favourable neuroendocrine profile than frusemide. However, in hypertensive patients, the blood pressure-lowering effect of candoxatril has been disappointing. This may be partly due to the non-specific nature of the enzyme NEP, which catalyses the degradation of several other peptides, including angiotensin II, in addition to natriuretic peptides. In practice, the clearance of angiotensin II is diminished by candoxatril and its vasopressor effects are enhanced.[50] In patients with heart failure who already have an activated renin–angiotensin system, this potentiation of the effects of angiotensin II may partially counteract the beneficial effects that are caused by increased natriuretic peptide activity during candoxatril treatment.

It is notable that in patients with heart failure who are treated with ACE inhibitors, the suppression of plasma angiotensin II and aldosterone levels is often incomplete. A report from the SOLVD investigators[51] has suggested that those patients taking enalapril who continue to deteriorate are those in whom the angiotensin II levels escape suppression. There is also growing evidence from animal and human studies of the potential detrimental effects of excessive aldosterone activity. A logical approach is therefore to combine ACE inhibition with another agent that will cause further neurohormonal suppression; this is the rationale for the addition of a neutral endopeptidase inhibitor to treatment with an ACE inhibitor. Novel drugs that combine both of these actions in a single molecule are currently undergoing clinical trials in patients with heart failure; ultimately they may replace the current standard treatment of a loop diuretic and an ACE inhibitor (Table 9.2).

Both ANP and BNP have been shown to have anti-ischaemic properties in humans, although as yet there are no reports of the treatment of angina with neutral endopeptidase inhibitors. Coexistent angina is common in patients with heart failure and its treatment can be problematic, owing to the negative inotropic effects of beta-blockers and calcium channel antagonists. In such patients, neutral endopeptidase inhibitors may be beneficial, and their effects on cardiac ischaemia merit further investigation.

As mentioned previously, the clearance of natriuretic peptides from the circulation is partly dependent on uptake by the C-receptor, and several authors have suggested that the blockade of this receptor might be a useful therapeutic method to boost the effects of

• Augmented suppression of renin–angiotensin–aldosterone system
• Coronary vasodilator effects
• Balanced reductions of preload and afterload
• Total number of tablets may be reduced
• Should avoid diuretic-related adverse reactions (e.g. gout, impaired glucose tolerance)

Table 9.2
Potential benefits of combined ACE inhibitor and neutral endopeptidase inhibitor against ACE inhibitor and loop diuretic combination in treatment of heart failure.

natriuretic peptides. However, there is uncertainty regarding the exact role of this receptor in man and as yet there are no reports of the use of C-receptor ligands in humans. Of greater interest is the development of non-peptide agonists for the A and B receptors (which are linked to guanylate cyclase); such agonists could potentially produce many of the desirable effects of natriuretic peptides after oral administration. These agents are at an early (non-clinical) stage of development. Other compounds that inhibit the metabolic degeneration of cGMP, the second messenger shared by the natriuretic peptides and nitric oxide, are under investigation. Further understanding of the biology of natriuretic peptide receptors and their relationship to biological effects is required to predict accurately the likely efficacy of such drugs, but there is clearly enormous therapeutic potential in agents that can augment the natriuretic, diuretic, vasodilatory, and possible anti-ischaemic properties of cGMP.

Conclusion

The natriuretic peptides form a complimentary cardiovascular control system, which powerfully modulates the activity of the renin–angiotensin–aldosterone cascade. Current knowledge of these peptides suggests that they may have important uses both as diagnostic markers of cardiac pathology and as therapeutic tools in the management of cardiovascular disease. During the next few years, the physiological, pathophysiological, and therapeutic roles of natriuretic peptides will be more clearly defined, and this period promises to yield significant reward for the intensive research that has been performed in this field.

References

1 Kangawa K, Matsuo H. Purification and complete amino acid sequence of alpha-human atrial natriuretic polypeptide (alpha-hANP). *Biochem Biophys Res Commun* 1984; **118**:131–139.

2 Richards AM. Atrial natriuretic factor administered to humans 1984–1988. *J Cardiovasc Pharmacol* 1989;**13(suppl 6)**:S69–S74.

3 Sudoh T, Kangawa K, Minamino N, Matsuo H. A new natriuretic peptide in porcine brain. *Nature* 1988;**332**:78–81.

4 Mukoyama M, Nakao K, Hosoda K, et al. Brain natriuretic peptide as a novel cardiac hormone in humans. *J Clin Invest* 1991;**87**:1402–1412.

5 Hunt PJ, Richards AM, Espiner EA, Nicholls MG, Yandle TG. Bioactivity and metabolism of C-type natriuretic peptide in normal man. *J Clin Endocrinol Metab* 1994;**78**:1428–1435.

6 Nakao K, Ogawa Y, Suga S, Imura H. Molecular biology and biochemistry of the natriuretic peptide system I: natriuretic peptides. *J Hypertens* 1992;**10**:907–912.

7 Kinnunen P, Vuolteenano O, Ruskoaho H. Mechanisms of atrial and brain natriuretic peptide release from rat ventricular myocardium: effect of stretching. *Endocrinology* 1993; **132**:1961–1970.

8 Yasue H, Yoshimura M, Sumida H, et al. Localization and mechanism of secretion of B-type natriuretic peptide in comparison with those of A-type natriuretic peptide in normal subjects and patients with heart failure. *Circulation* 1994;**90**:195–203.

9 Wei C, Heublein DM, Perrella MA, et al. Natriuretic peptide system in human heart failure. *Circulation* 1993;**88**:1004–1009.

10 Benedict CR, Johnstone DE, Weiner DH, et al. Relation of neurohormonal activation to clinical variables and degree of left ventricular dysfunction. *J Am Coll Cardiol* 1994; **23**:1410–1420.

11 Richards AM, Crozier IG, Yandle TG, Espiner EA, Ikram H, Nicholls MG. Brain natriuretic factor: regional plasma concentrations and correlations with haemodynamic state in cardiac disease. *Br Heart J* 1993;**69**:414–417.

12 Volpe M, Tritto C, DeLuca N, et al. Failure of atrial natriuretic factor to increase with saline load in patients with dilated cardiomyopathy and mild heart failure. *J Clin Invest* 1991; **88**:1481–1489.

13 Hasegawa K, Fujiwara H, Doyama K, et al. Ventricular expression of brain natriuretic peptide in hypertrophic cardiomyopathy. *Circulation* 1993;**88**:372–380.

14 Kohno M, Horio T, Yokokawa K, et al. Brain natriuretic peptide as a cardiac hormone in essential hypertension. *Am J Med* 1992; **92**:29–34.

15 Morita E, Yasue H, Yoshimura M, et al. Increased plasma levels of brain natriuretic peptide in patients with acute myocardial infarction. *Circulation* 1993;**88**:82–91.

16 Nakao K, Ogawa Y, Suga S, Imura H. Molecular biology and biochemistry of the natriuretic peptide system II: natriuretic peptide receptors. *J Hypertens* 1992;**10**:1111–1114.

17 Levin ER. Natriuretic peptide C-receptor: more than a clearance receptor. *Am J Physiol* 1993; **264**:E483–E489.

18 Wilcox JN, Augustine A, Goeddel DV, Lowe DG. Differential regional expression of 3 natriuretic peptide receptor genes within primate tissues. *Mol Cell Biol* 1991;**11**:3454–3462.

19 Kenny AJ, Bourne A, Ingram J. Hydrolysis of human and pig natriuretic peptides, urodilatin, C-type natriuretic peptide and some C-receptor ligands by endopeptidase-24.11. *Biochem J* 1993;**291**:83–88.

20 Yandle TG, Richards AM, Nicholls MG, Cuneo R, Espiner EA, Livesey J. Metabolic clearance rate and plasma half-life of alpha-human atrial natriuretic peptide in man. *Life Sci* 1986;**38**:1827–1833.

21 Holmes SJ, Espiner EA, Richards AM, Yandle TG, Frampton C. Renal, endocrine and haemo-

dynamic effects of human brain natriuretic peptide in normal man. *J Clin Endocrinol Metab* 1993;**76**:91–96.
22 Kurtz A, Della Bruna R, et al. Atrial natriuretic peptide inhibits renin release from juxtaglomerular cells by a cGMP mediated process. *Proc Natl Acad Sci U S A* 1986;**83**:4769–4773.
23 Kawaguchi H, Ito K, Takamura I. ANF inhibits ACE activity stimulated by endothelin. *J Hypertension* 1992;**10(suppl 4)**:S98.
24 Delkers W, Kleiner S, Bähr V. Effects of incremental infusions of atrial natriuretic factor on aldosterone, renin and blood pressure in humans. *Hypertension* 1988;**12**:462–467.
25. Kohno M, Yasunari K, Yokokawa K, Murakawa K, Horio T, Takeda T. Inhibition by atrial and brain natriuretic peptides of endothelin-1 secretion after stimulation with angiotensin II and thrombin of cultured human endothelial cells. *J Clin Invest* 1991; **87**:1999–2004.
26 Ebert TJ, Cowley AW Jr. Atrial natriuretic factor attenuates carotid baroreflex-mediated cardioacceleration in humans. *Am J Physiol* 1988; **254**:R590–R594.
27 Racz K, Kuchel O, Buu NT, Debinski W, Cantin M, Genest J. Atrial natriuretic factor, catecholamines and natriuresis. *N Engl J Med* 1989;**314**:321–322.
28 Raine AEG, Firth JG, Ledingham JGG. Renal actions of atrial natriuretic peptide. *Clin Sci* 1989;**76**:1–8.
29 Chu A, Morris KG, Kuehl WD, Cusma J, Navetta F, Cobb FR. Effects of atrial natriuretic peptide on the coronary arterial vasculature in humans. *Circulation* 1989;**80**:1627–1635.
30 Tanaka H, Yasue H, Yoshimura M, et al. Suppression of hyperventilation-induced attacks with infusion of atrial natriuretic peptide in patients with variant angina pectoris. *Am J Cardiol* 1993;**72**:128–133.
31 Porter JG, Catalano R, McEnroe G, Lewicki JA, Protter AA. C type natriuretic peptide inhibits growth factor-dependent DNA synthesis in smooth muscle cells. *Am J Physiol* 1992; **263**:C1001–C1006.
32 The SOLVD investigators. Effect of enalapril on mortality and the development of heart failure in asymptomatic patients with reduced left ventricular ejection fractions. *N Engl J Med* 1992;**321**:685–691.
33 The SAVE investigators. Effect of captopril on mortality and morbidity in patients with left ventricular dysfunction after myocardial infarction. *N Engl J Med* 1991;**327**:669–677.
34 Lerman A, Gibbons RJ, Rodeheffer RJ, et al. Circulating N-terminal atrial natriuretic peptide as a marker for symptomless left-ventricular dysfunction. *Lancet* 1993;**341**:1105–1109.
35 Motwani JG, McAlpine H, Kennedy N, Struthers AD. Plasma brain natriuretic peptide as an indicator for angiotensin-converting-enzyme inhibition after myocardial infarction. *Lancet* 1993;**341**:1109–1113.
36 Davidson NC, Naas A, Hanson J, Kennedy N, Coutie W, Struthers AD. A comparison of ANP, BNP and N-terminal pro ANP as indicators of LV systolic dysfunction. *Am J Cardiol* 1995.
37 Hall C, Rouleau JL, Moyè L, et al. N-terminal proatrial natriuretic factor. An independent predictor of long-term prognosis after myocardial infarction. *Circulation* 1994;**89**:1934–1942.
38 Tsutamoto T, Maeda Y, Wada A, Adachi T, Natamura Y, Kinoshita M. Plasma brain natriuretic peptide concentration as a prognostic predictor in patients with chronic congestive heart failure. *Circulation* 1993;**88(suppl 4:2)**:I26.
39 Horio T, Kohno M, Takeda T. Cosecretion of atrial and brain natriuretic peptides stimulated by endothelin-1 from cultured rat atrial and ventricular cardiocytes. *Metabolism* 1993; **42**:94–96.
40 McMurray JJ, Ray SG, Abdullal I, et al. Plasma endothelin in chronic heart failure. *Circulation* 1992;**85**:1374–1379.
41 Saito Y, Nakao K, Nishimura K, et al. Clinical application of atrial natriuretic polypeptide in patients with congestive heart failure: beneficial effects on left ventricular function. *Circulation* 1987;**76**:115–124.
42 Cody RJ, Atlas SA, Laragh JH, et al. Atrial natriuretic factor in normal subjects and heart failure patients. *J Clin Invest* 1986;**78**:1362–1374.
43 Nakamura M, Arakawa N, Yoshida H, Makita S, Hiramori K. Vasodilatory effects of C-type

natriuretic peptide on forearm resistance vessels are distinct from those of atrial natriuretic peptide in patients with chronic heart failure. *Circulation* 1994;**90**:1210–1214.

44 Garcia R, Bonhomme MC, Schiffrin EL. Divergent regulation of atrial natriuretic factor receptors in high-output heart failure. *Am J Physiol* 1992;**263**:H1790–H1797.

45 O'Connell JE, Jardine AG, Davies DL, McQueen J, Connell JM. Renal and hormonal effects of chronic inhibition of neutral endopeptidase in normal man. *Clin Sci* 1993;**85**:19–26.

46 Bevan EG, Connell JM, Doyle J, et al. Candoxatril, a neutral endopeptidase inhibitor: efficacy and tolerability in essential hypertension. *J Hypertens* 1992;**10**:607–613.

47 Lang CC, Motwani JG, Coutie WJ, Struthers AD. Influence of candoxatril on plasma brain natriuretic peptide in heart failure. *Lancet* 1991;**338**:255.

48 Richards AM, Crozier IG, Espiner EA, Yandle TG, Nicholls MG. Plasma brain natriuretic peptide and endopeptidase 24.11 inhibition in hypertension. *Hypertension* 1993;**22**:231–236.

49 Northridge DB, Jackson NC, Metcalfe MJ, McFarlane N, Dargie H. Effects of candoxatril, a novel endopeptidase inhibitor compared to frusemide in mild chronic heart failure. *Br J Clin Pharm* 1991;**32**:645.

50 Richards AM, Wittert GA, Espiner EA, Yandle TG, Ikram H. Effect of inhibition of neutral endopeptidase 24.11 on responses to angiotensin II in normal volunteers. *Circ Res* 1992; **71**:1501–1507.

51 Pouleur H, Konstam MA, Benedict CR, et al. Progression of left ventricular dysfunction during enalapril therapy: relationship with neurohormonal reactivation. *Circulation* 1993;**88**: I–293.

10

Endothelin in the pathophysiology of chronic heart failure

Michael P Love, John JV McMurray

The importance of chronic heart failure

Despite progressive advances in our understanding of its haemodynamic, neuroendocrine, and other pathophysiological mechanisms, chronic heart failure (CHF) continues to cause considerable cardiovascular morbidity and mortality on a worldwide scale. CHF affects between 0.4% and 2% of the population in Europe and the USA, and both its incidence and prevalence appear to be rising.[1] Modern vasodilator therapies undoubtedly improve symptoms and prolong survival,[2–5] but CHF, once established, still impairs quality of life more than most other chronic medical illnesses, and kills 60–70% of patients within 5 years of diagnosis. The economic impact of CHF is similarly disturbing, primarily related to the frequency with which CHF patients require hospitalization.[6] Recent analyses indicate that CHF accounts for approximately 10% of spending on diseases of the circulatory system and 1–2% of total health care expenditure in Europe and the USA.[6,7] Consequently, in addition to crucial preventive strategies, further improvement in our understanding of the complex and almost invariably progressive pathophysiology of CHF is essential if novel therapeutic strategies are to be developed to lessen its considerable human and financial burden.

Vasoconstriction as a fundamental mechanism in the pathophysiology of chronic heart failure

Impairment of ventricular performance in CHF of all aetiologies leads to activation of multiple neuroendocrine and systemic reflexes in an attempt to maintain cardiovascular homeostasis.[8,9] These reflexes initially serve to maintain cardiac output and tissue perfusion, but ultimately adversely influence cardiovascular haemodynamics by increasing systemic vascular resistance and reducing vascular compliance. The failing ventricle is particularly sensitive to alterations in afterload such that rising vascular resistance progressively impairs ventricular performance. Vasoconstriction of the skeletal muscle bed in CHF impairs vasodilating capacity during exercise, and is a major mechanism contributing to the cardinal symptoms of fatigue and poor exercise tolerance.[10] Chronically increased pulmonary vascular resistance compromises right ventricular function, promotes fluid retention and hepatic congestion, and ultimately leads to pulmonary hypertension. Systemic venoconstriction increases both preload and afterload, further exacerbating biventricular dysfunction. Renal vasoconstriction occurs early in the course of CHF and causes a proportionally greater reduction in renal blood flow than in any other vascular bed.[11] Reduced renal perfusion in turn further augments sodium and water retention, primarily via activation of the renin–angiotensin–aldosterone system.

The blood vessels as therapeutic targets in chronic heart failure

Drug therapies that decrease systemic and pulmonary vascular resistance in CHF lead to improvements in well-being and functional capacity.[2–5] Indeed, in terms of symptoms and survival, the most successful treatments for CHF to date have been vasodilator drugs that act directly on systemic and pulmonary resistance vessels to interrupt neuroendocrine vasoconstrictor reflexes. ACE inhibitors have undoubtedly had the greatest impact.[2–5] Their benefit was initially presumed to be related principally to reduced synthesis of the endogenous vasoconstrictor and mitogen angiotensin II. There is increasing evidence, however, that the beneficial effects of ACE inhibitors may be at least partly related to reduced degradation of bradykinin, which in turn enhances endothelial cell nitric oxide and prostaglandin release.[12] However, improvements in symptoms and prognosis in CHF have been extremely modest, at least in part because none of the vasodilator therapies currently available (including ACE inhibitors) achieve normalization of vascular resistance or exercise-associated vasodilatation in CHF. The blood vessels and the multiple vasoactive factors acting on them would seem to be the most obvious targets for any novel therapeutic intervention in CHF aimed at restoring endothelial function and achieving a greater reduction in vascular resistance than is possible with current agents.

The importance of the vascular endothelium in chronic heart failure

The vascular endothelium undoubtedly plays a pivotal role in the modulation of vascular tone in both health and disease states through local synthesis and release of various vasodilator (e.g. endothelium-derived relaxing factor, endothelium-derived hyperpolarizing factor, bradykinin, and prostacyclin I_2) and vasoconstrictor substances (e.g. angiotensin II, endothelium-derived contracting factor, and endothelin).[13] The increase in vasomotor tone that characterizes CHF is presumed to represent the net effect of the interaction of these locally produced factors with the other systemically activated vasoconstrictor reflexes, in particular the sympathetic nervous system and the renin–angiotensin–aldosterone system. The concept of endothelial dysfunction in CHF is now widely accepted[14] and, as already described, there is preliminary evidence that the benefit of ACE inhibitors may be partly related to improved endothelium-mediated vasodilatation, possibly by enhancing bradykinin-mediated release of nitric oxide and prostacyclin.[12] However, the relative contributions of either diminished endothelial synthesis of relaxing factors or enhanced synthesis of contracting factors to vasoconstriction in CHF remains to be established. Recent evidence suggests that basal release of endothelium-derived relaxing factor, presumed to be nitric oxide, is at least preserved in CHF and may even be enhanced, thus counteracting the various opposing constrictor influences.[14,15] Conversely, there is accumulating evidence that endothelial production of endothelin, the most potent vasoconstrictor substance known, may be enhanced in CHF and that endothelin may contribute to the pathophysiology of CHF.[16–24] In this chapter, the aim is to summarize current understanding

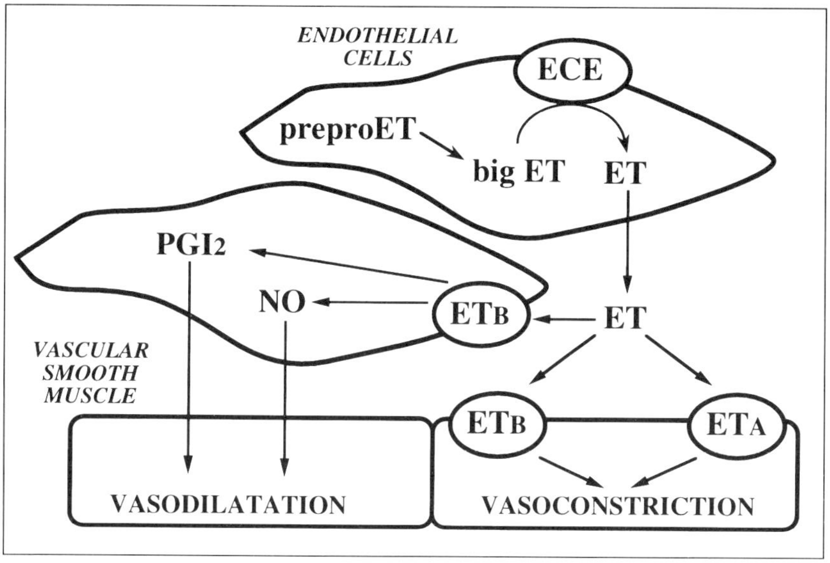

Fig. 10.1 *Diagrammatic representation of vascular ET synthesis and action. ET, endothelin; ECE, endothelin converting enzyme; NO, nitric oxide; PGI_2, prostacyclin.*

of the basic principles of endothelin physiology, to evaluate the evidence implicating endothelin in the pathophysiology of CHF, and to discuss the potential therapeutic relevance to human CHF.

The physiology of endothelin synthesis and action

In 1988, Yanagisawa et al[25] isolated and sequenced a 21-amino-acid peptide from cultured porcine aortic endothelial cells which they named 'endothelin' (ET). Since that original report, ET has been characterized as the most potent vasoconstrictor substance known and has been implicated as playing an important physiological role in cardiovascular regulation and a putative pathophysiological role in a range of disorders of the circulatory system.[26,27] A family of three structurally and functionally similar ET isopeptides exists (ET-1, ET-2, and ET-3), encoded by distinct genes on chromosomes 6, 1, and 20 respectively.[26] ET-1 is the predominant isoform expressed in the human vasculature and has approximately 10 times greater vasoconstrictor potency *in vitro* than angiotensin II.[25] ET-2 has been shown to have similar vasoconstrictor potency to ET-1.[26] Though its precursor proET-2 (or 'big ET-2') has been detected in cultured vascular endothelial cells, the mature form of the peptide is not detectable in human plasma.[28,29] ET-3, the least potent vasoconstrictor in the ET family, is detectable in human plasma but its major source and physiological role are unclear. Precursor mRNA for ET-3 has been detected in brain, lung, pancreas, kidney, and spleen but not in endothelial or cardiac tissues.[27]

Each ET isopeptide is derived in a two-stage process involving enzymatic proteolysis[25] (Fig. 10.1). The corresponding 200 or so residue prepropolypeptides are cleaved at sites that contain pairs of dibasic amino acids by specific endoproteases to form biologically inactive intermediate propeptides or 'big endothelins' (big ET-1, ET-2, and ET-3). The Trp^{21}–Val^{22} bonds in the carboxy terminal of these big ET molecules are subsequently cleaved by a highly specific novel metalloprotease, ET converting enzyme or ECE, to generate the 21 residue mature peptides.[30,31] Several proteases with ECE-like activity have been identified, but the major physiologically relevant form of the enzyme is probably ECE-1, a membrane bound Zn^{2+} metalloprotease expressed both intracellularly and on the surface of endothelial cells.[30] The physiological importance of ECE-1 is supported by the observations that the vascular endothelium is the predominant site of ECE-1 mRNA expression and that ECE-1 converts big ET-1 more efficiently than big ET-2 or big ET-3.[30] It is important to note that, despite remarkable structural similarity, ECE-1 is distinct from neutral endopeptidase (NEP), another important membrane-bound metalloprotease responsible for the degradation of various biologically active peptides including opioids, natriuretic peptides, angiotensin II, and ET-1 itself.[30]

Endothelial cells release ET-1 predominantly abluminally across their basement membrane, suggesting that it acts primarily in a paracrine fashion to alter vascular smooth muscle tone.[32] Thus, the increased serum ET-1 immunoreactivity seen in CHF (discussed below) and various other disease states may simply reflect overspill of local synthesis, such that measurement of circulating ET-1 may be poorly representative of local production and activity at the interface between endothelial cell and vascular smooth muscle. There is some evidence that circulating ET-1 may also have important biological activity, supporting a dual paracrine and hormonal role in the regulation of vascular tone.[33–35]

Cultured endothelial cells take around 30 minutes to release ET-1 after stimulation with various vasoactive agents, suggesting that endothelial ET-1 synthesis requires *de novo* gene expression and protein synthesis.[25] However, more rapid increases in plasma ET-1 have been demonstrated in response to upright tilt and the cold pressor test in healthy subjects, implying the existence of a non-endothelial 'storage pool' of ET-1 that can be rapidly released in response to specific physiological stimuli.[21,36–38] ET-1 immunoreactivity has been demonstrated in neuroendocrine cells of the lung and in granular form within the posterior pituitary.[39,40] These observations support a hormonal as well as paracrine role for ET-1 in cardiovascular homeostasis.

Two high affinity ET receptor subtypes, ET_A and ET_B, have been identified by *in vitro* expression of cloned human cDNA.[41,42] In humans, ET_A receptor mRNA is expressed primarily in vascular smooth muscle cells (particularly in aortic, cardiac, pulmonary, and renal tissues) but not in endothelial cells.[43] ET_A receptors have selective affinity for ET-1 (binding potency ET-1 > ET-2 $\gg$ ET-3), with approximately 100-fold greater affinity for ET-1 than ET-3.[44] ET_B receptors have equal affinity for each ET isoform (binding potency ET-1 = ET-2 = ET-3).[44] ET_B receptor mRNA has been shown to be highly expressed in endothelial cells,[45] and more recently has also been shown to be expressed in vascular smooth muscle obtained from human aorta, pulmonary artery, and coronary artery.[46] Endothelial ET_B receptor stimulation results in vasodilatation through release of nitric oxide or prostacyclin or both,[47] while vascular smooth muscle ET_B receptors mediate vasoconstriction.[48–50] This distribution helps to explain why the pressor effect of bolus injection of ET-1 in humans and animals is preceded by transient hypotension.[27] Recent functional studies, however, have indicated that there is probably a far greater diversity of ET_A and ET_B receptor subtypes than was initially believed, but at present there are insufficient data to extend the current receptor classification.[51] A third postulated ET_C receptor subtype with selective affinity for ET-3 has been identified in *Xenopus laevis* dermal melanophores but has yet to be cloned in humans or other mammalian tissues.[52]

In vitro studies have indicated considerable variation between species in vascular smooth muscle expression of constrictor ET_A and ET_B receptor subtypes as well as variation between vascular beds within the same species.[53,54] Studies with isolated healthy human vessels of over 400 μm diameter have suggested that the ET_A receptor is the main receptor subtype that mediates arterial vasoconstriction in humans, with little or no ET_B-mediated constriction.[54,55] The ET_A receptor also appears to be functionally more important in the human skin microcirculation.[56] However, as already described, ET_B receptor mRNA is detectable in the media of various human vessels[46] and there is increasing evidence that ET_B receptors are also functionally important in mediating vasoconstriction.[48–50] ET_B-mediated vasoconstriction may be relatively more important in smaller resistance vessels[50,54,57] and in the presence of low concentrations of ET-1.[49,53] Contractile ET_B receptors also appear to be functionally more important than contractile ET_A receptors in certain animal species.[53–55]

ET receptors belong to the G-protein-coupled family of receptors that trigger a complex series of diverse intracellular signalling pathways.[58] Elevation of intracellular calcium is understood to be the principal final event mediating ET-1 induced vasoconstriction. Receptor binding stimulates phospholipase C mediated synthesis of inositol triphosphate, which in turn facilitates calcium release from the sarcoplasmic reticulum.[59] The resulting elevation of intracellular calcium simultaneously activates a family of protein kinases involved in regulation of protein synthesis.[58]

In addition to releasing calcium from the sarcoplasmic reticulum, ET-1 opens dihydropyridine-sensitive voltage-operated calcium channels (probably indirectly) and allows calcium influx through other non-voltage-operated calcium channels.[27,58] Dihydropyridine calcium channel antagonists thus only interfere with one of the mechanisms mediating ET-1-induced vasoconstriction, which may limit their 'anti-ET' therapeutic potential. Phospholipase C activation also promotes release of diacylglycerol from the cell membrane, which in turn activates protein kinase C and enhances expression of mRNA for the growth-promoting proto-oncogenes c-*fos* and c-*myc*.[60,61] ET-1 may also activate phospholipase A_2 to release prostaglandin and thromboxane second messengers from arachidonic acid.[58] There is additional experimental evidence that ET-1 may activate various ion transporters (including ATP-sensitive potassium channels) and perhaps a membrane-bound guanylate cyclase.[58]

Biological activity of endothelin

ET-1 has characteristically potent and long-lasting vasopressor activity and probably acts both as a locally active paracrine factor and as a circulating hormone in the regulation of arterial and venous tone.[62–64] Local ECE inhibition and selective ET_A receptor blockade in the forearm vasculature of healthy volunteers substantially increases forearm blood flow, suggesting that endogenous generation of ET-1 contributes to maintenance of basal vascular tone in humans.[65] In addition to its direct arterial and venoconstrictor actions, ET-1 may augment the action of other vasoconstrictor and neuroendocrine mechanisms in CHF. There is experimental evidence that ET-1 may enhance conversion of angiotensin I to angiotensin II.[66] ET-1 has been shown to increase adrenal synthesis of both adrenaline[67] and aldosterone (probably by a direct mechanism)[68] and also to augment plasma renin activity.[62] Furthermore, angiotensin II and arginine vasopressin have been shown to increase ET-1 secretion from cultured endothelial cells,[69,70] and a significant correlation has been demonstrated between plasma levels of angiotensin II and ET-1 in patients with heart failure.[71] Thus, ET-1 secretion and activation of the renin–angiotensin–aldosterone system may potentiate each other and synergistically augment vasoconstriction and sodium retention in CHF. Subthreshold concentrations of ET-1 have been shown to potentiate contractile responses to catecholamines and serotonin.[72] ET-1 may therefore amplify vasoconstrictor reflexes and be of pathophysiological relevance even when plasma levels of peptide are not elevated. Interaction between ET-1 and the sympathetic nervous system is supported by the observation that sympathetically mediated venoconstriction is potentiated by ET-1 in hypertensive patients.[73] Conversely, there is evidence that nitric oxide and atrial natiuretic peptide (ANP) inhibit endothelial cell synthesis of ET-1 through formation of cyclic GMP and that they may act as physiological antagonists of ET-1.[74,75] ANP has also been shown to reverse ET-1 induced vasoconstriction *in vitro*.[74]

The renal vasculature is particularly sensitive to the vasoconstrictor effects of ET-1.[77] ET-1 constricts both afferent and efferent renal arterioles *in vitro*[78] (unlike the selective effect of angiotensin II on the efferent renal arteriole). There are approximately twice as many ET_B as ET_A receptors in the human kidney, with ET_A receptors apparently mainly localized to the renal vasculature and ET_B receptors concentrated in the renal medulla.[79] In animals, exogenously administered sub-pressor doses of ET-1 modestly reduce both renal plasma flow (RPF) and glomerular filtration rate (GFR), and minimally increase urinary sodium loss, at least in part via a direct nephron effect.[77] Higher pharmacological doses of ET-1 cause profound reductions in RPF and GFR such that marked sodium retention results.[62,77] There is a relative paucity of data regarding the renal effects of ET-1 in humans.[33,35,80] In contrast to the animal studies, it has been demonstrated that even low-dose exogenous ET-1 has antinatriuretic effects in the absence of significant changes in RPF or GFR when infused intravenously into healthy volunteers.[35] In this same study, it was shown that infusion of ET-1 at higher doses sufficient to increase circulating concentrations threefold (such as are seen in experimental and human CHF) causes more profound sodium retention and reductions in both RPF and GFR.[35] Endogenously generated ET-1 may therefore be pathophysiologically relevant to the alterations in renal function that are characteristic of CHF.

ET-1 has also been shown to have potent growth regulatory properties – it promotes cell division and hypertrophy and DNA synthesis in vascular smooth muscle cells and myocytes through induction of proto-oncogenes c-*fos* and c-*myc*.[81] Thus, as appears to be the case with angiotensin II, ET-1 may act as a growth factor in CHF and contribute to the processes of myocardial and vascular remodelling. ET-1 may also have significant direct cardiac effects in the setting of CHF, being positively inotropic and chronotropic at low doses, but causing cardiac output to fall at higher doses secondary to direct coronary vasoconstriction and increased systemic vascular resistance.[27,62] Again whether endogenously generated ET-1 plays a significant pathophysiological role in the modulation of myocardial contractility in CHF remains to be established.

Cumulatively, this (mainly circumstantial) evidence implicates ET-1 in the pathophysiology of CHF, in particular suggesting that ET-1 may contribute to vasoconstriction and

Reference	Aetiology of CHF	Elevation in plasma ET
Hiroe et al[16]	IDCM	× 4.4
McMurray et al[17]	IDCM, IHD, HT, valvular	× 2.3
Cody et al[18]	NS	× 2.5
Rodeheffer et al[19]	IDCM, IHD, HT, valvular	× 1.8
Lerman et al[20]	IDCM, IHD	× 1.7
Stewart et al[21]	IDCM, IHD	× 5
Pacher et al[22]	IDCM, IHD, HT	× 2.9
Cacoub et al[23]	IDCM, IHD, HT, valvular	× 1.75
Wei et al[24]	IDCM, IHD	≈ × 1.8

Table 10.1
Plasma endothelin in CHF. (ET – endothelin; IDCM – idiopathic dilated cardiomyopathy; IHD – ischaemic heart disease; HT – hypertension; NS – not specified.)

renal dysfunction while also depressing myocardial contractility and modulating ventricular and vascular remodelling. The pharmacological tools with which to address this issue further and clarify the role of ET-1 in CHF are now becoming available. This investigative work will help to establish whether agents that inhibit the generation or actions of ET-1 might be therapeutically beneficial in CHF.

Endothelin concentrations in CHF

The preferential abluminal secretion of ET-1 by vascular endothelial cells is often cited as an explanation for the observation that circulating levels of ET-1 in healthy humans and in various pathophysiological states are well below the threshold required to elicit vasoconstriction *in vitro*.[82] However, as already described, there is evidence that exogenously administered ET-1 has biological actions *in vivo* at the sort of plasma concentrations that are seen in pathophysiological states such as CHF.[33–35] Several groups have reported varying degrees of elevation in plasma ET-1 concentrations in various animal models of heart failure and in patients with CHF (Table 10.1).[16–24] Immunoassay antibodies with varying selectivity for ET-1 have tended to be used in these studies, with the result that some of the variability in plasma ET-1 levels is likely to have arisen from cross-reactivity with other ET and big ET peptides. On average, total circulating immunoreactive (IR) ET-1 appears to be increased two to three fold in CHF of all aetiologies in proportion to the symptomatic and haemodynamic severity of the syndrome (see below). Two groups[22,24] have suggested that there may be a predominant increase in circulating big ET-1 in CHF, which suggests that either big ET-1 synthesis or secretion is enhanced or that cleavage of big ET-1 to mature ET-1 by ECE is diminished. Circulating big ET-1 has negligible biological activity but represents a potential source of mature ET-1. Whether or not vascular ECE activity is altered in CHF is not yet known.

Haemodynamic parameters	r	*p* value
Left ventricular ejection fraction	−0.52	0.0001
Mean arterial pressure	−0.44	0.001
Right arterial pressure	0.51	0.0001
Pulmonary artery pressure	0.35	0.01
Pulmonary capillary wedge pressure	0.43	0.001

Table 10.2
Correlation of plasma endothelin immunoreactivity with haemodynamic parameters in CHF. (Adapted from reference 22.)

The principal trigger for the increase in circulating IR ET-1 in CHF is not known, but several neurohormonal and physical factors probably contribute. Catecholamines, angiotensin II, arginine vasopressin, glucocorticoids, cytokines, tumour necrosis factor, free radicals, hypoxia, and shear stress have all been shown to increase endothelial cell production of ET-1 *in vitro*, and all of these factors could be relevant in the setting of CHF.[25,27] It is presumed that the vascular endothelium is the main source of circulating ET-1 in CHF. There is some evidence to suggest that the main source of circulating ET-1 in CHF is the pulmonary vascular bed.[83] It has also been shown that circulating mononuclear cells from patients with CHF but not from healthy volunteers synthesize ET-1 spontaneously, suggesting that these cells may also be an important source of circulating ET-1 in CHF.[84]

Endothelin and the severity of chronic heart failure

Plasma ET-1 concentrations are greatest in those CHF patients with the poorest ventricular function and the most abnormal systemic and (especially) pulmonary haemodynamics.[16,18,19,22–24] ET-1 levels have been shown to correlate positively with the severity of pulmonary hypertension in CHF,[18,22,23] a unique observation not seen with other markers of neurohormonal activity in CHF. A similar correlation has been seen in patients with primary pulmonary hypertension and secondary pulmonary hypertension not due to CHF;[85] however, whether the elevation in plasma ET-1 is simply a marker of the occurrence of pulmonary hypertension or is of true pathophysiological importance remains speculative. Plasma ET-1 has also been shown to correlate positively with NYHA clinical class[16,19,22,23] (Fig. 10.2) and inversely with left ventricular ejection fraction (Table 10.2).[19,22,24] As with other neuroendocrine systems, the severity of haemodynamic disturbance in CHF appears to be a major determinant of plasma ET-1.

Plasma endothelin and prognosis in chronic heart failure

Measurement of plasma big ET-1 in patients with CHF has been shown to be of prognostic value. A high plasma concentration predicts a greater chance of clinical deterioration, need for

Clinical course	Big ET-1 concentration (fmol/ml)
stable (n = 33)	2.7 ± 0.9
transplanted (n = 11)	5.8 ± 3.0 ($p < 0.001$ vs concentration in stable cases)
died (n =9)	5.4 ± 1.7 ($p < 0.001$ vs concentration in stable cases)

Table 10.3
Plasma big endothelin-1 and prognosis in CHF. (Adapted from reference 22.)

cardiac transplantation, or of risk of death (Table 10.3).[22] Similar observations have been made with other markers of neuroendocrine activation in CHF. For example, activation of the renin–angiotensin–aldosterone system is most marked in those patients who are most ill, who have the greatest haemodynamic derangement, and who have the worst prognosis. It is in these patients with the greatest renin–angiotensin–aldosterone system activation that ACE inhibition has been shown to be of most benefit. It is tempting to speculate that those CHF patients with the highest circulating ET-1 concentrations will derive the greatest benefit from any novel anti-ET therapies.

Endothelin receptor regulation in chronic heart failure

Changes in receptor density and affinity secondary to chronic neuroendocrine activation are characteristic features of human CHF. This is

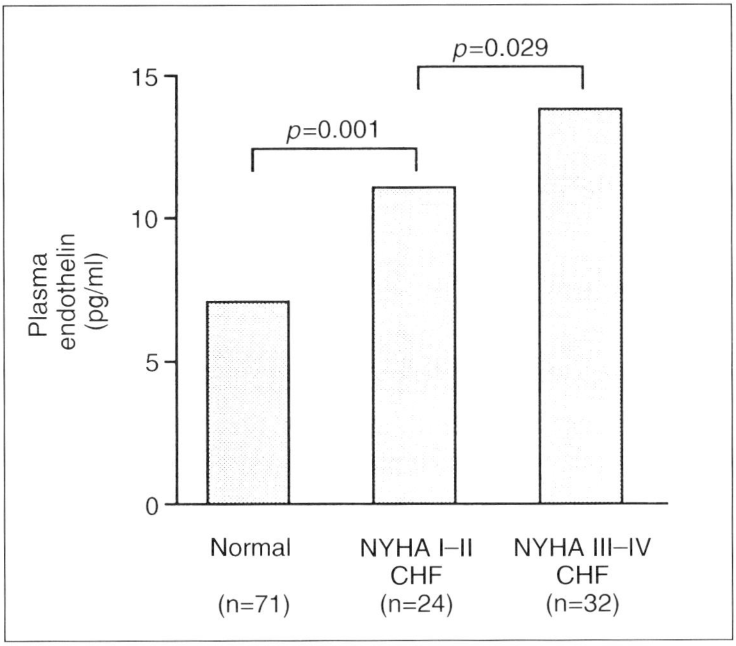

Fig. 10.2
Plasma endothelin and NYHA clinical class. (Adapted from reference 19.)

Reference	Model	Tissue type	Density	Affinity	Response
Gauquelin et al[89]	rat (aortocaval shunt)	glomerular	↓	–	–
Fu et al[90]	rat	mesenteric artery	↓	↑	↓
	(coronary ligation)	ventricle	↔	↔	–
Löffler et al[91]	rabbit	renal	↓	↑	–
	(aortic stenosis and incompetence)	myocardial	↓	↔	–
Calderone et al[92]	dog		–	–	↓
	(rapid pacing)	coronary artery			

Table 10.4
Endothelin receptor regulation in experimental CHF.

particularly true for adrenergic, angiotensin II, and ANP receptors. Autocrine ET-1 production and other endocrine factors known to be increased in CHF (e.g. angiotensin II) have been shown to change ET receptor density and affinity.[86–88] It is not surprising, therefore, that altered ET receptor regulation has been described in various experimental models of CHF (Table 10.4).[89–92] In an aorto-caval shunt rat model of CHF, renal glomerular ET receptor density is reduced.[89] In a rat coronary ligation model of CHF, ventricular ET receptor density and affinity are unchanged while mesenteric arterial ET receptor density is reduced and affinity increased.[90] In a rabbit model of CHF, renal and myocardial receptor density are reduced with an associated increase in renal but not myocardial receptor affinity.[91] In coronary arteries from dogs with CHF induced by rapid ventricular pacing, basal and ET-1-stimulated generation of the second messenger inositol triphosphate are reduced, suggesting desensitization of the ET-1 signalling pathway.[92] The systemic haemodynamic response to intravenous infusion of ET-1 in the rat coronary ligation model of CHF is also of interest. The initial vasodilator response (presumed to be due to endothelial ET_B receptor stimulation) is preserved, whereas the pressor response (vascular smooth muscle constrictor $ET_A \pm ET_B$ receptor-mediated) is attenuated compared to controls.[90]

This in turn suggests that endothelial ET_B receptor expression is unaffected in CHF but that there may be down-regulation of constrictor $ET_A \pm ET_B$ receptors. There is further experimental evidence that ET_A and ET_B receptors may be differentially regulated in CHF. Angiotensin II (circulating levels of which are increased in CHF, even in patients on long-term treatment with an ACE inhibitor) increases ET_B (but not ET_A) mRNA expression in cultured cardiomyocytes.[87] Interestingly, angiotensin II also increases ET-1 mRNA expression and ET-1 secretion in cultured vascular smooth muscle cells.[93] Treatment with an ACE inhibitor, however, has been shown to have no effect on circulating ET-1 levels in patients with CHF.[94]

Preliminary evidence that anti-endothelin strategies may be of therapeutic benefit in chronic heart failure

As discussed above, the role of ET_A and ET_B receptor subtypes may be altered in CHF, though whether this is the case in humans remains to be established. Clearly this is important in terms of developing the most appropriate anti-ET therapeutic strategy for CHF, which may involve selective ET_A or ET_B receptor antagonism, non-selective receptor antagonism, or ECE inhibition. The potential of such agents is demonstrated by a recent report that administration of a non-selective ET receptor antagonist (bosentan) to rats with CHF significantly reduces cardiac afterload, with an additive effect observed in animals concurrently treated with an ACE inhibitor.[95] However, the potential disadvantage of endothelial ET_B receptor blockade (with resultant loss of endothelial release of nitric oxide and prostacyclin) is illustrated by the observation that administration of a selective ET_B receptor antagonist (IRL 1038) to dogs with CHF significantly increases systemic vascular resistance.[96] The authors have recently shown that brachial artery infusion of an ECE inhibitor increases forearm blood flow by about 50% in CHF patients already treated with a diuretic, digoxin, and ACE inhibitor.[97] We have also shown that brachial artery infusion of BQ-123, a selective ET_A receptor antagonist, increases forearm blood flow by about 30% in similarly treated CHF patients.[97] Collectively, these preliminary studies indicate that ET-1 contributes importantly to vascular resistance in CHF and suggest that anti-ET agents may be therapeutically useful.

Further studies are obviously required to establish the systemic effects of selective and non-selective endothelin receptor antagonists as well as to determine whether the disadvantage of blocking endothelial ET_B receptors may be overshadowed by the benefit of blocking constrictor ET_B receptors on vascular smooth muscle. The ongoing development of ET receptor antagonists with differential selectivity for constrictor and dilator ET_B receptor subtypes should allow this issue to be specifically addressed.

Conclusion

The endothelins are a family of peptides with potent vascular, cardiac, and renal actions which may be of pathophysiological importance in the setting of CHF. Human studies with selective and non-selective ET receptor antagonists are required to clarify their role in the pathophysiology of CHF and to establish whether anti-ET drugs may be therapeutically useful.[98] The impact of ACE inhibitors on the management of CHF has been such that, for any new treatment to be of value, it will have to offer haemodynamic benefit over and above that already obtained with an ACE inhibitor; anti-ET agents seem to have this potential.[95,97] The recent formal cloning and characterization of ECE should hasten the development of specific and selective ECE inhibitors and thus provide an alternative investigative, and perhaps therapeutic, tool.[30,31] Morbidity and mortality from CHF remain unacceptably high even in patients receiving conventional maximal medical therapy, including an ACE inhibitor. Blockade of either the generation (through ECE inhibition) or actions (through receptor blockade) of ET-1 warrant further investigation as potential new therapeutic strategies.

References

1 Dargie HJ, McMurray JJV. Diagnosis and management of heart failure. *BMJ* 1994;**308**:321–328.

2 Cohn JN, Archibald DG, Ziesche S, et al. Effect of vasodilator therapy on mortality in chronic congestive heart failure. *N Engl J Med* 1986;**314**:1547–1552.

3 The CONSENSUS Trial Study Group. Effects of enalapril on mortality in severe congestive heart failure: results of the Cooperative North Scandinavian Enalapril Survival Study. *N Engl J Med* 1987;**316**:1429–1435.

4 The SOLVD Investigators. Effect of enalapril on survival in patients with reduced left ventricular ejection fractions and congestive heart failure. *N Engl J Med* 1991;**325**:293–302.

5 Cohn JN, Johnson G, Ziesche S, et al. A comparison of enalapril with hydralazine-isosorbide dinitrate in the treatment of chronic congestive heart failure. *N Engl J Med* 1991;**325**:303–310.

6 McMurray J, Hart W, Rhodes G. An evaluation of the cost of heart failure to the National Health Service in the UK. *Br J Med Econ* 1993;**6**:91–98.

7 Kannel WB, Ho K, Thom T. Changing epidemiological features of cardiac failure. *Br Heart J* 1994;**72(suppl 2)**:S3–S9.

8 Francis GS, Goldsmith SR, Levine TB, Olivari MT, Cohn JN. The neurohumoral axis in congestive heart failure. *Ann Intern Med* 1984;**101**:370–377.

9 Packer M. The neurohormonal hypothesis; a theory to explain the mechanisms of disease progression in heart failure. *J Am Coll Cardiol* 1992;**20**:248–254.

10 Zelis R, Longhurst J, Capone RJ, Mason DT. A comparison of regional blood flow and oxygen utilization during dynamic forearm exercise in normal subjects and patients with congestive heart failure. *Circulation* 1974;**50**:137–143.

11 Vanhoutte PM. Adjustments in the peripheral circulation in chronic heart failure. *Eur Heart J* 1983;**4(suppl A)**:67–83.

12 Drexler H. Endothelial dysfunction in heart failure and potential for reversal by ACE inhibition. *Br Heart J* (suppl 3) 1994;**72**:11–14.

13 Vane JR, Anggard EE, Botting RM. Regulatory functions of the vascular endothelium. *N Engl J Med* 1990;**323**:27–36.

14 Drexler H, Hayoz D, Munzel T, et al. Endothelial function in chronic congestive heart failure. *Am J Cardiol* 1992;**69**:1596–1601.

15 Habib F, Dutka D, Crossman D, Oakley C, Cleland JGF. Enhanced basal nitric oxide production in heart failure: another failed counter-regulatory vasodilator mechanism? *Lancet* 1994;**344**:371–373.

16 Hiroe M, Hirata Y, Fujita N, et al. Plasma endothelin-1 levels in idiopathic dilated cardiomyopathy. *Am J Cardiol* 1991;**68**:1114–1115.

17 McMurray JJ, Ray SG, Abdullah I, Dargie HD, Morton JJ. Plasma endothelin in chronic heart failure. *Circulation* 1992;**85**:1374–1379.

18 Cody RJ, Haas GJ, Binkley PF, Capers Q, Kelly R. Plasma endothelin correlates with the extent of pulmonary hypertension in patients with chronic heart failure. *Circulation* 1992;**85**:504–509.

19 Rodeheffer RJ, Lerman A, Heublein DM, Burnett JC Jr. Increased plasma concentrations of endothelin in chronic heart failure in humans. *Mayo Clin Proc* 1992;**67**:719–724.

20 Lerman A, Kubo SH, Tschumperlin LK, Burnett JC Jr. Plasma endothelin concentrations in humans with end-stage heart failure and after heart transplantation. *J Am Coll Cardiol* 1992;**20**:849–853.

21 Stewart DJ, Cernacek P, Costello KB, Rouleau JL. Elevated endothelin-1 in heart failure and loss of normal response to postural change. *Circulation* 1992;**26**:510–517.

22 Pacher R, Bergler-Klein J, Globits S, et al. Plasma big endothelin-1 concentrations in congestive heart failure patients with or without

systemic hypertension. *Am J Cardiol* 1993;**71**: 1293–1299.
23 Cacoub P, Dorent R, Nataf P, et al. Plasma endothelin and pulmonary pressures in patients with congestive heart failure. *Am Heart J* 1993;**126**:1484–1488.
24 Wei C-M, Lerman A, Rodeheffer RJ, et al. Endothelin in human congestive heart failure. *Circulation* 1994;**89**:1580–1586.
25 Yanagisawa M, Kurihara H, Kimura S, et al. A novel potent vasoconstrictor peptide produced by vascular endothelial cells. *Nature* 1988;**332**:411–415.
26 Inoue A, Yanagisawa M, Kimura S, et al. The human endothelin family: three structurally and pharmacologically distinct isopeptides predicted by three separate genes. *Proc Natl Acad Sci U S A* 1989;**86**:2863–2867.
27 Haynes WG, Webb DJ. The endothelin family of peptides: local hormones with diverse roles in health and disease? *Clin Sci* 1993;**84**:485–500.
28 Suzuki N, Matsumoto H, Kitada C, Masaki T, Fujino M. A sensitive sandwich-enzyme immunoassay for human endothelin. *J Immunol Methods* 1989;**118**:245–250.
29 Howard PG, Plumpton C, Davenport AP. Anatomical localisation and pharmacological activity of mature endothelins and their precursors in human vascular tissue. *J Hypertens* 1992;**10**:1379–1386.
30 Xu D, Emoto N, Giaid A, et al. ECE-1: a membrane bound metalloprotease that catalyzes the proteolytic activation of big endothelin-1. *Cell* 1994;**78**:473–485.
31 Shimada K, Takahashi M, Tanzawa K. Cloning and functional expression of endothelin-converting enzyme from rat endothelial cells. *J Biol Chem* 1994;**269**:1–5.
32 Wagner OF, Christ G, Wojta J, et al. Polar secretion of endothelin-1 by cultured endothelial cells. *J Biol Chem* 1992;**267**:16066–16068.
33 Vierhapper H, Wagner O, Nowotny P, Waldhäusl W. Effects of endothelin-1 in man. *Circulation* 1990;**81**:1415–1418.
34 Lerman A, Hildebrand FL Jr, Aarhus LL, Burnett JC Jr. Endothelin has biological actions at pathophysiological concentrations. *Circulation* 1991;**83**:1808–1814.
35 Rabelink TJ, Kaasjager KAH, Boer P, Stroes EG, Braam B, Koomans HA. Effects of endothelin-1 on renal function in humans: implications for physiology and pathophysiology. *Kidney Int* 1994;**46**:376–381.
36 Kaufmann H, Oribe E, Oliver JA. Plasma endothelin during upright tilt: relevance for orthostatic hypotension. *Lancet* 1991;**338**: 1542–1545.
37 Shichiri M, Hirata Y, Ando K, et al. Postural change and volume expansion affect plasma endothelin levels. *JAMA* 1990;**263**:661.
38 Fyhrquist F, Saijonmaa O, Metsarrine K, et al. Raised plasma endothelin-1 concentration following cold pressor test. *Biochem Biophys Res Commun* 1990;**169**:217–221.
39 Giaid A, Polak JM, Vivekanand G, et al. Distribution of endothelin-like immunoreactivity and mRNA in the developing and adult human lung. *Am J Respir Cell Mol Biol* 1991;**4**:50–58.
40 Yoshizawa T, Shinmi O, Giaid A, et al. Endothelin: a novel peptide in the posterior pituitary system. *Science* 1990;**247**:462–464.
41 Arai H, Hori S, Aramori I, Ohkubo H, Nakanishi S. Cloning and expression of a cDNA encoding an endothelin receptor. *Nature* 1990;**348**:730–733.
42 Sakurai T, Yanagisawa M, Takuwa Y, et al. Cloning of a cDNA encoding a non-isopeptide selective subtype of the endothelin receptor. *Nature* 1990;**348**:732–735.
43 Hosoda K, Nakao K, Hiroshi A, et al. Cloning and expression of human endothelin-1 receptor cDNA. *FEBS Lett* 1991;**287**:23–26.
44 Williams DL, Jones KL, Colton CD, Nutt RF. Identification of high affinity endothelin-1 receptor subtypes in human tissues. *Biochem Biophys Res Commun* 1991;**180**:475–480.
45 Ogawa Y, Nakao K, Arai H, et al. Molecular cloning of a non-isopeptide-selective human endothelin receptor. *Biochem Biophys Res Commun* 1991;**178**:248–255.
46 Davenport AP, O'Reilly G, Molenaar P, et al. Human endothelin receptors characterized using reverse transcriptase-polymerase chain reaction, in-situ hybridization, and subtype-selective ligands BQ123 and BQ3020: evidence for expression of ET_B receptors in human

vascular smooth muscle. *J Cardiovasc Pharmacol* 1993;**22**(**suppl** 8):S22–S25.
47 Haynes WG, Webb DJ. Endothelium dependent modulation of responses to endothelin-1 in human veins. *Clin Sci* 1993;**84**:427–433.
48 White DG, Garratt H, Mundin JW, Sumner MJ, Vallance PJ, Watts IS. Human saphenous vein contains both endothelin ET_A and ET_B contractile receptors. *Eur J Pharmacol* 1994;**257**:307–310.
49 Seo B, Oemar BS, Siebenmann R, von Segesser L, Lüscher TF. Both ET_A and ET_B receptors mediate contraction to endothelin-1 in human blood vessels. *Circulation* 1994;**89**:1203–1208.
50 Haynes WG, Strachan FE, Webb DJ. Endothelin ET_A and ET_B receptors cause vasoconstriction of human resistance and capacitance vessels *in vivo*. *Circulation* 1995;**92**: 357–363.
51 Bax WA, Saxena PR. The current endothelin receptor classification: time for reconsideration? *Trends Pharmacol Sci* 1994;**15**:379–386.
52 Karne S, Jayawickreme CK, Lerner MR. Cloning and characterization of an endothelin-3 specific receptor (ET_C receptor) from *Xenopus laevis* dermal melanophores. *J Biol Chem* 1993;**268**:19126–19133.
53 Yanagisawa M. The endothelin system. A new target for therapeutic intervention. *Circulation* 1994;**89**:1320–1322.
54 Davenport AP, Maguire JJ. Is endothelin-induced vasoconstriction mediated only by ET_A receptors in humans? *Trends Pharmacol Sci* 1994;**15**:9–11.
55 Riezebos J, Watts IS, Vallance JTP. Endothelin receptors mediating functional responses in human small arteries and veins. *Br J Pharmacol* 1994;**111**:609–615.
56 Wenzel RR, Noll G, Lüscher TF. Endothelin receptor antagonists inhibit endothelin in human skin microcirculation. *Hypertension* 1994;**23**:581–586.
57 Ekelund U, Adner M, Edvisson L, Mellander S. Effects of selective ET_B receptor stimulation on arterial, venous and capillary functions in cat skeletal muscle. *Br J Pharmacol* 1994;**112**: 887–894.
58 Simonson MS, Dunn MJ. The molecular mechanisms of cardiovascular and renal regulation by endothelin peptides. *J Lab Clin Med* 1992;**119**:622–639.
59 Resink TJ, Scott-Burden T, Buhler FR. Endothelin stimulates phospholipase C in cultured vascular smooth muscle cells. *Biochem Biophys Res Commun* 1988;**157**:1360–1368.
60 Griendling KK, Tsuda T, Alexander RW. Endothelin stimulates diacylglycerol accumulation and activates protein kinase C in cultured vascular smooth muscle cells. *J Biol Chem* 1989;**264**:8237–8240.
61 Simonson MS, Wann S, Mene P, et al. Endothelin stimulates phospholipase C, Na^+/K^+ exchange, c-*fos* expression, and mitogenesis in rat mesangial cells. *J Clin Invest* 1989; **83**:708–712.
62 Miller WL, Redfield MM, Burnett JC Jr. Integrated cardiac, renal and endocrine actions of endothelin. *J Clin Invest* 1989;**83**:317–320.
63 Clarke JG, Benjamin N, Larkin SW, et al. Endothelin is a potent long-lasting vasoconstrictor in men. *Am J Physiol* 1989;**257**: H2033–H2035.
64 Haynes WG, Clarke JG, Cockcroft JR, Webb DJ. Pharmacology of endothelin-1 *in vivo* in humans. *J Cardiovasc Pharmacol* 1991;**17** (**suppl** 7):284–286.
65 Haynes WG, Webb DJ. Contribution of endogenous generation of endothelin-1 to basal vascular tone. *Lancet* 1994;**344**:852–854.
66 Kawaguchi H, Sawa H, Yasuda H. Endothelin stimulates angiotensin I to angiotensin II conversion in cultured pulmonary artery endothelial cells. *J Mol Cell Cardiol* 1990;**22**:839–842.
67 Boarder MR, Marriot DB. Characterization of endothelin-1 stimulation of catecholamine release from adrenal chromaffin cells. *J Cardiovasc Pharmacol* 1989;**13**(**suppl** 5):223–224.
68 Cao L, Banks RO. Cardiorenal actions of endothelin, part 1: effects of converting enzyme inhibition. *Life Sci* 1990;**46**:577–583.
69 Emori T, Hirata Y, Ohta K, et al. Cellular mechanisms of endothelin-1 release by angiotensin and vasopressin. *Hypertension* 1991; **18**:165–170.
70 Bakris GL, Fairbanks R, Traish AM, Akerstorm V, Kern S. Arginine vasopressin stimulates human mesangial production of endothelin. *J Clin Invest* 1991;**87**:1158–1164.

71 Good JM, Nihoyannopoulos P, Ghatel MA, et al. Elevated plasma endothelin concentrations in heart failure: an effect of angiotensin II? *Eur Heart J* 1994;**15**:1634–1640.
72 Yang Z, Richard V, von Segesser L, et al. Threshold concentrations of endothelin-1 potentiate contractions to norepinephrine and serotonin in human arteries. *Circulation* 1990;**82**:188–195.
73 Haynes WG, Hand MF, Johnstone H, Padfield PL, Webb DJ. Direct and sympathetically mediated venoconstriction in essential hypertension. *J Clin Invest* 1994;**94**:1359–1364.
74 Boulanger C, Lüscher TF. Release of endothelin from the porcine aorta: inhibition by endothelium-derived nitric oxide. *J Clin Invest* 1990;**85**:587–590.
75 Saijonmaa O, Ristimäki A, Fyrquist F. Atrial natriuretic peptide, nitroglycerine, and nitroprusside reduce basal and stimulated endothelin production from cultured endothelial cells. *Biochem Biophys Res Commun* 1990; **173**:514–520.
76 Bonhomme MC, Cantin M, Garcia R. Relaxing effect of atrial natriuretic factor on endothelin-precontracted strips. *Proc Soc Exp Med Biol* 1989;**191**:309–315.
77 Kohan DE. Endothelins in the kidney: physiology and pathophysiology. *Am J Kid Dis* 1993;**22**:493–510.
78 Edwards RM, Trizna W, Ohlstein EH. Renal microvascular effects of endothelin. *Am J Physiol* 1990;**259**:F217–F221.
79 Davenport AP, Kuc RE, Hoskins SL, Karet FE, Fitzgerald F. [^{123}I]-PD151242: a selective ligand for endothelin ET_A receptors in human kidney which localises to renal vasculature. *Br J Pharmacol* 1994;**113**:1303–1310.
80 Gasic S, Wagner O, Vierhapper H, Nowotny P, Waldhäusl W. Regional hemodynamic effects and clearance of endothelin-1 in humans: renal and peripheral tissues may contribute to the overall disposal of the peptide. *J Cardiovasc Pharmacol* 1992;**19**:176–180.
81 Battistini B, Chailler P, D'Orléans-Juste P, Brière N, Sirois P. Growth regulatory properties of endothelins. *Peptides* 1993;**14**:385–399.
82 Frelin C, Guedin D. Why are circulating concentrations of endothelin-1 so low? *Cardiovasc Res* 1994;**28**:1613–1622.
83 Tsutamoto T, Wada A, Maeda Y, Adachi T, Kinoshita M. Relation between endothelin-1 spillover in the lungs and pulmonary vascular resistance in patients with chronic heart failure. *J Am Coll Cardiol* 1994;**23**:1427–1433.
84 Krum H, Itescu S. Spontaneous endothelin production by circulating mononuclear cells from patients with chronic heart failure but not from normal subjects. *Clin Exp Pharmacol Physiol* 1994;**21**:311–313.
85 Stewart DJ, Levy RD, Cernacek P, Langleben D. Increased plasma endothelin-1 in pulmonary hypertension: marker or mediator of disease? *Ann Intern Med* 1991;**114**:464–469.
86 Clozel M, Löffler BM, Breu V, Hilfiger L, Maire JP, Butscha B. Downregulation of endothelin receptors by autocrine production of endothelin-1. *Am J Physiol* 1993;**265**: C188–C192.
87 Kanno K, Hirata Y, Tsujino M, et al. Up-regulation of ET_B receptor subtype mRNA by angiotensin II in rat cardiomyocytes. *Biochem Biophys Res Commun* 1993;**194**:1282–1287.
88 Roubert P, Gillard V, Plas P, Guillon JM, Chabrier PE, Braquet P. Angiotensin II and phorbol-esters potently down-regulate endothelin (ET-1) binding sites in vascular smooth muscle cells. *Biochem Biophys Res Commun* 1989;**164**:809–815.
89 Gauquelin G, Thibault G, Garcia R. Renal glomerular endothelin receptors in rats with high output heart failure. *Regulatory Peptides* 1991;**35**:73–79.
90 Fu L, Sun X, Hedner T, et al. Decreased density of mesenteric arteries but not of myocardial endothelin receptors and function in rats with chronic ischaemic heart failure. *J Cardiovasc Pharmacol* 1993;**22**:177–182.
91 Löffler BM, Roux S, Kalina B, Clozel M, Clozel JP. Influence of chronic heart failure on endothelin levels and receptors in rabbits. *J Mol Cell Cardiol* 1993;**25**:407–416.
92 Calderone A, Rouleau JL, de Champlain J, Belichard P, Stewart DJ. Regulation of the endothelin-1 transmembrane signalling pathway: the potential role of agonist-induced desensitization in the coronary artery of the

rapid ventricular pacing-overdrive dog model of heart failure. *J Mol Cell Cardiol* 1993;**25**:895–903.

93 Hahn AWA, Resink TJ, Scott-Burden T, Powell JS, Dohi Y, Bühler FR. Stimulation of endothelin mRNA and secretion in rat vascular smooth muscle cells: a novel autocrine function. *Cell Regul* 1990;**1**:649–659.

94 Towend J, Doran J, Jones S, Davies M. Effect of angiotensin converting enzyme inhibition on plasma endothelin in chronic heart failure. *Int J Cardiol* 1994;**43**:299–304.

95 Teerlink JR, Löffler BM, Hess P, Maire J-P, Clozel M, Clozel JP. Role of endothelin in the maintenance of blood pressure in conscious rats with chronic heart failure. *Circulation* 1994;**90**:2510–2518.

96 Wada A, Maeda Y, Tsutamoto T, Matsuda Y. Comparison with ET_A and ET_B receptor mediated cardiorenal and endocrine functions of endogenous endothelin in congestive heart failure. *Circulation* 1994;**90**:I173.

97 Love MP, Haynes WG, Webb DJ, McMurray JJV. Anti-endothelin therapy is of potential benefit in heart failure. *Circulation* 1994;**90**:I547.

98 Clozel M, Breu V, Burri K, et al. Pathophysiological role of endothelin revealed by the first orally active endothelin receptor antagonist. *Nature* 1993;**365**:759–761.

11

Aldosterone in chronic heart failure: have we forgotten it?

Allan D Struthers

Introduction

It is well established that activation of the renin–angiotensin–aldosterone system correlates with mortality in chronic heart failure.[1] The V-HeFT II results shows that the beneficial effects of ACE inhibitors are due to neurohormonal suppression as well as their vasodilator effects. Until recently, the traditional view was that it was angiotensin II which is the principal culprit in the renin–angiotensin–aldosterone system. However, this has turned out to be an over-simplification and it is now beginning to be appreciated that aldosterone is a second culprit and that the harmful effects of aldosterone are very similar to the harmful effects of angiotensin II.

It might initially be considered that differentiating the adverse effects of angiotensin II from those of aldosterone was rather academic, since ACE inhibitors reduce both substances. However this has also turned out to be a misconception. ACE inhibitors do undoubtedly produce an acute decrease in aldosterone but the chronic suppressive effects of ACE inhibitors on aldosterone levels are weak, variable, and unsustained.

The relatively poor suppressive effect of ACE inhibitors on plasma aldosterone was shown by Cleland et al,[2] where the median plasma aldosterone level after 6 weeks of treatment was 224 pmol/litre (range 56–1568) on captopril compared to 280 pmol/litre (range 84–2072) on placebo. In fact, this amounts to only a 20% fall on average, which is not statistically significant and which appears from the ranges presented to be very variable from one patient to the next. Clearly the important clinical point is that, if aldosterone is independently harmful, then there is plenty of residual aldosterone around after an ACE inhibitor for this to be a potential problem. It is also a potentially reversible problem, since spironolactone is an aldosterone antagonist that could, with due caution, be added to an ACE inhibitor in chronic heart failure (CHF). It should be pointed out that Cleland et al[2] found that angiotensin II levels behaved similarly to aldosterone in that they were also not suppressed very effectively by captopril ten hours after dosing.

Effects of aldosterone

What therefore are the harmful effects of aldosterone and which of these effects are not shared by angiotensin II? There are basically five such adverse effects. These five effects are interlinked, but for clarity each will be discussed in turn (Fig. 11.1).

Magnesium loss

Firstly, aldosterone independently causes magnesium loss from the body by increasing urine magnesium output. This is well established but what is less well appreciated is that angiotensin II *per se* has the opposite effect, causing a fall in urinary magnesium output.[3] So, curiously, the renin–angiotensin–aldosterone system appears

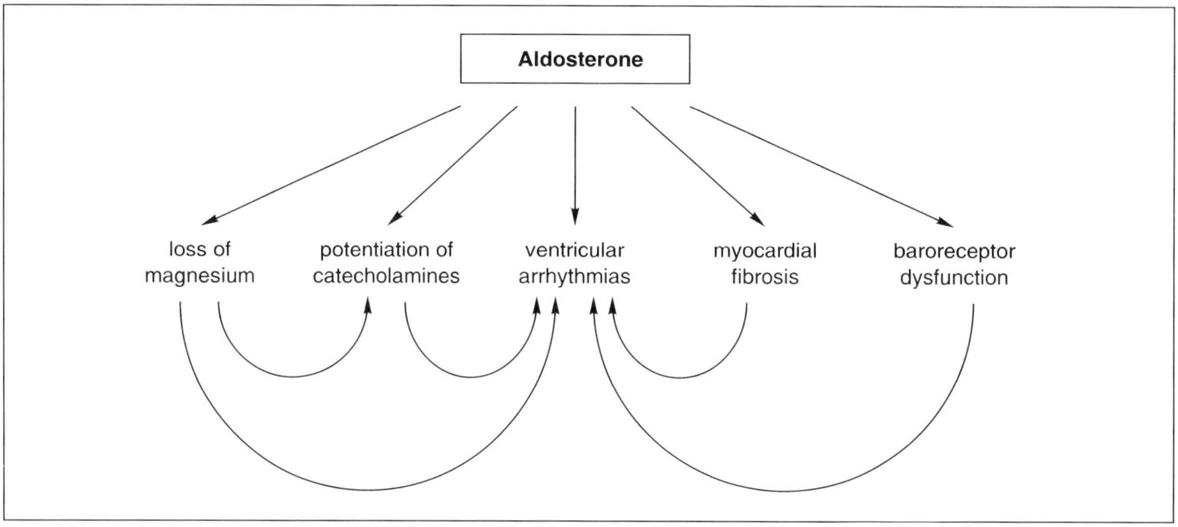

Fig. 11.1
Potentially adverse effects of aldosterone in CHF.

to have a biphasic effect on magnesium output. This may be why in CHF, ACE inhibitors have had a surprisingly small effect on serum magnesium levels. The increase in serum magnesium after an ACE inhibitor in CHF is of the order of only 2%.[4] This should be viewed along with the fact that serum magnesium starts at a low baseline in CHF, owing to diuretic therapy and activation of the renin–angiotensin–aldosterone system. The prevalence of magnesium deficiency in CHF is said to be found in between 7% and 37% of patients.[5]

The precise biological significance of magnesium in cardiovascular disease has been obscured somewhat by the recent contradictory results from the LIMIT and ISIS-4 post myocardial infarction (MI) studies. However, in contrast to the situation in MI patients, magnesium deficiency retains an important role in chronic heart failure patients. This difference between MI patients and CHF patients is not surprising, since the CHF patients are under the chronic magnesuric influence of diuretic therapy, whereas MI patients are not. A low serum magnesium is clearly associated with an increase in ventricular ectopy, both in CHF[5] and even in normal subjects.[6] Furthermore, magnesium replacement by either the intravenous route or by oral supplementation causes a fall in ventricular arrhythmias in CHF.[7,8]

All this is strong evidence to link magnesium deficiency to ventricular arrhythmias in CHF. In fact, magnesium is an essential cofactor of ATPase for the generation of contraction. Increases in cytosolic magnesium should therefore block inward calcium currents, reduce outward sodium transport and act on potassium channels to modify the duration of action potentials. Any or all of these effects could well be the basis of the antiarrhythmic effect of magnesium. A further interesting possibility that has been demonstrated recently in the dog is that magnesium deficiency may not act alone to cause arrhythmias, but rather it may well increase the arrhythmogenic response to adrenaline.[9] The possibility of aldosterone and magnesium interacting with catecholamines is a relatively new concept, which will be discussed in more detail below.

There are many caveats to be mentioned in discussing the link between magnesium and arrhythmias. Firstly, serum magnesium levels relate poorly to myocardial magnesium levels.[10] Secondly, it is always difficult to separate the effect of magnesium deficiency from potassium deficiency, since they commonly coexist. Indeed, in some studies, both magnesium and potassium replacement are required to decrease diuretic-induced ventricular ectopy.[11] However, since aldosterone increases excretion of both magnesium and potassium, differentiating between them is less essential when discussing aldosterone. Thirdly, although there is a clear link between magnesium and arrhythmias, a link between magnesium deficiency and mortality is controversial even in CHF patients.[5,12] This could be because, in severe CHF, coincidental renal dysfunction starts to normalize low serum magnesium values or because, as has been suggested, ventricular arrhythmias on Holter tapes are a poor indicator of those at risk of sudden death in CHF.[13]

Catecholamine potentiation

The second harmful effect of aldosterone relates to its ability to potentiate the effects of catecholamines. The precise mechanism of this effect is not established but one major component of it could be that aldosterone blocks catecholamine uptake in tissues. After noradrenaline is released from nerve terminals, its disposal and inactivation is largely achieved by reuptake, both into neurones (uptake$_1$) and into extraneuronal tissues (uptake$_2$). Both uptake$_1$ and uptake$_2$ are present in the myocardium. Uptake$_1$ is a low capacity, high affinity system that is blocked by desipramine. Uptake$_2$ is a high capacity, low affinity system that is blocked by corticosterone. Since corticosterone is the classical inhibitor of uptake$_2$ and since the chemical structure of corticosterone and aldosterone are similar, it would not be too surprising if aldosterone acted similarly to block the uptake$_2$ process.

The present evidence in this area certainly suggests that aldosterone potentiates the effect of catecholamines and that part of this potentiation is due to its blocking noradrenaline uptake. However it remains unknown whether this is specifically an effect on the uptake$_2$ process. It is also unknown whether aldosterone has some additional effects on the process of noradrenaline release itself. Angiotensin II has long been known to potentiate the release of noradrenaline from sympathetic nerve terminals, but whether aldosterone has similar effects is currently unknown.

What, therefore, are the biological consequences of aldosterone potentiating catecholamines? In vascular smooth muscle, aldosterone potentiates the constrictor effects of catecholamines.[14] In CHF, both aldosterone and catecholamines are elevated, so that an interaction of this kind in vascular tissue could well increase afterload. Of even more importance, however, would be a similar phenomenon in myocardial tissue. In a recent animal experiment, it was found that aldosterone did indeed block noradrenaline uptake in the heart *in vivo*. It has also been shown that spironolactone increased myocardial noradrenaline uptake in patients with CHF, as shown by m-iodobenzylguanidine (mIBG) scanning.[14a] The biological consequences of aldosterone's reducing myocardial noradrenaline uptake in CHF need to be explored further but, since catecholamines are undoubtedly harmful overall in CHF, it is likely that their potentiation by aldosterone would be similarly harmful.

The fact that catecholamines are harmful in CHF can be inferred from several observations. Plasma noradrenaline levels are linked closely to a poor prognosis in CHF.[15] Recent data with beta-blockers in CHF shows that sympathetic activation is not simply a marker of disease severity but rather that it contributes to acceleration of the CHF disease process.[16] This has been confirmed by the Metoprolol in Dilated Cardiomyopathy (MDC) trial, in which metoprolol improved symptoms and reduced disease progression, although surprisingly it did not alter either the total death rate or the sudden death rate.[17]

Therefore, aldosterone could well potentiate the adverse effects of catecholamines on vasoconstriction, on exercise limitation and on progression of the CHF disease process. It is tempting to speculate even further and suggest that because catecholamines are arrhythmogenic, their potentiation by aldosterone may increase arrhythmias and hasten death. This is still a hypothesis in need of testing, although the lack of effect of metoprolol on sudden death in the MDC trial is a strong pointer against the simplistic notion that catecholamines cause sudden death in CHF by way of provoking arrhythmias.

Induction of ventricular arrhythmias

The third harmful effect of aldosterone could be the induction of ventricular arrhythmias. The hypothesis that aldosterone might cause arrhythmias by potentiating catecholamines has been discussed above. There is, however, another possibility, which is that aldosterone causes arrhythmias by some as yet undefined, non-catecholamine mechanism. This was first suggested in 1962 by the work of Arora and Somani,[18] who performed coronary artery ligation in dogs and then studied the ventricular arrhythmias produced when adrenaline or aldosterone were infused. Adrenaline was arrhythmogenic as expected, but somewhat surprisingly aldosterone alone displayed a striking arrhythmogenic effect that followed a clear dose–response relationship. This study was not placebo controlled, but the arrhythmogenic effect of aldosterone was more pronounced and more prolonged than that produced by exogenous adrenaline. Furthermore, in this experiment, the arrhythmogenic effect of aldosterone was of rapid onset, which makes magnesium and potassium depletion an unlikely mechanism.

Myocardial fibrosis

The fourth adverse effect of aldosterone is its ability to stimulate fibrosis in the myocardium. This is one of the adverse effects that appears to be attributable not only to aldosterone but also to angiotensin II. Nevertheless a separate effect of aldosterone does appear to exists.[19] Brilla et al[19] showed that aldosterone induces biventricular fibrosis in the rat and that myocardial fibrosis could be prevented by spironolactone at a dose that was too low to alter the blood pressure itself.[20] This observation has been extended to show that aldosterone acts independently of haemodynamic factors to induce mRNA for collagen in both the left and right ventricle.[21]

Fibrosis in the myocardium is likely to be a key process in the production of myocardial stiffness (diastolic dysfunction), and it may also be relevant to the production of malignant ventricular arrhythmias. Experimentally at least, myocardial fibrosis causes anisotropic re-entry, repolarization inhomogeneity, and a decreased threshold for ventricular fibrillation. This also seems to occur in human CHF, since it was recently found that QTc dispersion identifies CHF patients who are at risk of dying suddenly and unexpectedly at a relatively early stage of the CHF disease process.[22] It is likely that the underlying pathological basis of QTc dispersion is widespread, patchy myocardial fibrosis. However, aldosterone is clearly not the only cause of myocardial fibrosis in CHF, since past ischaemia or infarction along with LV dilatation or hypertrophy are also liable to cause fibrosis. How important aldosterone is in the genesis of myocardial fibrosis in CHF remains to be established, but there is enough evidence to suggest that this is worthy of further investigation. One of the difficulties in studying the causes of myocardial fibrosis is that fibrosis may be a mechanism to prevent left ventricular dilatation, which means that there is unlikely to be simple direct correlation by which fibrosis increases as left ventricular dilatation also increases.

From the above, it is at least possible that aldosterone is one cause of patchy myocardial fibrosis and that this lowers the threshold for malignant ventricular arrhythmias in CHF.

Baroreflex function

The fifth potentially harmful effect of aldosterone is its ability to blunt the baroreflex. As with fibrosis, this is an effect shared with angiotensin II,[23] but recent data suggest that aldosterone has an independent effect in this regard. In an elegant study, Wang et al.[24] showed that perfusion of the carotid sinus with aldosterone reduced maximum baroreceptor discharge. Barr and Struthers[25] found a similar effect in humans in that aldosterone blunted the reflex bradycardic response to noradrenaline. Baroreflex function is well known to be impaired in clinical CHF and to be an independent marker of poor prognosis, at least in a post-MI population.[26,27]

The reason why baroreflex dysfunction and prognosis are related is not known, but it is thought that intact vagal function might oppose the arrhythmogenic effect of sympathetic tone even though vagal stimulation itself has little intrinsic effect on myocardial excitability.[28] Aldosterone may therefore disturb this crucial balance between the parasympathetic and the sympathetic nervous system, decreasing the influence of the former and increasing the influence of the latter. It is therefore possible to speculate that, even after an ACE inhibitor in CHF, there is enough residual aldosterone to blunt baroreflex function and that this could contribute directly or indirectly to the poor prognosis.

Other traditional effects of aldosterone

There are of course other well-known effects of aldosterone, which could be harmful. These include its ability to cause sodium retention and its ability to increase blood pressure. Both of these effects are also operative in CHF. Van Vliet et al[29] showed clearly that spironolactone exhibits a natriuretic effect in CHF even in the presence of a loop diuretic and an ACE inhibitor – a natriuresis was induced by 100 mg spironolactone in 81% of CHF patients who were otherwise resistant to high dose diuretic therapy. This effect varies from one patient to the next.[30] Aldosterone also increases blood pressure, not only from its ability to retain sodium but also by way of a vasoconstrictor effect, the mechanism of which may be potentiation of noradrenaline.

These effects of aldosterone on ventricular arrhythmias, catecholamine potentiation, myocardial fibrosis, and baroreflex function have been described only relatively recently. Along with this mini revolution in our understanding of the physiological effects of aldosterone, there is a parallel revolution in our understanding of the biochemistry of aldosterone action.[31] Aldosterone's effects are now divided into rapid effects (within minutes – so called non-genomic effects) and later, genomic effects, which require transcription and translation within cells. Many tissues (kidney, smooth muscle, and lymphocytes) appear to exhibit both genomic and non-genomic effects. How these issues relate to the clinical significance of aldosterone in CHF has not yet been explored. Understanding these issues could be important if better ways of blocking the effects of aldosterone are to be developed.

Conclusion

There are many potentially harmful effects of aldosterone in CHF. These effects are magnesium loss, catecholamine uptake inhibition, and the production of ventricular arrhythmias, myocardial fibrosis, and baroreflex malfunction. It is possible that even with standard diuretic and ACE inhibitor therapy in CHF, there is enough residual aldosterone to cause at least some of these effects. We have examined the effects of spironolactone added to diuretics and ACE inhibitors in CHF.[14a] Spironolactone did indeed cause magnesium retention, an increase in myocardial noradrenaline uptake, and a fall in ventricular arrhythmias. These data suggest that spironolactone has the potential to produce a mortality benefit over and above the well-described mortality reduction seen with ACE inhibitors. This crucial issue is being addressed by the Randomized Aldactone Evaluation Study, now abbreviated to RALES.[32] This study will finish around 1997 and its results are eagerly awaited, especially by those who feel that even after ACE inhibitors there is still more therapeutic mileage in CHF to be gained from neuroendocrine suppression.

References

1 Swedberg K, Eneroth P, Kjekshus J, Wilhemsen L, for the CONSENSUS Trial Study Group. Hormones regulating cardiovascular function in patients with severe congestive heart failure and their relation to mortality. *Circulation* 1990;**82**:1730–1736.

2 Cleland JGF, Dargie HJ, Hodsman GP, et al. Captopril in heart failure. A doubled blind controlled trial. *Br Heart J* 1984;**52**:530–535.

3 Rahman ARA, Lang CC, Nicoll G, Fraser CG, Struthers AD. Angiotensin II and aldosterone have opposite effects on urine magnesium output [abstract]. *Scott Med J* 1992;**37**:157–158.

4 Cleland JGF, Dargie JH, Ball SG, et al. Effects of enalapril in heart failure: a double blind study of effects on exercise performance, renal function, hormones and metabolic rate. *Br Heart J* 1985;**54**:305–312.

5 Eichhom EJ, Tandon PK, Di Bianco R, et al. Clinical and prognostic significance of serum magnesium concentration in patients with severe CHF: the PROMISE study. *J Am Coll Cardiol* 1993;**21**:634–640.

6 Tsuji H, Venditti FJ Jr, Evans JC, Larson MG, Levy D. The association of serum potassium and magnesium levels with occurrence of complex or frequent ventricular arrhythmias. *Circulation* 1993;**88**:I354.

7 Gottlieb SS, Baruch L, Kuklin ML, et al. Prognostic importance of the serum magnesium concentration in patients with congestive heart failure. *J Am Coll Cardiol* 1990; **16**:827–831.

8 Bashir Y, Sneddon JF, Staunton A, et al. Effects of oral magnesium chloride replacement in CHF secondary to coronary artery disease. *Am J Cardiol* 1993;**72**:1156–1162.

9 Bean BL, Varghese PL. Role of magnesium deficiency in the pressor and arrhythmogenic response to epinephrine in the intact dog. *Am Heart J* 1994;**127**:96–102.

10 Ralston MA, Murname MR, Kelley RE, et al. Magnesium content of serum, circulating mononuclear cells, skeletal muscle and myocardium in CHF. *Circulation* 1989;**80**:573–580.

11 Helfant RH. Short and long term mechanisms of sudden cardiac death in CHF. *Am J Cardiol* 1990;**65**:41K–43K.

12 Gottlieb S, Fischer ML, Pressel MD, Pattern RD, Weinberg M, Greenberg N. Effects of intravenous magnesium sulphate on arrhythmias in patients with CHF. *Am Heart J* 1993; **125**:1645–1650.

13 Packer M. Lack of relation between ventricular arrhythmias and sudden death in patients with chronic heart failure. *Circulation* 1992;**85**:I50–I56.

14 Weber MA, Purdy RE. Catecholamine mediated constrictor effects of aldosterone on vascular smooth muscle. *Life Sci* 1982; **30**:2009–2117.

14a Barr CS, Lang CC, Hanson J, Arnott M, Kennedy N, Struthers AD. Effects of adding spironalactone to an ACE inhibitor in chronic congestive heart failure secondary to coronary artery disease. *Am J Cardiol* 1995 (in press).

15 Cohn JN, Levine B, Olivari MT, et al. Plasma norepinephrine as a guide to prognosis in patients with CHF. *N Engl J Med* 1984; **311**:819–823.

16 Fisher ML, Gottlieb SS, Plotnick GD, et al. Beneficial effects of metoprolol in heart failure associated with coronary artery disease: a randomised trial. *J Am Coll Cardiol* 1994;**23**:943–950.

17 Waagstein F, Bristow MR, Swedberg K, et al, for the MDC Group. Beneficial effects of metoprolol in idiopathic dilated cardiomyopathy. *Lancet* 1993;**342**:1441–1446.

18 Arora RB, Somari P. Ectopic arrhythmia provoking action of aldosterone. *Life Sci* 1962; **5**:215–218.

19 Brilla CG, Matsubara LS, Weber KT. Antialdosterone treatment and the prevention of myocardial fibrosis in primary and secondary hyperaldosteronisin. *J Mol Cell Cardiol* 1993; **25**:563–575.

20 Brilla CG, Weber KT. Reactive and reparative myocardial fibrosis in arterial hypertension in the rat. *Cardiovasc Res* 1992;**26**:671–676.

21 Robert V, van Theim N, Cheav SL, Mouas C, Swynghedau B, Delcayre C. Increased cardiac types I and III collagen mRNAs in aldosterone salt hypertension. *Hypertension* 1994;**24**:30–36.

22 Barr CS, Naas A, Freeman M, Lang CC, Struthers AD. QT dispersion and sudden unexpected death in chronic heart failure. *Lancet* 1994;**343**:327–329.

23 Mace PJE, Watson RDS, Skan W, Littler WA. Inhibition of the baroreceptor heart rate reflex by angiotensin II in normal man. *Cardiovasc Res* 1985;**19**:525–527.

24 Wang W, McClaim JM, Zucker IH. Aldosterone reduces baroreceptor discharge in the dog. *Hypertension* 1992;**19**:270–277.

25 Barr CS, Struthers AD. Aldosterone blunts the reflex baroreceptor response but not the pressor response to noradrenaline in healthy man. *Br Heart J* 1994;**71**:P96.

26 Rea RF, Berg WJ. Abnormal baroreflex mechanisms in congestive heart failure: recent insights. *Circulation* 1990;**81**:2026–2027.

27 Kjellgren O, Gomes JA. Heart rate variability and baroreflex sensitivity in myocardial infarction. *Am Heart J* 1993;**125**:204–215.

28 Myers RW, Pearlman AS, Hyman RM, et al. Beneficial effects of vagal stimulation and bradycardia during experimental acute myocardial ischaemia. *Circulation* 1974;**49**:943–947.

29 van Vilet AA, Donker AJM, Nauta JJP, Verheugt FWA. Spironolactone in CHF refractory to high dose loop diuretic and low dose ACE inhibitor. *Am J Cardiol* 1993;**71**:21A–28A.

30 Sanders LL, Melby JC. Aldosterone and the edema of congestive heart failure. *Arch Intern Med* 1964;**113**:331–341.

31 Wehling M, Christ M, Gerzer R. Aldosterone-specific membrane receptors and related rapid, non-genomic effects. *Trends Pharmacol Sci* 1993;**14**:1–4.

32 Garg R, Yusuf S. Current and ongoing randomized trials in heart failure and left ventricular dysfunction. *J Am Coll Cardiol* 1993; **22(suppl A)**:194A–197A.

SECTION IV

INVESTIGATION

12

Which exercise test, if any?

TP Chua, Andrew JS Coats

Introduction

Chronic heart failure (CHF) is a common and debilitating illness with a high annual mortality. Whilst recent trials have shown that certain therapies, especially angiotensin converting enzyme (ACE) inhibitors, have improved the survival of such patients, the symptoms of CHF remain limiting. These symptoms, which include dyspnoea and muscle fatigue, manifest especially during exertion. Although indices such as left ventricular ejection fraction, left ventricular dimensions, and haemodynamic measurements reflect the degree of cardiac dysfunction, there is little correlation between these and exercise capacity.[1–3] Dysfunction and pathological changes occur in the lungs,[4] skeletal muscle,[5,6] peripheral resistance vessels[7,8] and the vascular endothelium[9] as a complication of CHF, and these may intervene to become the major factors limiting daily exercise and causing unpleasant symptoms in the treated patient with chronic heart failure. Exercise testing allows an objective assessment of the functional capacity of patients with chronic heart failure,[10–13] and, when combined with electrocardiographic, haemodynamic, respiratory gas exchange, and metabolic monitoring, can help determine the factors limiting an individual patient. The assessment of respiratory gas exchange during maximal exercise testing has been shown to provide a more reproducible and objective test of the functional status of chronic heart failure patients than exercise capacity alone.[10,13,14]

Physiology of exercise

According to the Fick principle,[15] cardiac output is equal to oxygen consumption divided by the arteriovenous oxygen difference. The arteriovenous oxygen difference represents oxygen extraction by the peripheral tissues and averages 40 ml oxygen/litre. During exercise, this increases to its maximum (5–10 times resting). From the Fick equation, it can be seen that, as the arteriovenous oxygen difference reaches a constant value during peak exercise, the total body oxygen consumption becomes a function of cardiac output. Therefore, not only does cardiopulmonary exercise testing help assess functional capacity, but it also reflects cardiac output during maximal exercise, provided that maximal oxygen extraction by the exercising muscles has been achieved.

In theory, any part of the pathway for the delivery of oxygen from ambient air to skeletal muscle mitochondrial oxidative enzymes, and the removal of metabolic byproducts such as carbon dioxide and acid from the mitochondria to the expired air or urine might be a limiting step to the maintenance of muscular exercise. In most normal subjects, lung function is rarely the limiting factor, and the maximum capacity of the heart to pump blood is considered the commonest limitation to exercise. Thus, maximal oxygen consumption is considered a good estimate of maximal integrated cardiopulmonary function, usually reflecting cardiac reserve capacity.

It was natural, therefore, for the medical community to assume that, in heart failure, where there is a specific and severe limitation to the maximal pumping capacity of the heart, the cardiac function would be the limiting factor. If changes occur in response to CHF, however, in other components of the pathway, these could supervene to limit exercise and cause symptoms even at a level of exercise below that sustainable by the maximal pumping capacity of the heart. These factors include respiratory muscle function,[16] oxygen diffusing capacity of the alveolar membrane,[17,18] peripheral vascular function, and the delivery of blood to the muscles,[19] extraction of oxygen by muscle,[20] oxidative capacity of muscle mitochondria,[5] the extraction of lactate and carbon dioxide,[21] and the tolerance by the patient of dyspnoea and fatigue signals carried to the cortex as a result of sensory signals from all these components.[22] Abnormalities in all the above areas have been described as being both operative and important in CHF, so that in an individual patient, cardiopulmonary exercise testing may tell us not only about the extent of exercise limitation, but also its cause.

Despite the correlation between oxygen consumption and work rate both in normal subjects[23] and in chronic heart failure patients,[10] the relation between the two is not constant enough to estimate oxygen consumption accurately, especially after the onset of anaerobic metabolism due to variations in oxygen uptake kinetics.[24] Despite this, some laboratories estimate oxygen consumption from the work rate achieved by assuming a certain relationship between the two variables and expressing this in terms of metabolic equivalents (METs). Each MET is equivalent to approximately 3.5 ml/minute per kg and is derived from the resting oxygen consumption of a 40-year-old, 70 kg man.[25] Although this circumvents the need for measuring respiratory gas exchange, estimating oxygen consumption from work rate may lead to gross inaccuracy. External work rate may fail to predict oxygen consumption in instances such as failure to reach a steady state (which takes 3 minutes to reach if below the anaerobic threshold or longer if above) or in the presence of cardiopulmonary disease, where there is not always a linear relationship between oxygen consumption and work rate.[24]

Although in theory there is a point of maximal oxygen uptake (where further increase in exercise intensity leads to no further increase in oxygen uptake, but merely to an increase in accumulated oxygen debt), in practice a true maximal oxygen consumption is rarely reached. The alternative measure of peak achieved oxygen uptake is what is normally measured for patients with CHF. Provided the onset of some degree of anaerobic metabolism has been ensured by an increase in the respiratory exchange ratio by at least 0.2 and to at least 1.0, then peak oxygen consumption is a valid estimate of the true maximal oxygen consumption.[26]

The value of exercise testing in CHF

One of the most difficult aspects of managing a patient with heart failure is the assessment of the severity of the disease and the progress of the patient's condition. Routine examination can detect signs of congestion, which can be treated by adjustment in the dose of diuretics. It is much more difficult to assess the dose of ACE inhibition, especially as it is not yet known whether the high doses used in the large mortality trials are necessary for all the beneficial effects of this drug class. The symptoms reported by the patient are poorly reproducible and highly subjective, so that it is difficult to use these to gauge whether a patient is improving with treatment. The objectivity of an assessment of exercise capacity can assist in this evaluation. This has advantages in individual patient management as well as for risk stratification, selection for transplantation, assessment of new treatments, and clinical research.

Exercise capacity has been shown to be predictive of survival in CHF, with predictive capacity independent of the severity of left ventricular impairment or the apparent symptomatic status of the patient.[27–30] Thus there are strong arguments for the utility of some form of exercise capacity assessment for patients with chronic heart failure.

The choice of exercise test in CHF

Informal exercise tests are frequently used in practice to assess the ability of a patient to perform simple daily tasks or to walk at different speeds or up and down stairs. These can be combined with simple physiological monitoring, such as heart rate or respiratory rate. They can be useful in estimating a patient's capacity quickly and inexpensively, but the information obtainable is limited as there is little standardization of test procedures.

Numerous formal exercise protocols exist, utilizing a variety of different exercise modes. The choice of test depends on the test objectives – for maximal capacity assessment, a progressive, incremental test is used; if physiological responses are to be measured a constant load test may be more useful as a steady state can be achieved. Whatever the purpose, standardization of the test is crucial to ensure the value of repeated testing of one patient and to enable comparisons between patients, centres, and different treatment effects. In the assessment of CHF and left ventricular dysfunction, levels of exercise capacity varying from less than 10 ml/kg per minute to over 40 ml/kg per minute in peak oxygen consumption can be expected. As a result, no single protocol is likely to be equally useful in all patients. A young patient with asymptomatic left ventricular dysfunction needs high workloads and rapidly incremental loads to reach maximal capacity in the optimal time of around 12 minutes, whereas a patient with severe heart failure will need a much gentler load.

Incremental tests

To measure maximal capacity requires an incremental test. Although individual muscle groups can be tested for strength and resistance to fatigue, the most relevant exercise tests for patients with CHF are those that demand a sustained high cardiac output (i.e. dynamic exercise with the body's large muscle groups). Theoretically, walking, swimming, running, rowing, cycling, or stepping would all be suitable, but in practice treadmill walking test and stationary cycling are the two most popular. Treadmill testing is the most common in the UK. Some of the treadmill protocols most widely employed to determine this quantity are shown in Table 2.1.

The level of exercise load achieved depends on the mode of exercise, the bulk of muscle used in performing the exercise, and the rate of load increment during the test; the more rapid the increment the higher the final load achieved. A treadmill test achieves the greater cardiovascular challenge because it involves a larger muscle mass and achieves higher levels of oxygen consumption. On the other hand, there may be greater security for the patient with cycle ergometry; the patient is seated and can stop with safety at any time. Treadmill walking is vastly

Bruce protocol

Stage	Speed (mph)	Grade (%)	Stage length (min)	Metabolic equivalent (MET)
1	1.7	10	3	5
2	2.5	12	3	7
3	3.4	14	3	9
4	4.2	16	3	11
5	5.0	18	3	13

Modified Bruce (Sheffield)

Stage	Speed (mph)	Grade (%)	Stage length (min)	MET
1	1.7	0	3	2.3
2	1.7	5	3	3.5
3	1.7	10	3	4.8
4	2.5	12	3	6.6
5	3.4	14	3	8.4
6	4.2	16	3	10.2

Modified Bruce (National Heart Hospital, London)

Stage	Speed (mph)	Grade (%)	Stage length (min)	MET
1	1.7	5	3	3.5
2	1.7	10	3	4.8
3	2.5	12	3	6.6
4	3.4	14	3	8.4
5	4.2	16	3	10.2

Balke

Stage	Speed (mph)	Grade (%)	Stage length (min)	MET
1	3	0	3	3
2	3	2	3	4
3	3	5	3	5
4	3	7.5	3	6
5	3	10	3	7
6	3	12.5	3	8

Table 12.1
Commonly used treadmill protocols with MET values for each stage or minute interval completed.

different from free walking and patients may feel that they are unstable and that they have less control over the test. The use of hand rails diminishes these problems but of course decreases the work done and therefore the oxygen uptake; this leads to underestimation of capacity and to loss of standardization. External work rate can be determined on a cycle ergometer, whereas in treadmill testing this depends on the weight of the subject.

Peak heart rates during cycle ergometry are similar to those seen in treadmill exercise; however oxygen consumption is about 5–10% lower and systolic blood pressure tends to be somewhat higher, possibly owing to the isometric contractions of the arm muscles in gripping the handlebars. Blood lactate concentrations tend to be higher during exercise of a given proportion of peak oxygen consumption during cycling compared to treadmill exercise.[31]

Cycle ergometer protocols usually begin with an 'unloaded' stage, followed by progressive increments of between 25 and 50 watts, every 2–3 minutes, although there has been increasing use of 1 minute 10 watt incremental stages for heart failure patients. On isokinetic ergometers (usually electrically braked), work rate is independent of pedal frequency, with the load being modified depending on cycling frequency. On mechanical ergometers, the frequency of pedalling must be controlled if the test is to be standardized. A constant pedal frequency of 50–60 rpm is comfortable for most patients.

Where neither a treadmill nor a cycle ergometer is available, externally paced stepping or walking are alternatives for which a degree of standardization is possible. The same principles of testing apply; the test should be graded, with short or longer test stages according to objectives.

Whether the levels of an incremental exercise test should increase in a stepwise manner or continuously depends on the purpose of the test; for the measurement of the physiological responses to exercise, longer stages (at least 4 minutes) allow steady-state conditions to develop, but this is longer than the stages in any of the commonly used protocols; if the test function is purely to evaluate functional capacity, then either shorter stages or a continuously increasing intensity is preferable. Excessively long tests should be avoided because they are poorly reproducible and because local muscle fatigue may cause the test to be ended prematurely before the true peak in oxygen consumption is attained. The rate of load increment has an effect on both the achieved peak oxygen consumption and even the symptom-limiting exercise.[32]

Although it is unlikely that there is a single protocol ideally suited to all the uses of exercise testing, it does appear that a progressive test lasting between 8 and 15 minutes is close to ideal for evaluation of peak oxygen consumption. One test less frequently used in the assessment of cardiac patients than the protocols listed in Table 12.1 is the STEEP test,[33] in which 1 minute incremental loads starting from 2 METs and increasing by 15% per minute, leads to progressive absolute load increments and a narrower range of total exercise durations. Its relative role compared to the more conventional protocols remains to be established.

Endurance tests

Although maximal exercise performance remains a useful measurement, an alternative and important aspect of exercise capacity is endurance or stamina, the ability to sustain exercise, which represents a high proportion of personal peak exercise capacity. Stamina is also probably more relevant to the exercise demands of everyday life of most patients with CHF. It is independent of peak oxygen consumption, depending mainly on the metabolic 'quality' of the muscles. Endurance is ideally measured as the maximum time for which a patient can maintain exercise at around 60–70% of maximal capacity. If the test is performed at too low an exercise intensity (relative to peak oxygen uptake), an excessively long test will result, leading to poorly reproducible results with boredom contributing to the reasons for termination; if too great a load is used, maximal performance rather than stamina will be assessed.

An alternative to conventional endurance tests is to examine the changes over time in the physiological responses to preset submaximal levels of exercise by measuring ventilation, heart rate, and blood lactate concentrations. This will give a reasonable indication of whether the patient could have sustained the studied intensity of exercise for a prolonged period; if 'steady state' responses are seen without lactate accumulation, then exercise is probably sustainable; if progressive increases are evident over 5–10 minutes, then endurance at this exercise load would be restricted.

Endurance tests allow objective monitoring of physiological responses to a constant submaximal work load comparable to many of the activities of daily living, but to be worthwhile they require prior assessment of functional capacity. Most commonly, these tests are performed on a treadmill or cycle ergometer, but are less commonly used in practice because of the potentially very long duration of 30 minutes or more.

Other exercise tests

Another increasingly popular form of exercise test involves timed task completion, or tasks completed within a preset time. These include such assessments as the distance which can be walked in a specified time, e.g. 6 or 12 minute walk tests,[34] or the time taken to complete a set task, e.g. the corridor walk test; it is important to remember, however, that they measure integrated exercise performance, which of course depends on both functional capacity and endurance.

Whatever mode of exercise is chosen, the patient must be familiarized with both the mode of exercise and any equipment to be used for expired air collection. Familiarization to treadmill walking should include experience of stopping, starting and of changes in grade and speed. Time spent doing this should be regarded as an investment to secure good data.

Cardiopulmonary exercise testing

During the cardiopulmonary exercise test, the patient wears a nose clip and breathes through a respiratory valve that separates inspired and expired air. Measurements of oxygen consumption (VO_2) and carbon dioxide production (VCO_2) are made either breath-by-breath using either rapid gas analysers or respiratory mass spectrometer, or by use of a mixing chamber.[35] A third respiratory parameter, the rate of air flow, is also measured by use of a flow meter linked to the respiratory valve. From the air flow and the duration per breath, the volume of air expired per minute (minute ventilation, $\dot{V}_E$) is worked out. Electrocardiographic monitoring is essential and pulse oximetry is often helpful.

From the measured parameters – oxygen consumption, carbon dioxide production, minute ventilation, and heart rate – a whole series of derivatives can be obtained on line. These include the ratio of carbon dioxide production to oxygen consumption (respiratory exchange ratio, RER or RQ), anaerobic threshold, ventilatory equivalent for oxygen ($\dot{V}_E/\dot{V}O_2$ ratio) and carbon dioxide ($\dot{V}_E/\dot{V}CO_2$ ratio), $\dot{V}_E/\dot{V}CO_2$ regression slope, oxygen pulse, and dead space–tidal volume ratio.

Maximal oxygen consumption

This may be defined as the oxygen consumption that has reached a plateau despite increases in work rate. As mentioned above, this reflects the cardiac output. As expected, the maximal

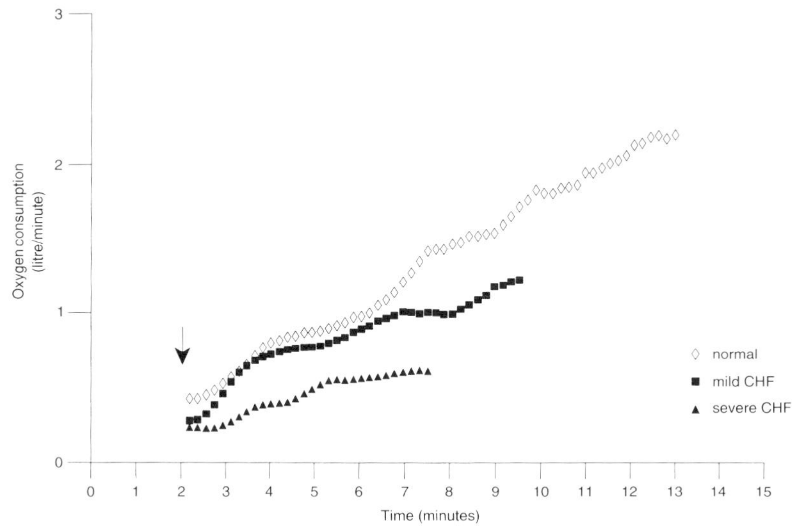

Fig. 12.1
Plot of oxygen consumption of two patients with CHF and an age-matched normal patient during incremental exercise. Arrow denotes start of exercise.

oxygen consumption is reduced in CHF compared to a normal subject. Patients with a maximal oxygen consumption of 16–20 ml/minute per kg are considered to have mild to moderate functional impairment of cardiac reserve; those with a value of 10–16 ml/minute per kg have moderate to severe functional impairment; and those with a maximal oxygen consumption of less than 10 ml/minute per kg have severe functional impairment; on a similar basis, they may also be categorized into groups A–D according to their maximal oxygen consumption.[12] Fig. 12.1 shows a graph of oxygen consumption during incremental exercise of two patients with different severities of CHF compared with an age-matched normal subject. It is not always clear whether the oxygen consumption has reached a plateau, especially in normal subjects[36] and in patients with mild disease. In such instances, other additional criteria may be useful. These additional criteria include the attainment of predicted maximal heart rate and a respiratory exchange ratio of over 1.1.

Extrapolated maximal oxygen consumption

Buller and Poole-Wilson[37] have suggested a mathematical model relating $\dot{V}O_2$ and $\dot{V}CO_2$ to derive an estimate of maximal oxygen consumption that is independent of exercise duration. They have termed this the 'extrapolated maximal oxygen consumption' (EMOC). This is particularly useful in instances when a true plateau in oxygen consumption is not seen. If this value is close to the maximal oxygen consumption, then the patient has exercised to a maximum. If otherwise, then it is likely that exercise is limited by some factors other than cardiac functional reserve. It appears to be more reliable than anaerobic threshold.[26]

Anaerobic threshold

In 1964, Wasserman and McIlroy[38] introduced the concept of anaerobic threshold to measure cardiopulmonary capacity. This may be defined as the level of oxygen consumption above which aerobic energy production is supplemented by anaerobic mechanisms. According to this concept, above this threshold there is a sustained rise in blood lactate, owing to increased production by exercising muscle, with an associated increase in ventilation, and the blood lactate is buffered by plasma bicarbonate, which causes an increase in carbon dioxide production. Because the anaerobic threshold is usually reached at 60–70% of maximal oxygen consumption, it may be used as a marker that the patient is on the way to a maximal cardiopulmonary test, and that it could, therefore, be used as an objective end-point for assessing patients and treatments. If anaerobic threshold is not reached during exercise, then the corollary applies (i.e. maximal oxygen consumption has not been attained at peak exercise, and the limitation in exercise is less likely to be cardiac in origin). The limitation in this situation is probably due to a ventilatory or musculoskeletal disorder or to poor motivation.

In chronic heart failure, the level of exercise load at which anaerobic threshold occurs is associated with the severity of the condition. Thus in mild CHF the anaerobic threshold may be greater than 12 ml/minute per kg; in moderate CHF, this may be between 9 and 10 ml/minute per kg; and in severe CHF as little as 6 ml/minute per kg.[12] The anaerobic threshold can be determined non-invasively by observing the disproportionate increase in carbon dioxide output and ventilation in relation to oxygen consumption (Fig. 12.2); there is also

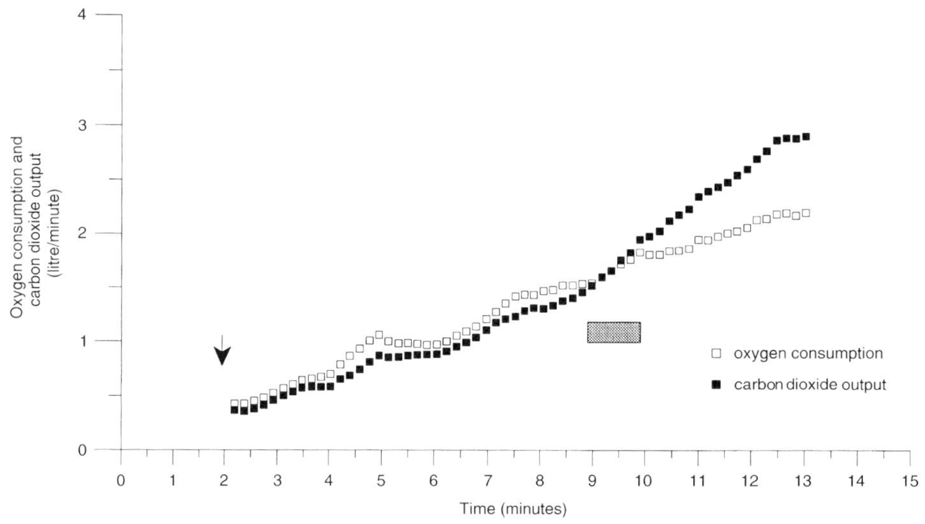

Fig. 12.2
Oxygen consumption and carbon dioxide output of a normal subject during incremental exercise. Arrow denotes start of exercise. During early exercise, oxygen consumption and carbon dioxide output increase at the same rate. The grey zone indicates a period of transition as carbon dioxide output rises disproportionately relative to oxygen consumption. This period includes the transition to anaerobic metabolism, although a clearly defined point may not always be seen.

a concomitant rise in the respiratory exchange ratio and in end-tidal oxygen concentration caused by the disproportionate increase in ventilation. There may be a large range of reviewer variability using the visual method of analysis[39] but more reliable methods have been introduced.[40,41]

The anaerobic threshold may also be assessed invasively by determining the onset of blood lactate accumulation, although some investigators have been unable to establish the phenomenon of blood lactate accumulation,[39] and others question whether this is related to a lack in delivery of oxygen rather than a defect in muscular uptake of oxygen.[42] This has led to the whole concept of a detectable point of anaerobic threshold and its linkage to lactate accumulation being questioned. Furthermore, lactate production is known to occur in aerobic conditions, and anaerobic metabolism can also be present at rest.[43] In addition to the lack of total agreement on the physiological basis of anaerobic threshold, the threshold determined by analysis of the shapes of the respiratory gas exchange data (termed the 'ventilatory anaerobic threshold') is not always seen as a clearly defined point during incremental exercise. Its use in cardiopulmonary exercise testing is, therefore, not universally accepted.

Respiratory exchange ratio

The resting respiratory exchange ratio is about 0.8. During early exercise, oxygen consumption and carbon dioxide output increase at the same rate, as seen in Fig. 12.2. At about 60–70% of maximal oxygen consumption, carbon dioxide output and minute ventilation begin to increase at a greater rate than oxygen consumption, heralding the onset of anaerobic threshold, as mentioned above, and the respiratory exchange ratio also increases accordingly.

Minute ventilaton

Minute ventilation increases in proportion to both oxygen consumption and carbon dioxide production during incremental exercise until the onset of anaerobic threshold. In fact, for work increments of 1 minute, it increases in proportion to carbon dioxide output for about 2 minutes after anaerobic threshold; this period is also known as the isocapnic buffering period.

There is also a more linear and less variable relationship between ventilation and carbon dioxide output than oxygen consumption.[23] An index of ventilatory drive can be obtained by correlating ventilation and carbon dioxide production using linear regression analysis.[44] In normal subjects, this $\dot{V}_E/\dot{V}CO_2$ slope is about 20.[45] Patients with CHF who have an excessive exercise ventilatory response have a steeper slope. The $\dot{V}_E/\dot{V}CO_2$ slope is also inversely related to maximal oxygen consumption and is itself a measure of the severity of CHF.[44] The relationship between minute ventilation and the rate of carbon dioxide production of two patients with CHF of different severity compared with a normal subject is shown in Fig. 12.3, which also illustrates a steeper $\dot{V}_E/\dot{V}CO_2$ slope in the more severely affected patient.

If the $\dot{V}_E/\dot{V}CO_2$ ratio at a particular instant in time (i.e. the ventilatory equivalent for carbon dioxide) is plotted against work rate, $\dot{V}_E/\dot{V}CO_2$ is seen to decrease until a plateau in normal subjects and in patients with mild CHF.[46] This is thought to be due to a reduction in dead space ventilation consequent to improved perfusion of hitherto poorly perfused regions of the lungs during incremental exercise. In those with more severe CHF, this $\dot{V}_E/\dot{V}CO_2$ ratio may decrease initially but it continues to rise at the end of exercise.[46] This may be due to increased dead space ventilation[3] but a non-carbon dioxide drive to ventilation is also plausible.[47] This

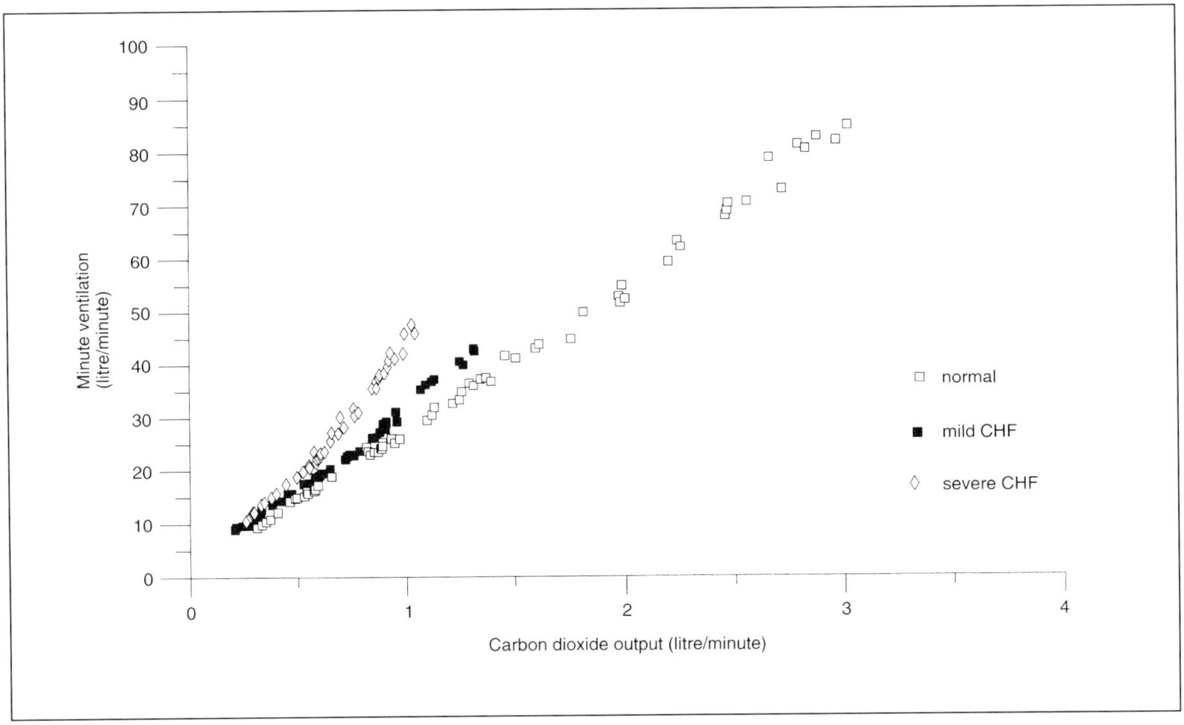

Fig. 12.3
The relationship between minute ventilation and carbon dioxide output in a normal subject and two patients with CHF. Note the steeper slope in the patient with the more severe CHF.

might be mediated by a cortical spill-over from the perception of effort, from abnormal release of ventilatory stimulants (e.g. potassium, adenosine), or from hypoxic sensitivity.[17]

Dead space ventilation

The dead space–tidal volume (VD/VT) ratio is an index of ventilation–perfusion matching and can be worked out from the parameters measured using the Bohr equation, which is as follows:

$$\frac{VD}{VT} = \frac{FACO_2 - FECO_2}{FACO_2}$$

where $FACO_2$ and $FECO_2$ are fractional concentration of carbon dioxide in the alveolar space and expired air respectively. $FACO_2$ may be estimated from the end-tidal fractional concentration of carbon dioxide measured at the mouth; VT is obtained by dividing minute ventilation by respiratory rate.

In normal subjects, the VD/VT ratio decreases from 0.35 or more, to 0.2 during exercise, owing to improvement of lung perfusion.[48] In patients with CHF, this ratio remains higher than normal during all stages of exercise, although it follows a similar declining trend during exercise,[3] which is suggestive of increased dead space ventilation compared with normal subjects. This may be partly due to an altered pattern of ventilation in heart failure with a reduced tidal volume and an increase in respiratory frequency. Although this cannot completely explain the excess ventilatory response to exercise in heart failure, studies should account for this increased proportionate dead space ventilation in assessing ventilatory responses in heart failure. As heart failure patients start with improved ventilation–perfusion matching because of increased perfusion of the upper zones of the upright lung, there may be less room for improvement with progressive exercise.

Oxygen kinetics

Changes in oxygen uptake with changing work rates are delayed in patients with chronic heart failure.[24] This may be due to delayed increases in leg blood flow or to alterations in the biochemical function of skeletal muscle in CHF. In either case, it could lead to increased symptomatic exercise limitation and is best detected by specially designed exercise protocols with measurements of respiratory gas exchange. In addition, recovery from exercise is also delayed.[24] As yet, little is known of the cause or best management of these altered oxygen consumption dynamics.

Arterial oxygen saturation

Pulse oximetry is often useful during cardiopulmonary exercise testing. Various investigators have not found any significant arterial oxygen desaturation during exercise in patients with CHF.[11,49,50] In contrast, there may be arterial oxygen desaturation in patients whose shortness of breath is due to pulmonary disorders.[51] This area remains, however, one of controversy, because some reports describe a higher rate of oxygen desaturations in heart failure occurring at rest and during sleep using predominantly transcutaneous oximetry.[52,53] Despite this, if significant arterial oxygen desaturation on direct arterial blood gas measurement is seen during cardiopulmonary exercise testing, then an alternative non-cardiac cause of shortness of breath should be sought. The typical patterns of respiratory gas exchange during exercise in CHF are listed in Table 12.2.

Maximal VO_2	Reduced
Anaerobic threshold	Reduced
V_E–VCO_2 regression slope	Increased
VD/VT	Increased
Oxygen pulse	Reduced
Arterial oxygen desaturation	None (?)

Table 12.2
Summary of observed patterns of respiratory gas exchange during exercise in chronic heart failure.

Ratings of perceived exertion

In assessing the response to exercise, it can be useful to know the level of perception of effort or symptomatic distress of the subject. This can be assessed as an 'all embracing" measure or it can be assessed separately for fatigue, dyspnoea, or chest pain. The rating of perceived exertion (RPE) scale described by Borg[54] (Table 12.3) is a useful way to quantify the subjective responses to exercise, and it has proved both reproducible and reasonably correlated with objective measures of physiological stress, such as the percentage of peak oxygen consumption which the exercise elicits. Most patients can use the scales appropriately, rating 60–75% of peak performance as 'somewhat hard' or 'hard' (RPE 13–16). As with any rating scale, it is important to give patients standardized instructions before their use, and reliability increases with repeat testing. Anxious patients may overestimate the stress early in the test, but this can be improved in later exercise tests.

6	
7	very, very light
8	
9	very light
10	
11	fairly light
12	
13	somewhat hard
14	
15	hard
16	
17	very hard
18	
19	very, very hard
20	

Table 12.3
Scale for ratings of perceived exertion (RPE). (From reference 54.)

The value of maximal oxygen consumption in CHF

Lipkin[10] found that maximal oxygen consumption was related to functional class as assessed by the NYHA criteria, although other investigators found a poorer association.[11] The discrepancy may be attributable to the definition of NYHA criteria as used in the studies. Franciosa[11] suggested that the lack of correlation between NYHA functional class II and III and maximal oxygen consumption in his study indicated that cardiopulmonary exercise testing was more discriminating in categorizing patients according to functional impairment than the NYHA classification was. It may also be that they are measuring different aspects of symptomatology, as poor correlations have been found between maximal oxygen consumption and detailed quality of life scores, estimates of habitual daily activity, or even different types of exercise testing such as submaximal endurance tests.

Effects of interventions

Maximal oxygen consumption can be used as an objective end-point of trials that are aiming at improving clinical status in CHF. For obvious reasons, this is easier than establishing an effect on mortality and more relevant than changes in ejection fraction or haemodynamics. In normal subjects, physical training may increase the maximal oxygen consumption by up to 33%, depending on the level of activity of subjects before training.[55,56] This is due to an increase in cardiac output (particularly stroke volume, since maximal heart rate remains unchanged or decreases with training) and also an increase in extraction of oxygen from the blood by the tissues. In CHF, physical training has also been shown to increase maximal oxygen consumption by 15–20% and in some (but not all) studies has been shown to generate a small increase in cardiac output at matched workloads and peak exercise.[57,58] It also causes a decrease in minute ventilation and in $\dot{V}_E/\dot{V}CO_2$ slope. Physical deconditioning may therefore in part explain the abnormal patterns of respiratory gas exchange that are seen in CHF.

Conclusion

Exercise testing has been used not only in the research setting but also clinically in order to assess the functional capacity of patients with CHF. Data obtained from such testing are both reproducible and objective, especially when combined with an analysis of respiratory gas exchange. Exercise testing has also been used to assess response to medical therapy and exercise training in CHF. Cardiopulmonary exercise testing will continue to play an important role in the management of CHF and it remains an allied tool in its future research.

References

1 Franciosa JA, Park M, Levine TB. Lack of correlation between exercise capacity and indexes of resting left ventricular performance in heart failure. *Am J Cardiol* 1981;**47**:33–39.

2 Higginbotham MB, Morris KG, Conn EH, Coleman ER, Cobb FR. Determinants of variable exercise performance among patients with severe left ventricular dysfunction. *Am J Cardiol* 1983;**51**:52–60.

3 Sullivan MJ, Higginbotham MB, Cobb FR. Increased exercise ventilation in patients with chronic heart failure: intact ventilatory control despite hemodynamic and pulmonary abnormalities. *Circulation* 1988;**77**:552–559.

4 Chua TP, Coats AJS. The lung in chronic heart failure. *Eur Heart J* 1995 (in press).

5 Drexler H, Riede U, Münzel T, König H, Funke E, Just H. Alterations of skeletal muscle in chronic heart failure. *Circulation* 1992;**85**: 1751–1759.

6 Clark A, Coats A. Mechanisms of exercise intolerance in cardiac failure; abnormalities of skeletal muscle and pulmonary function. *Curr Opin Cardiol* 1994;**9**:305–314.

7 Wilson JR, Martin JL, Schwartz D, Ferraro N. Exercise intolerance in patients with chronic heart failure: role of impaired nutritive flow to skeletal muscle. *Circulation* 1984;**69**:1079–1087.

8 Katz SD, Jondeau G, Galvao M, Sonnenblick EH, LeJemtel TH. Peripheral vascular abnormalities and peak aerobic capacity in patients with chronic heart failure [abstract]. *Circulation* 1991;**84(suppl II)**:11–73.

9 Lindsay DC, Jiang C, Brunotte F, et al. Impairment of endothelium dependent responses in a rat model of chronic heart failure: effects of an exercise training protocol. *Cardiovasc Res* 1992;**26**:694–697.

10 Lipkin DP, Perrins J, Poole-Wilson PA. Respiratory gas exchange in the assessment of patients with impaired ventricular function. *Br Heart J* 1985;**54**:321–328.

11 Franciosa JA. Exercise testing in chronic congestive heart failure. *Am J Cardiol* 1984;**53**:1447–1450.

12 Weber KT. Janicki JS. Cardiopulmonary exercise testing for evaluation of chronic heart failure. *Am J Cardiol* 1985;**55**:22A–31A.

13 Wasserman K. Measures of functional capacity in patients with chronic cardiac failure. *Circulation* 1990;**81(suppl II)**: II-1–II-4.

14 Elborn JS, Riley M, Stanford CF, Nicholls DP. Anaerobic threshold in patients with chronic cardiac failure due to ischaemic heart disease. *Presse Med* 1994;**23**:367–371.

15 Fick A. *Über die Messung des Blutquantums in den Herzventrikeln.* Sitz der Physik Med Gesellschaft, Würzburg, 1870.

16 Mancini D, Henson D, Rein A, Levine S. Respiratory muscle strength is an important determinate of dyspnea in patients with chronic heart failure [abstract]. *Circulation* 1991; **84(suppl II)**:II–73.

17 Moore DP, Weston AR, Hughes JM, Oakley CM, Cleland JG. Effects of increased inspired oxygen concentrations on exercise performance in chronic heart failure. *Lancet* 1992;**339**:850–853.

18 Puri S, Baker BL, Oakley CM, Hughes JM, Cleland JG. Increased alveolar/capillary membrane resistance to gas transfer in patients with chronic heart failure. *Br Heart J* 1994;**72**:140–144.

19 Zelis R, Nellis SH, Longhurst J, Lee G, Mason DT. Abnormalities in the regional circulations accompanying congestive heart failure. *Prog Cardiovasc Dis* 1975;**18**:181–199.

20 Wilson JR, Mancini DM, Dunkman WB. Exertional figures due to skeletal muscle dysfunction in patients with heart failure. *Circulation* 1993;**87**:470–475.

21 Wasserman K. The peripheral circulation and lactic acid metabolism in heart, or cardiovascular, failure. *Circulation* 1989;**80**:1084–1086.

22 Adams L, Guz A. Dyspnea on exertion. In: Whipp BJ, Wasserman K, eds. *Exercise.*

Pulmonary Physiology and Pathophysiology. Marcel Dekker, New York, 1991:449–494.
23 Wasserman K, Whipp BJ. Exercise physiology in health and disease. *Am Rev Respir Dis* 1975;**112**:219–249.
24 Sietsema KE, Ben Dov I, Zhang YY, Sullivan C, Wasserman K. Dynamics of oxygen uptake for submaximal exercise and recovery in patients with chronic heart failure. *Chest* 1994;**105**: 1693–1700.
25 Balke B, Ware RW. An experimental study of physical fitness of Air Force personnel. *US Armed Forces Med J* 1959;**10**:673–688.
26 Clark AL, Poole-Wilson PA, Coats AJS. Effects of motivation of the patient on indices of exercise capacity in chronic heart failure. *Br Heart J* 1994;**71**:162–165.
27 Szlachic J, Massie BM, Kramer BL, Topic N, Tubau J. Correlates and prognostic implication of exercise capacity in chronic congestive heart failure. *Am J Cardiol* 1985;**55**:1037–1042.
28 Roul G, Moulichon ME, Bareiss P, et al. Exercise peak VO_2 determination in chronic heart failure: is it still of value? *Eur Heart J* 1994;**15**:495–502.
29 Madsen BK, Hansen JF, Stokholm KH, Brons J, Husum D, Mortensen LS. Chronic congestive heart failure. Description and survival of 190 consecutive patients with a diagnosis of chronic congestive heart failure based on clinical signs and symptoms. *Eur Heart J* 1994;**15**:303–310.
30 Parameshwar J, Keegan J, Sparrow J, Sutton GC, Poole-Wilson PA. Predictors of prognosis in severe chronic heart failure. *Am Heart J* 1992;**123**:421–426.
31 Page E, Cohen Solal A, Jondeau G, et al. Comparison of treadmill and bicycle exercise in patients with chronic heart failure. *Chest* 1994;**106**:1002–1006.
32 Lipkin DP, Canepa-Anson R, Stephens MR, Poole-Wilson PA. Factors determining symptoms in heart failure: comparison of fast and slow exercise tests. *Br Heart J* 1986;**55**:439–445.
33 Northridge DB, Grant S, Henderson E, Ray S, McMurray JJ, Dargie HJ. A novel exercise protocol suitable for use on a treadmill or a bicycle ergometer. *Br Heart J* 1990;**64**:313–316.
34 Sparrow J, Parameshwar J, Poole-Wilson PA. Assessment of functional capacity in chronic heart failure: time-limited exercise on a self-powered treadmill. *Br Heart J* 1994;**71**:391–394.
35 Davies N, Denison DM. The measurement of metabolic gas exchange and minute ventilation by mass spectrometry alone. *Respir Physiol* 1979;**36**:261–267.
36 Myers J, Walsh D, Buchanan N, Froelicher VF. Can maximal cardiopulmonary capacity be recognized by a plateau in oxygen uptake? *Chest* 1989;**96**:1312–1315.
37 Buller NP, Poole-Wilson PA. Extrapolated maximum oxygen consumption: a new method for objective analysis of respiratory gas exchange during exercise. *Br Heart J* 1988; **59**:212–217.
38 Wasserman K, McIlroy MB. Detecting the threshold of anaerobic metabolism in cardiac patients during exercise. *Am J Cardiol* 1964;**14**:844–852.
39 Yeh MP, Gardner MR, Adams TD, Tanowitz FG, Crapo RO. 'Anaerobic threshold': problems of determination and validation. *J Appl Physiol* 1983;**55**:1178–1186.
40 Beaver WL, Wasserman K, Whipp BJ. A new method for detecting anaerobic threshold by gas exchange. *J Appl Physiol* 1986;**60**:2020–2027.
41 Hossack KF, Eldridge JE, Ades PA, Giansiracusa RF, Jones RH. Computer analysis of oxygen consumption and minute ventilation for the detection of lactate threshold. *Cardiology* 1988;**75**:123–132.
42 Yamabe H, Itoh K, Yasaka Y, Takata T, Yokoyama M. Lactate threshold is not an onset of insufficient oxygen supply to the working muscle in patients with chronic heart failure. *Clin Cardiol* 1994;**17**:391–394.
43 Brooks GA. Anaerobic threshold: review of the concept and directions for future research. *Med Sci Sports Exerc* 1985;**17**:19–31.
44 Buller NP, Poole-Wilson PA. Mechanism of the increased ventilatory response to exercise in patients with chronic heart failure. *Br Heart J* 1990;**63**:281–283.
45 Clark AL, Coats AJS. Relationship between ventilation and carbon dioxide production in normal subjects with induced changes in anatomical dead space. *Eur J Clin Invest* 1993;**23**: 428–432.

46 Clark AL, Poole-Wilson PA, Coats AJS. Relation between ventilation and carbon dioxide production in patients with chronic heart failure. *J Am Coll Cardiology* 1992;**20**:1326–1332.
47 Clark A, Coats A. The mechanisms underlying the increased ventilatory response to exercise in chronic stable heart failure. *Eur Heart J* 1992;**13**:1698–1708.
48 Wasserman K, Van Kessel AL, Burton GG. Interaction of physiological mechanisms during exercise. *J Appl Physiol* 1967;**22**:71–85.
49 Rubin SA, Brown HV, Swan HJC. Arterial oxygenation and arterial oxygen transport in chronic myocardial failure at rest, during exercise and after hydralazine treatment. *Circulation* 1982;**66**:143–148.
50 Clark AL, Coats AJ. Usefulness of arterial blood gas estimations during exercise in patients with chronic heart failure. *Br Heart J* 1994;**71**:528–530.
51 Loke J. Distinguishing cardiac versus pulmonary limitation in exercise performance. *Chest* 1983;**83**:441–442.
52 Munger MA, Stanek EJ, Nara AR, Strohl KP, Decker MJ, Nair RN. Arterial oxygen saturation in chronic congestive heart failure. *Am J Cardiol* 1994;**73**:180–185.
53 Davies SW, John LM, Wedzicha JA, Lipkin DP. Overnight studies in severe chronic left heart failure: arrhythmias and oxygen desaturation. *Br Heart J* 1991;**65**:77–83.
54 Borg GA. Perceived exertion: a note on history and methods. *Med Sci Sports Exerc* 1975;**5**:90–93.
55 Saltin B, Blomqvist G, Mitchell JH, Johnson RLJr, Wildenthal K, Chapman CB. Response to exercise after bed rest and after training. *Circulation* 1968;**38(suppl 7)**:1–78.
56 Astrand PO, Rodahl K. *Textbook of Work Physiology. Physiological Bases of Exercise.* McGraw–Hill, New York, 1986.
57 Coats AJS, Adamopoulos S, Radaelli A, et al. Controlled trial of physical training in chronic heart failure: exercise performance, hemodynamics, ventilation and autonomic function. *Circulation* 1992;**85**:2119–2131.
58 Sullivan MJ, Higginbotham MB, Cobb FR. Exercise training in patients with chronic heart failure delays ventilatory anaerobic threshold and improves submaximal exercise performance. *Circulation* 1989;**79**:324–329.

Section V

TREATMENT

13

Arrhythmias and sudden death in heart failure: can we prevent them?

Andrew C Rankin, Stuart M Cobbe

Introduction

Cardiac arrhythmias are common in patients with heart failure, but different arrhythmias have different clinical importance. Ventricular premature beats are virtually universal in heart failure and are usually asymptomatic.[1] Atrial fibrillation occurs in between 15% and 20% of patients with heart failure[2] and, while rarely life-threatening, may provoke haemodynamic decompensation. Most seriously, patients with heart failure are at risk from ventricular tachycardia or ventricular fibrillation, which can result in sudden death (usually defined as within 1 hour in patients who were clinically stable).[3]

It is these malignant ventricular arrhythmias, in particular, that present the greatest challenge. The question therefore is: is it possible to identify those patients who are at high risk of sudden arrhythmic death and, if so, are treatments available which might prevent it?

Sudden death and heart failure

Heart failure is a lethal condition. Death from heart failure can be due to progressive haemodynamic deterioration secondary to pump failure or it may be sudden, without prior increase in symptoms. The Framingham Study reported the development of heart failure in 461 patients during a 30-year follow-up of over 5000 patients.[4] Within 4 years of diagnosis of heart failure, 55% of men and 24% of women had died. Approxmately 50% of these deaths were sudden. Analysis of the mechanism of 568 deaths in the Vasodilator-Heart Failure Trials (V-HeFT I and II) reported 40% were sudden deaths, 31.5% were due to progressive heart failure, and a further 15% were sudden, though in the context of worsening cardiac symptoms (Fig. 13.1).[5]

Overall mortality has been found to increase exponentially with increasing severity of heart failure, but the proportion of sudden deaths decreases. Annual mortality rates increase from 10–15% in NYHA class I and II to over 60% in class IV, whereas sudden death accounts for over 50% of deaths in class I and II and less than 30% in class IV.[6] Similarly, increasing severity of left ventricular dysfunction is associated with increased mortality but with a lowered proportion of sudden deaths (Fig. 13.2).[7]

Sudden death is often caused by fatal ventricular arrhythmias.[8] However, sudden death may be due to mechanisms other than ventricular fibrillation, and assessment of the role of fatal ventricular arrhythmias in heart failure is important before consideration can be given to strategies for arrhythmia prevention. In about two thirds of patients with out-of-hospital cardiac arrest, the presenting rhythms are

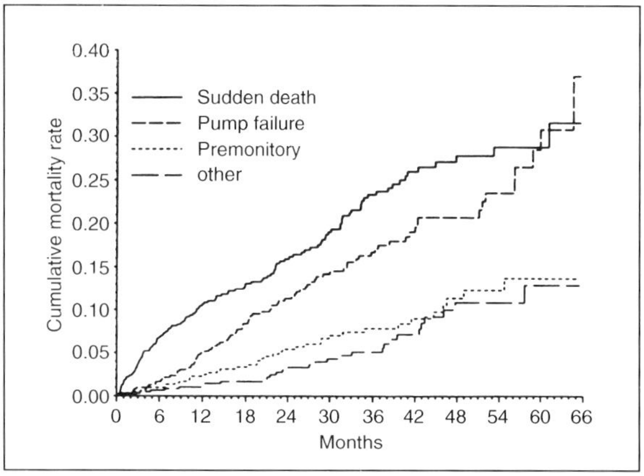

Fig. 13.1
Mechanisms of death in heart failure. Cumulative mortality by cause of death in the Vasodilator-Heart Failure Trial I. During follow-up, 283 of 642 patients died. (From Goldman et al,[5] with permission: © American Heart Association 1993.)

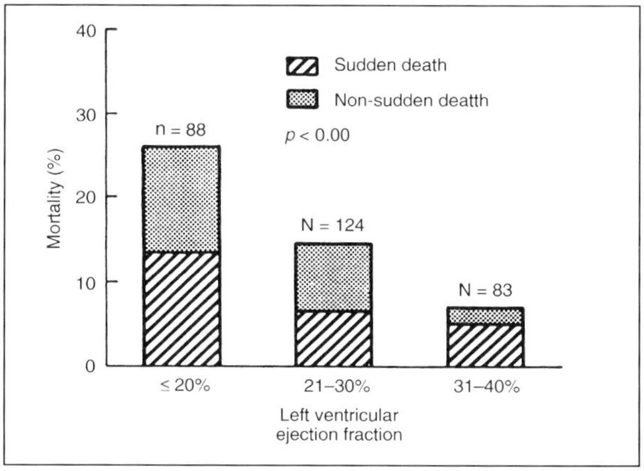

Fig. 13.2
*Relation between left ventricular ejection fraction and subsequent mortality rate. The average follow-up period was 16 months. (Reproduced with permission from the American College of Cardiology (*Journal of the American College of Cardiology *1989;14:567).*

ventricular tachyarrhythmias that are amenable to shock treatment.[8,9] Many of these patients, however, have their cardiac arrest in the context of acute myocardial infarction or ischaemia and not heart failure. In a review of 157 patients who died suddenly while undergoing ambulatory rhythm recording, the majority of whom did not have cardiac failure, the cause of death was malignant ventricular arrhythmias in 84% of cases and bradyarrhythmia in 16%.[10] By contrast, in 20 patients with severe heart failure the mechanism of unexpected cardiac arrest was severe bradycardia or electromechanical dissociation in 62% and ventricular tachyarrhythmia in only 38%.[11]

It has been recognized that sudden death may not be due to arrhythmia and that arrhythmic deaths may not fall within the definition of sudden death.[12,13] The classification of deaths as arrhythmic or non-arrhythmic after myocardial infarction may be particularly difficult in patients with long-standing symptoms of congestive heart failure.[13] The exact incidence of fatal ventricular arrhythmias in heart failure is therefore unknown, but the evidence points to a substantial proportion of deaths being due to primary ventricular arrhythmias,[14] and to the risk of arrhythmic death existing even in patients with mild to moderate heart failure.[7] Even when patients with heart failure have shown clear evidence of haemodynamic deterioration requiring hospital admission, the immediate mechanism of death is often arrhythmic.[5] This observation suggests that patients may be more prone to lethal arrhythmia during periods of haemodynamic decompensation.

Arrhythmogenic mechanisms in heart failure

A number of different mechanisms of cardiac arrhythmias have been identified[15] and there are arrhythmogenic factors associated with heart failure which may predispose to each (Table 13.1).[16,17] Re-entrant mechanisms are believed to underlie many sustained tachyar-

Mechanisms of arrhythmia	Arrhythmogenic factors
Re-entry	Scarring and fibrosis Regions of slow conduction Myocardial ischaemia
Triggered activity	
Delayed after depolarizations	Calcium overload Digoxin toxicity Myocardial ischaemia
Early after depolarizations	Prolonged repolarization Increased catecholamines Hypokalaemia Hypomagnesaemia
Increased automaticity	Increased catecholamines

Table 13.1
Mechanisms of arrhythmias and arrhythmogenic factors in heart failure.

rhythmias, including ventricular tachycardia and ventricular fibrillation. This is particularly the case in patients with coronary artery disease and prior myocardial infarction, in whom regions of abnormal slow conduction at the border zone of the scar provide the potential for re-entry circuits. Therefore, many patients with heart failure secondary to myocardial infarction have the potential myocardial substrate for re-entrant arrhythmias.

A second mechanism for arrhythmias is triggered activity, where after-depolarizations are triggered by the preceding beat. These may be delayed after-depolarizations, occurring after repolarization of the action potential and caused by intracellular calcium overloading. These abnormalities may underlie arrhythmias in heart failure.[18] Another form of triggered activity, early after-depolarizations, occurs before repolarization of the action potential, and may result from abnormalities of repolarization in heart failure.[19] These may be induced by the effects of mechanically induced changes in electrophysiology.[20] Other factors that predispose to arrhythmia include electrolyte abnormalities, such as diuretic-induced hypokalaemia or hypomagnesaemia,[21] and increased catecholamines.[22]

Identification of risk of arrhythmia

Treatment strategies to prevent arrhythmia or sudden death would be best applied to those patients at highest risk, and efforts have been directed at identifying these patients.

Prior cardiac arrest

Patients with left ventricular dysfunction who have previously survived an episode of ventricular tachycardia or fibrillation are at high risk of recurrent malignant ventricular arrhythmia.[23] The prognostic impact of prior cardiac arrest has been reported in 458 patients with severe heart failure, of whom 53 patients

(12%) had survived cardiac arrest.[24] Thirty-one had had primary cardiac arrest and 22 had cardiac arrest secondary to an identifiable cause (acute heart failure in 11, drug-induced torsade de pointes in 10, and hypokalaemia in 1 patient). Despite treatment of these underlying causes, the 1-year sudden death risk was 39%, and the 1-year total mortality was 54%. In the 31 patients with primary cardiac arrest, most of whom received antiarrhythmic treatments (amiodarone in 17, class I antiarrhythmic drugs in 8 and an implantable cardioverter defibrillator in 5 patients), the 1-year sudden death risk was 17% and total mortality rate was 24%, which were similar to those patients without prior cardiac arrest (17% sudden death and 30% mortality). With available treatments, therefore, patients with primary cardiac arrest had a prognosis similar to those without prior cardiac arrest, but secondary arrest was indicative of high risk despite attempts to control the precipitating factors.

Left ventricular dysfunction

The severity of heart failure, whether assessed by symptoms, functional capacity, or measures of left ventricular dysfunction, is a major predictor of total mortality and also of sudden death.[5,7]

Ventricular arrhythmias

Spontaneous chronic ventricular arrhythmias detected during ambulatory monitoring might be considered to be evidence of likelihood of more serious arrhythmia, either as manifestations of an arrhythmic focus or as triggers for re-entrant tachyarrhythmias. The prevalence of ventricular arrhythmias increases with increasing severity of heart failure and is associated with overall prognosis, but not specifically with the risk of sudden death.[6,25] Frequency of non-sustained ventricular tachycardia is independently associated with both total mortality and sudden death.[7]

Late potentials

The signal-averaged electrocardiogram (SAECG) is a technique that allows the identification of low amplitude late potentials occurring after the standard QRS complex on a surface ECG (Fig. 13.3).[26] Late potentials indicate the

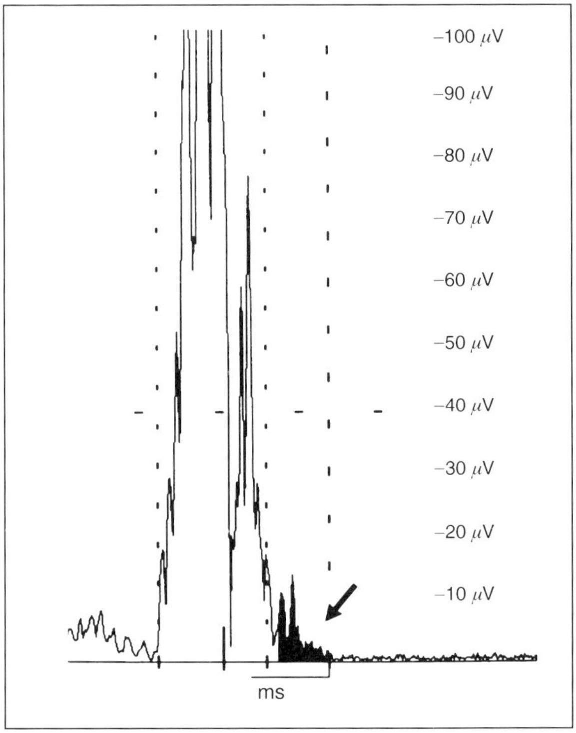

Fig. 13.3
Signal-averaged electrocardiogram. The high amplitude deflection corresponds to the QRS complex, with the last 40 ms shaded in black. There is a low amplitude 'late potential' (arrow). The standard QRS duration was 85 ms, the total QRS (filtered 40–250 Hz) was 135 ms, the duration under 40 μV was 62 ms, and the RMS voltages in the last 40 ms were 5.5 μV. Criteria for late potentials include a total filtered QRS of >114 ms, a duration of low amplitude signal (less than 40 μV) of >38 ms, and terminal (last 40 ms) voltages of <25 μV.

presence of areas of slow conduction in the diseased myocardium which may represent potential substrates for re-entrant arrhythmias.[27] In patients with left ventricular dysfunction secondary to coronary artery disease, the presence of late potentials has a weak positive predictive accuracy of arrhythmic events but their absence is a strong negative predictor, with very low likelihood of arrhythmia in patients with normal SAECG, even in the presence of ventricular dysfunction.[28] In 114 patients with non-ischaemic cardiomyopathy the presence of an abnormal SAECG was a marker of past and future arrhythmic events and was an independent predictor of outcome.[29] The 1-year survival was 95% in patients with normal SAECG and only 39% in 20 patients with an abnormal SAECG.

Heart rate variability

If the SAECG is an indication of arrhythmia substrate, and ventricular premature beats may be the triggers that initiate sustained arrhythmia, then autonomic tone may be the environment which allows their interaction. Heart rate variability can be measured from Holter recordings and is a measure of autonomic tone. Reduced heart rate variability has been shown to be associated with adverse outcome following myocardial infarction.[30,31] In congestive heart failure the decrease in heart rate variability has been shown to be not an indicator of severity of disease but rather a marker of sympathetic excitation, as assessed by muscle sympathetic nerve activity and plasma noradrenaline.[32] Such autonomic influences may be important in the initiation of sustained arrhythmias.[33]

Induction of tachyarrhythmia

Invasive electrophysiological studies may induce sustained arrhythmias by electrical stimulation of the ventricles. The majority of patients who have had spontaneous monomorphic ventricular tachycardia will have a similar tachycardia induced by stimulation studies. This especially applies to patients with prior myocardial infarction and scar-related re-entrant tachycardias. The responses of induced arrhythmia at electrophysiology study is of value in guiding selection of therapy in patients with prior ventricular tachycardia or fibrillation.[23] In patients with recent myocardial infarction who have never had spontaneous arrhythmia, induction of sustained ventricular tachycardia is predictive of subsequent arrhythmic events.[34] In these patients, the negative predictive accuracy is high (98%), with a lower positive predictive accuracy (30%).

This may not be the case in patients with heart failure. In a study of 72 patients with severe heart failure, ventricular tachycardia was inducible in nine (13%) patients, of whom one died suddenly. However, 13 of 63 patients in whom arrhythmias were not inducible died suddenly, and the actuarial risk of sudden death in non-inducible patients was 30% at 6 months.[35] Similarly, survivors of out-of-hospital cardiac arrest with no inducible ventricular tachycardia are still at risk of recurrent arrhythmia; this is particularly so for patients with left ventricular dysfunction and dilated cardiomyopathy.[36] Inducible arrhythmias were found to be of predictive value in patients with severe heart failure awaiting cardiac transplantation, in whom sustained ventricular tachyarrhythmias were induced in 13 of 37 patients (35%).[37] The positive predictive value for sudden death or non-fatal ventricular arrhythmia of induced tachyarrhythmia was 38%; this increased to 50% when combined with an abnormal SAECG. Induction of ventricular arrhythmia, therefore, is an indicator of risk, but it lacks sensitivity, particularly in patients with dilated cardiomyopathy.[38]

Treatment of heart failure and arrhythmias

Vasodilator therapy and risk of arrhythmia

Medical treatment might improve some of the arrhythmogenic factors in heart failure, such as raised filling pressures and increased wall tension. If medical treatment does reduce the likelihood of arrhythmia, it might alter the markers of arrhythmia risk. Ventricular late potentials, however, are unaltered by ventricular pressure reduction in heart failure.[39] Despite the marked reduction in pulmonary capillary wedge pressure and the increase in cardiac output in response to intravenous nitroprusside and diuretics, there was no significant change in the SAECG in 27 patients with heart failure (mean left ventricular ejection fraction 20%). Changes in haemodynamic state also have little acute effect on cardiac electrophysiology and arrhythmia induction. In 12 patients with left ventricular dysfunction secondary to coronary artery disease, acute haemodynamic improvement due to nitroprusside, with a reduction in left ventricular size, did not affect induction of ventricular tachycardia.[40] Similarly, neither captopril or hydralazine combined with nitrate altered arrhythmia induction in eight patients with left ventricular dysfunction due to prior myocardial infarction and inducible ventricular tachycardia.[41] Conversely, acute haemodynamic decompensation in nine patients with dilated cardiomyopathy did not predispose to arrhythmia induction.[42] Despite lack of inducible tachycardia in this study, there were three sudden deaths during follow-up, confirming the lack of predictive value of ventricular stimulation in dilated cardiomyopathy.[38] These observations would be consistent with the lack of reduction in sudden death, despite the improved total mortality, produced by vasodilator therapy in V-HeFT I using hydrallazine–isosorbide combination.[5]

Angiotensin converting enzyme inhibitors and sudden death

The beneficial effects of angiotensin-converting enzyme (ACE) inhibitors on mortality in patients with heart failure are now well established,[43–45] but the mechanism is still debated.[46] Despite the lack of effect of captopril on ventricular tachycardia induction, captopril did prolong ventricular refractory period and repolarization, which are potentially beneficial electrophysiological effects.[41] The frequency of ventricular premature beats, couplets and non-sustained ventricular tachycardia in patients with heart failure are reduced by captopril[47] or enalapril.[48,49] Early studies with small numbers of patients indicated a reduction in sudden death compared to placebo.[50,51] Larger controlled studies, however, have shown no significant reductions in sudden death with enalapril in moderate[44] or severe[43] heart failure, or with captopril in patients with left ventricular dysfunction after myocardial infarction.[52] This apparent lack of benefit of ACE inhibitors in preventing sudden death in the presence of asymptomatic left ventricular dysfunction[52] or moderate heart failure[44] may be partially attributable to the definitions of sudden death in these studies. Thus arrhythmic deaths occurring during periods of haemodynamic decompensation were regarded as 'haemodynamic' rather than 'arrhythmic' in origin.

Reduction in sudden deaths in patients treated with captopril and enalapril have been observed in studies in which they were compared to hydrallazine–isosorbide combinations.[45,53] The Hy-C study showed a reduction in sudden death in 117 patients with advanced heart failure evaluated for cardiac transplantation in whom the drugs were titrated to produce equivalent haemodynamic improvements.[53] The actuarial incidence of sudden death at 1 year was 5% in the captopril-treated group and 37% in the hydralazine-treated group. In V-HeFT II, which studied 804 men with moderate heart failure, the improved survival with enalapril compared to hydralazine–isosorbide was due to a lower incidence of sudden death with or without premonitory worsening.[45] Much of this benefit was seen in the patients with relatively better left ventricular function.[5] In patients with left ventricular ejection fractions of less than 0.35 treated with enalapril, there were 37 sudden deaths without premonitory symptoms and 12 with premonitory symptoms, compared to 46 and 22, respectively, with hydrallazine–isosorbide combination. In those with better left ventricular function (ejection fraction of less than 0.35), there were fewer sudden deaths, but proportionally greater benefit (in the enalapril group, three sudden deaths without and one with premonitory symptoms; in the hydrallazine–isosorbide group, 13 sudden deaths without and five with premonitory symptoms).

The cause of the apparent discrepancy between the improvement in sudden death with ACE inhibitors in the Hy-C and V-HeFT studies[45,53] and the lack of reduction in sudden death or arrhythmic events with enalapril in the CONSENSUS and SOLVD trials[43,44] and with captopril in the SAVE study[52] is not known. Explanations include different patient populations, severity of heart failure, classifications of sudden death, and the beneficial effect of hydrallazine–isosorbide on pump failure, with a consequent proportional increase in importance of sudden death.[5,46] However, it would appear that there is a real benefit from ACE inhibitors with respect to sudden death, although this is only one aspect of their actions.

A further certainty is that the problem of sudden death in heart failure persists despite ACE inhibition, accounting for between 11% of deaths in CONSENSUS (where the majority of deaths were non-sudden or due to pump failure) and 37% in V-HeFT II. Other drug treatments for heart failure are not promising for further reductions in sudden death. Vesnarinone, an oral inotropic agent, produced a 50% risk reduction with improvements in sudden and cardiac mortality, but it was associated with neutropenia and had a narrow therapeutic window with increased mortality with a higher dose.[54] Other inotropic drugs (e.g. milrinone, a phophodiesterase inhibitor) have also been associated with increased mortality of unknown cause – proarrhythmia has been suspected.[55]

Antiarrhythmic drugs and heart failure

Safety of class I antiarrhythmic drugs

In view of the failure of conventional drug therapy to achieve substantial reduction in the risk of sudden death in heart failure, the possibility that specific antiarrhythmic treatment might further reduce arrhythmic deaths must be considered. Ventricular arrhythmias in patients with heart failure are associated with sudden death,[7] and antiarrhythmic drug treatment may reduce the frequency of ventricular ectopy, but will this also improve mortality?

There are reasons to believe that this may not be the case with most antiarrhythmic drugs, particularly those with class I actions (sodium channel blockade). In patients with sustained ventricular tachycardia or ventricular fibrillation, antiarrhythmic drugs are less effective in patients with severe left ventricular dysfunction, both during short-term assessment[56–58] and long-term follow-up.[59,60] Many antiarrhythmic drugs have negative inotropic effects[61] and heart failure may be caused or exacerbated by their use.[62,63] There is additional concern that in patients with heart failure class I drugs are not only relatively ineffective at suppressing ventricular arrhythmias but that they may also cause harm by increasing the susceptibility to fatal arrhythmia.

This was most powerfully demonstrated by the Cardiac Arrhythmia Suppression Trial (CAST) in which mortality was increased by the class I drugs encainide and flecainide compared to placebo (8.5% versus 4%) in over 1000 patients with left ventricular dysfunction following myocardial infarction and asymptomatic ventricular arrhythmia.[64] There was a greater absolute increase in the risk of death or cardiac arrest associated with antiarrhythmic therapy in the subgroup of patients with radionuclide left ventricular ejection fractions of less than 0.30.

Concern regarding the safety of class I agents is supported by the observation that there was increased mortality in patients with heart failure who had been treated with antiarrhythmic drugs for atrial fibrillation rather than for ventricular arrhythmias.[65] Drugs with class I antiarrhythmic action, therefore, are of little value and are likely to be harmful in heart failure.[66]

Amiodarone in heart failure

Amiodarone, a drug with class III effect (prolongation of the refractory period) has few detrimental haemodynamic actions[67] and is generally tolerated by patients with heart failure. It reduces the incidence of ventricular premature beats and non-sustained ventricular tachycardia in patients with heart failure.[68] Initial studies had pointed to beneficial effects of amiodarone in heart failure, with arrhythmia reduction but no clear benefit on mortality.[68–70] A recent study from Argentina (GESICA) of 516 patients with severe heart failure with or without documented arrhythmia has shown a 28% risk reduction in mortality with amiodarone, 300 mg daily.[71] The benefit was due to an early (30 day) decrease in sudden death and a late reduction in mortality from progressive heart failure (Fig. 13.4). The beneficial effect of amiodarone was equal in patients with or without non-sustained ventricular tachycardia at baseline. The concern with amiodarone is its potential for non-cardiac side-effects, including dermatological, pulmonary, endocrine and neurological,[72] but in this study side-effects were reported in only 6.1% of patients. Longer follow-up of patients taking amiodarone, however, may reveal more problems. In a report of 589 patients treated with amiodarone for arrhythmias only 32% of patients were still taking amiodarone after 5 years.[73] Despite the encouraging results of the GESICA study, the Veterans Administration study (CHF STAT) of amiodarone in 633 patients with heart failure and more than 10 ventricular ectopic beats an

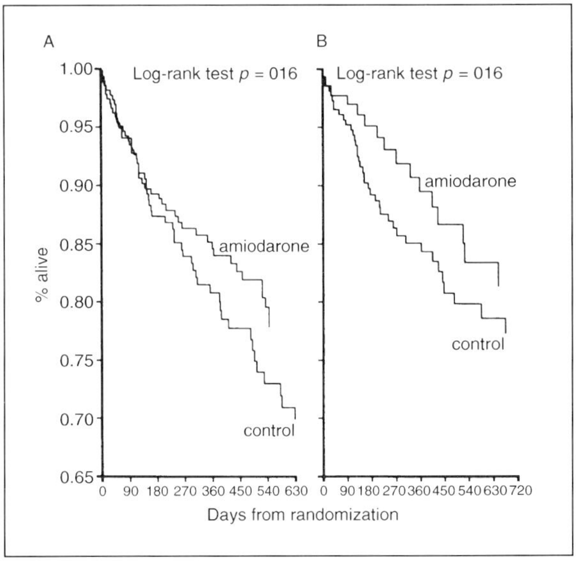

Fig. 13.4
Improved survival with amiodarone in heart failure (GESICA). Survival curves of 256 patients with heart failure in the control group and 260 patients in the amiodarone group. (A) Death from progressive heart failure; (B) Sudden death. (From Doval et al,[71] with permission: © The Lancet.)

hour on ambulatory monitoring failed to demonstrate any significant reduction in mortality despite suppression of ventricular arrhythmias.[74]

Amiodarone may be of benefit in patients following myocardial infarction.[75] The Basel Antiarrhythmic Study of Infarct Survival (BASIS) showed benefit of low-dose amiodarone (200 mg) compared to other antiarrhythmic drugs or no antiarrhythmic therapy in survivors of myocardial infarction with asymptomatic complex ventricular arrhythmias.[76] This benefit, however, was confined to patients with preserved left ventricular function.[77] By contrast, benefit has been shown in a study of 368 patients with left ventricular dysfunction and asymptomatic ventricular arrhythmias in which there was lower mortality with amiodarone 200 mg/day compared to metoprolol.[78]

The European Myocardial Infarct Amiodarone Trial (EMIAT) will study patients after myocardial infarction who have left ventricular dysfunction, whether or not they have ventricular arrhythmia,[79] and the Canadian Myocardial Infarction Amiodarone Trial (CAMIAT) will assess the effect of amiodarone in postinfarction patients with frequent ventricular premature beats.[80] These further studies will help to clarify the role of amiodarone in patients with left ventricular dysfunction and heart failure, but the evidence available at present suggests that the survival benefit achieved by amiodarone therapy may not be linked directly to its class III antiarrhythmic actions, and that its non-competitive alpha- and beta-adrenoceptor antagonist properties may be important. This hypothesis is supported by recent findings of the SWORD trial, in which d-sotalol, a class III agent with minimal beta-blocking activity, was found to increase mortality in patients with impaired left ventricular function or cardiac failure after previous myocardial infarction.[81]

Beta-blockers and heart failure

Raised catecholamines have been considered to be arrhythmogenic in heart failure.[17] Beta-blockade might therefore be beneficial, and has been reported to be associated with prognostic benefit in patients with ventricular tachycardia and left ventricular dysfunction[82] and in survivors of cardiac arrest.[83] In patients with heart failure, beta-blockers sometimes exacerbate the failure, but if used with caution they sometimes paradoxically result in improvement.[84,85] Randomized studies of patients with heart failure secondary to a variety of causes, including ischaemic heart disease and cardiomyopathy, have shown haemodynamic benefit but have been inconclusive concerning mortality.[86,87] In particular, no reduction in sudden death has been demonstrated.[87]

Implantable cardioverter defibrillators and heart failure

The recognition of the limitation of antiarrhythmic drug treatment for patients with ventricular arrhythmias and survivors of cardiac arrest has been paralleled by the development of non-pharmacological therapy, in particular the implantable cardioverter defibrillator (ICD). This device monitors the cardiac rhythm, and it responds to rapid ventricular tachyarrhythmias by delivering a direct current shock to the heart (Fig. 13.5). It has been highly successful in preventing sudden death in such high-risk patients.[88,89] The original systems used intrathoracic patches around the heart to deliver the shocks, and implantation, including thoracotomy, was associated with a perioperative mortality of 3–5%. The development of non-thoracotomy systems that use transvenous leads has reduced the perioperative mortality

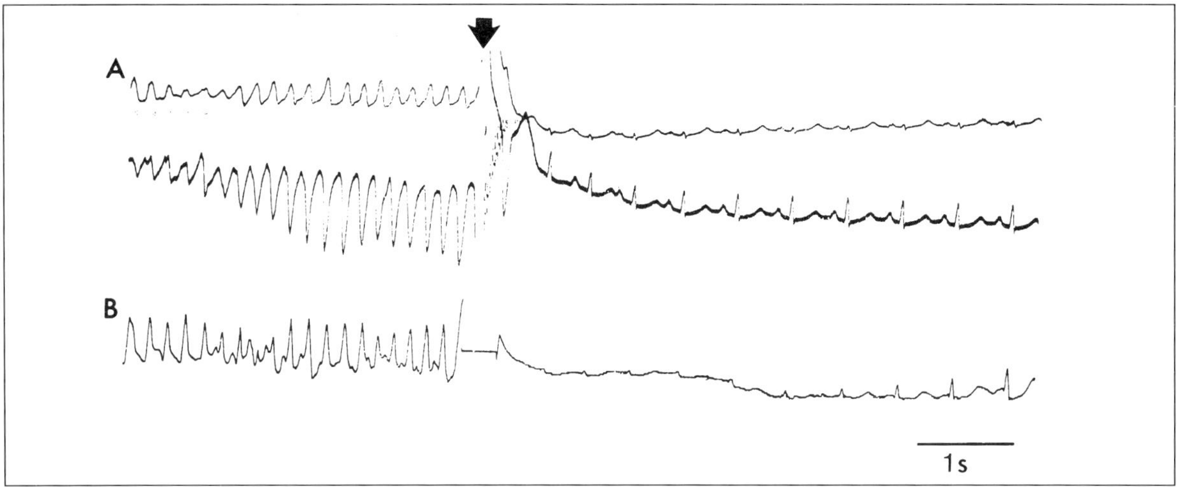

Fig. 13.5
Defibrillation from ventricular fibrillation by an implanted cardioverter defibrillator (ICD). A shock of 20 Joules delivered via a transvenous endocardial lead restored sinus rhythm. The upper tracings (A) show surface electrograms, I and aVf, during a test of the device which detected induced ventricular fibrillation and delivered a shock (arrow). The lower trace (B) shows intracardiac electrograms of the same event retrieved from the memory of the device.

to less than 1% and therefore increased the potential use of such therapy even in high-risk patients with severe cardiac disease.[90,91]

In patients who have survived episodes of life-threatening ventricular arrhythmias, the implantation of an ICD virtually eliminates sudden death[88,89] and may improve total mortality, even in patients with left ventricular dysfunction.[92–94] Powell et al[94] reported the outcome of 331 survivors of out-of-hospital cardiac

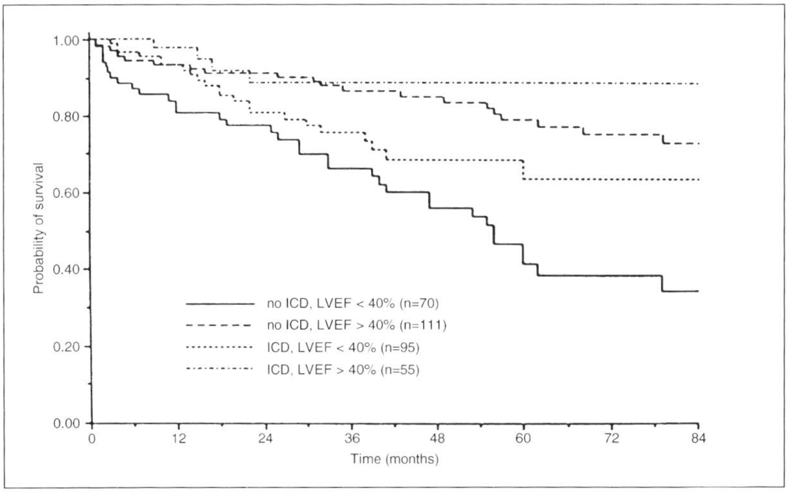

Fig. 13.6
Influence of an implantable cardioverter–defibrillator (ICD) and the degree of left ventricular dysfunction on total mortality in survivors of out-of-hospital cardiac arrest. Probability of survival with and without an ICD stratified by left ventricular ejection fraction (LVEF). (From Powell et al,[94] with permission: © American Heart Association 1993.)

Trial	Patients	Treatment variable
Survivors of arrhythmic events		
CASH (Cardiac Arrest Study Hamburg)	SCD	ICD *vs* amiodarone or metoprolol, or propafenone
CIDS (Canadian Internal Defibrillator Study)		
AVID (Antiarrhythmics versus Implantable	SCD, VT (syncope)	ICD *vs* amiodarone
Defibrillator)	SCD, VT (syncope, hypotension), LVEF < 40%	ICD *vs* Amiodarone or sotalol
Primary prophylaxis in high risk groups		
MADIT (Multicenter Automatic Defibrillator Implantation Trial)	CAD, LVEF < 35%, NSVT, inducible VT	ICD *vs* EP-guided drug therapy
MUSTT (Multicenter Unstained Tachycardia Trial)	CAD, LVEF < 40%, NSVT, inducible VT	EP-guided therapy (including ICD) *vs* no drug
CABG PATCH	CABG, LVEF < 35%, late potential, NSVT	ICD *vs* no antiarrhythmic drug
DEFIBRILAT (Defibrillator as Bridge to Later Transplant)	CHF awaiting heart transplant, NSVT, ind VT	ICD *vs* no antiarrhythmic drug
CAT (Cardiomyopathy Trial)	DCM, LVEF < 30%, CHF (NYHA II or III)	ICD *vs* no antiarrhythmic therapy

Table 13.2
Randomized trials of ICD therapy. (SCD – sudden cardiac death; VT – ventricular tachycardia; LVEF – left ventricular ejection fraction; ICD – implantable cardioverter defibrillator; NSVT – non-sustained VT; DCM – dilated cardiomyopathy; CABG – coronary artery bypass graft; CHF – chronic heart failure; EP – electrophysiological testing.)

arrest. Implantable defibrillators were placed in 150 patients and the remaining 181 patients were treated with drugs or surgery or both. The 1- and 5-year probabilities of survival free of cardiac mortality in patients with left ventricular ejection fractions of less than 0.40 were 94.3% and 69.6% with a defibrillator, and 82.1% and 45.3% without a defibrillator (Fig. 13.6). It has been recommended that survivors of cardiac arrest with severe left ventricular dysfunction (left ventricular ejection fraction of less than 30%) should receive an ICD regardless of responses to electrophysiological testing or apparent short-term responses to antiarrhythmic drug treatment.[95] However, there has been no randomized controlled study of the use of the ICD, and available data on the potential impact on prognosis is based on historical[94] or matched controls,[93] or on projected mortality based on device shocks indicating potential sudden death.[92] Even in reports on improved outcome with ICD therapy the absolute improvement in total mortality during long-term follow-up is modest;[92,93] particularly those patients with left ventricular dysfunction have a continuing substantial cardiac mortality rate due to the underlying cardiac disease, in addition to arrhythmia-related but non-sudden deaths.[96]

The main determinant of prognosis in patients with ICD therapy is the severity of left ventricular dysfunction.[94,96–98] Device therapy is expensive and there is continuing debate about the prognostic benefits and the cost-efficacy of the ICD.[99] The role of device therapy may be clarified by the results of on-going prospective randomized trials of the ICD (Table 13.2), both as secondary prevention in survivors of arrhythmic events and as primary prophylaxis in high-risk patients, including those with post-infarction left ventricular dysfunction, dilated cardiomyopathy, and heart failure (as a bridge to transplant).[95,99–102] At present, patients with controlled heart failure and life-threatening ventricular arrhythmias should be assessed for available therapies, which may include surgical revascularization or an ICD, or both.

Conclusion

Cardiac arrhythmias contribute to the high mortality in patients with cardiac failure. High risk patients can be identified, but the optimal treatments are still being assessed by clinical trials. It is clear that antiarrhythmic drug treatment can be detrimental because of deterioration in cardiac function and because they sometimes cause pro-arrhythmia. Conversely, there is recent evidence that amiodarone may improve survival in patients with heart failure by reducing both sudden death and death due to pump failure. Optimal medical treatment of the heart failure, including ACE inhibition, improves mortality, and this benefit may be partly due to reduction in sudden death. Patients with heart failure who have survived a cardiac arrest should be considered for ICD implantation. Device therapy will reduce mortality from recurrent cardiac arrest but it may not alter the long-term outcome, which will be determined by the severity of the heart disease.

References

1 Chakko CS, Gheorghiade M. Ventricular arrhythmias in severe heart failure: incidence, significance, and effectiveness of antiarrhythmic therapy. *Am Heart J* 1985;**109**:497–504.
2 Carson PE, Johnson GR, Dunkman WB, et al. The influence of atrial fibrillation on prognosis in mild to moderate heart failure. The V-HeFT studies. *Circulation* 1993;**87(suppl VI)**:102–110.
3 Kottkamp H, Budde T, Lamp B, Haverkamp W, Borggrefe M, Breithardt G. Clinical significance and management of ventricular arrhythmias in heart failure. *Eur Heart J* 1994; **15(suppl D)**:155–163.
4 Kannel WB, Plehn JF, Cupples LA. Cardiac failure and sudden death in the Framingham Study. *Am Heart J* 1988;**115**:869–875.
5 Goldman S, Johnson G, Cohn JN, et al. Mechanisms of death in heart failure. The Vasodilator-Heart Failure Trials. *Circulation* 1993;**87(suppl VI)**:24–31.
6 Kjekshus J. Arrhythmias and mortality in congestive heart failure. *Am J Cardiol* 1990; **65**:42I–48I.
7 Gradman A, Deedwania P, Cody R, et al. Predictors of total mortality and sudden death in mild to moderate heart failure. *J Am Coll Cardiol* 1989;**14**:564–570.
8 Demirovic J, Myerburg RJ. Epidemiology of sudden coronary death: an overview. *Prog Cardiovasc Dis* 1994;**37**:39–48.
9 Sedgwick ML, Dalziel K, Watson J, Carrington DJ, Cobbe SM. Performance of an established system of first responder out-of-hospital defibrillation. The results of the second year of the Heartstart Scotland Project in the 'Utstein Style'. *Resuscitation* 1993;**26**:75–88.
10 De Luna AB, Coumel P, Leclerq JF. Ambulatory sudden cardiac death: mechanisms of production of fatal arrhythmia on the basis of data from 157 cases. *Am Heart J* 1989;**117**:151–159.
11 Luu M, Stevenson WG, Stevenson LW, Baron K, Walden J. Diverse mechanisms of unexpected cardiac arrest in advanced heart failure. *Circulation* 1989;**80**:1675–1680.
12 Goldstein S, Friedman L, Hutchinson R, et al. Timing, mechanism and clinical setting of witnessed deaths in postmyocardial infarction patients. *J Am Coll Cardiol* 1984;**3**:1111–1117.
13 Greene HL, Richardson DW, Barker AH, et al. Classification of deaths after myocardial infarction as arrhythmic or nonarrhythmic (the Cardiac Arrhythmia Pilot Study). *Am J Cardiol* 1989;**63**:1–6.
14 Stevenson WG, Stevenson LG, Middlekauff HR, Saxon LA. Sudden death prevention in patients with advanced ventricular dysfunction. *Circulation* 1993;**88**:2953–2961.
15 The Task Force of the Working Group on Arrhythmias of the European Society of Cardiology. The 'Sicilian Gambit'. A new approach to the classification of antiarrhythmic drugs based on their actions an arrhythmogenic mechanisms. *Circulation* 1991;**84**:1831–1851.
16 Pye MP, Cobbe SM. Mechanisms of ventricular arrhythmias in cardiac failure and hypertrophy. *Cardiovasc Res* 1992;**26**:740–750.
17 Campbell RWF. Electrophysiological disturbances in heart failure. *Br Heart J* 1994; **72(suppl)**:S31–S35.
18 Pogwizd SM, Corr PB. Biochemical and electrophysiological alterations underlying ventricular arrhythmias in the failing heart. *Eur Heart J* 1994;**15(suppl D)**:145–154.
19 Tomaselli GF, Beuckelmann DJ, Calkins HG, et al. Sudden cardiac death in heart failure. The role of abnormal repolarisation. *Circulation* 1994;**90**:2534–2539.
20 Dean JW, Lab MJ. Arrhythmia in heart failure: role of mechanically induced changes in electrophysiology. *Lancet* 1989;**i**:1309–1312.
21 Storstein L. Electrophysiological impact of diuretics in heart failure. *Br Heart J* 1994; **72(suppl)**:54–46.
22 Francis GS. Neuroendocrine manifestations of congestive heart failure. *Am J Cardiol* 1988; **62**:9A–13A.

23 Wilber DJ, Garan H, Finkelstein D, et al. Out-of-hospital cardiac arrest: use of electrophysiologic testing in the prediction of long-term outcome. *N Engl J Med* 1988;**318**:19–24.
24 Stevenson WG, Middlekauf HR, Stevenson LW, Saxon LA, Woo MA, Moser D. Significance of aborted cardiac arrest and sustained ventricular tachycardia in patients referred for treatment therapy of advanced heart failure. *Am Heart J* 1992;**124**:123–130.
25 Cleland JGF, Dargie HJ, Ford I. Mortality in heart failure: clinical variables of prognostic value. *Br Heart J* 1987;**58**:572–582.
26 Vester EG, Strauer BE. Ventricular late potentials: state of the art and future perspectives. *Eur Heart J* 1994;**15(suppl C)**:34–48.
27 Hood MA, Pogwizd SM, Peirick J, Cain ME. Contribution of myocardium responsible for ventricular tachycardia to abnormalities detected by analysis of signal-averaged ECGs. *Circulation* 1992;**86**:1888–1901.
28 Kuchar DL, Thorburn CW, Sammel NL. Prediction of serious arrhythmic events after myocardial infarction: signal-averaged electrocardiogram, holter monitoring and radionuclide ventriculography. *J Am Coll Cardiol* 1987;**9**:531–538.
29 Mancini DM, Wong KL, Simson MB. Prognostic value of an abnormal signal-averaged electrocardiogram in patients with nonischemic congestive cardiomyopathy. *Circulation* 1993;**87**:1083–1092.
30 Kleiger RE, Miller JP, Bigger JT, et al. Decreased heart rate variability and its association with increased mortality after acute myocardial infarction. *Am J Cardiol* 1987;**59**:256–262.
31 Cripps TR, Malik M, Farrell TF, Camm AJ. Prognostic value of reduced heart rate variability after myocardial infarction: clinical evaluation of an new analysis method. *Br Heart J* 1991;**65**:14–19.
32 Kienzle MG, Ferguson DW, Birkett CL, Myers GA, Berg WJ, Mariano J. Clinical, hemodynamic and sympathetic neural correlates of heart rate variability in congestive heart failure. *Am J Cardiol* 1992;**69**:761–767.
33 Coumel P, Leenhardt A, Leclerq JF. Autonomic influences on ventricular arrhythmias in myocardial hypertrophy and heart failure. *Circulation* 1993;**87(suppl VII)**:84–91.
34 Richards DAB, Byth K, Ross DL, Uther JB. What is the best predictor of spontaneous ventricular tachycardia and sudden death after myocardial infarction? *Circulation* 1991;**83**: 756–763.
35 Stevenson WG, Stevenson LW, Weiss J, Tillisch JH. Inducible ventricular arrhythmias and sudden death during vasodilator therapy of severe heart failure. *Am Heart J* 1988;**16**:1447–1454.
36 Sager PT, Choudhary R, Leon C, Rahimtoola SH, Bhandari AK. The long-term prognosis of patients with out-of-hospital cardiac arrest but no inducible ventricular tachycardia. *Am Heart J* 1990;**120**:1334–1342.
37 Lindsay BD, Osborn JL, Schechtman KB, Kenzora JL, Ambos HD, Cain ME. Prospective detection of vulnerability to sustained ventricular tachycardia in patients awaiting cardiac transplantation. *Am J Cardiol* 1992;**69**:619–624.
38 Chen X, Shenasa M, Borggrefe M, et al. Role of programmed ventricular stimulation in patients with idiopathic dilated cardiomyopathy and documented sustained ventricular tachyarrhythmias: inducibility and prognosis value in 102 patients. *Eur Heart J* 1994;**15**:76–82.
39 Stevenson WG, Woo MA, Moser DK, Stevenson LW. Late potentials are unaltered by ventricular filling pressure reduction in heart failure. *Am Heart J* 1991;**122**:473–477.
40 Carlson MD, Schoenfeld MH, Garan H, et al. Programmed ventricular stimulation in patients with left ventricular dysfunction and ventricular tachycardia: effects of acute hemodynamic improvement due to nitroprusside. *J Am Coll Cardiol* 1989;**14**:1744–1752.
41 Bashir Y, Sneddon JF, O'Nunain S, et al. Comparative electrophysiological effects of captopril or hydralazine combined with nitrate in patients with left ventricular dysfunction and inducible ventricular tachycardia. *Br Heart J* 1992;**67**:355–360.
42 Kulick DL, Bhandari AK, Hong R, Petersen R, Leon C, Rahimtoola SH. Effect of acute hemodynamic decompensation on electrical inducibility of ventricular arrhythmia in patients with dilated cardiomyopathy and complex

nonsustained ventricular arrhythmias. *Am Heart J* 1990;**119**:878–883.

43 The CONSENSUS Trial Study Group. Effects of enalapril on mortality in severe congestive heart failure. Results of the Cooperative North Scandinavian Enelapril Survival Study (CONSENSUS). *N Engl J Med* 1987; **316**: 1429–1435.

44 The SOLVD Investigators. Effect of enalapril on survival in patients with reduced left ventricular ejection fractions and congestive heart failure. *N Engl J Med* 1991;**325**:293–302.

45 Cohn JN, Johnson G, Ziesche S, et al. A comparison of enalapril with hydralazine–isosorbide dinitrate in the treatment of chronic congestive heart failure. *N Engl J Med* 1991; **325**:303–310.

46 Cleland JGF, Puri S. How do ACE inhibitors reduce mortality in patients with left ventricular dysfunction with and without heart failure: remodelling, resetting, or sudden death? *Br Heart J* 1994;**72(suppl)**:81–86.

47 Cleland JGF, Dargie HJ, Hodsman GP, et al. Captopril in heart failure. A double blind controlled trial. *Br Heart J* 1984;**52**:530–535.

48 Webster MWI, Fitzpatrick A, Nicholls G, Ikram H, Wells JE. Effect of enalapril on ventricular arrhythmias in congestive heart failure. *Am J Cardiol* 1985;**56**:566–569.

49 Fletcher RD, Cintron GB, Johnson G, et al. Enalapril decreases prevalence of ventricular tachycardia in patients with chronic congestive heart failure. *Circulation* 1993;**83(suppl VI)**: 49–55.

50 Captopril Multi-center Research Group. A placebo-controlled trial of captopril in refractory chronic congestive heart failure. *J Am Coll Cardiol* 1983;**2**:755–766.

51 Newman TJ, Maskin CS, Dennick LG, Meyer JH, Hallows BG, Cooper WH. Effects of captopril on survival in patients with heart failure. *Am J Med* 1988;**84(suppl 3A)**:140–144.

52 Pfeffer MA, Braunwald E, Moyé LA, et al. Effect of captopril on mortality and morbidity in patients with left ventricular dysfunction after myocardial infarction. Results of the Survival and Ventricular Enlargement Trial. *N Engl J Med* 1992;**327**:669–677.

53 Fonarow GC, Chelimsky-Fallick C, Stevenson LW, et al. Effect of direct vasodilation with hydralazine versus angiotensin-converting enzyme inhibition with captopril on mortality in advanced heart failure: the Hy-C Trial. *J Am Coll Cardiol* 1992;**19**:42–50.

54 Feldman AM, Bristow MR, Parmley WW, et al. Effects of vesnarinone on morbidity and mortality in patients with heart failure. *N Engl J Med* 1993;**329**:149–155.

55 Packer M, Carver JR, Rodeheffer RJ, et al. Effect of oral milrinone on mortality in severe chronic heart failure. *N Engl J Med* 1991; **325**:1468–1475.

56 Kuchar DL, Rottman J, Berger E, Freeman CS, Garan H, Ruskin JN. Prediction of successful suppression of sustained ventricular tachyarrhythmias by serial drug testing from data derived at the initial electrophysiological study. *J Am Coll Cardiol* 1988;**12**:982–988.

57 Meissner MD, Kay HR, Horowitz LN, Spielman SR, Greenspan AM, Kutalek SP. Relation of acute antiarrhythmic drug efficacy to left ventricular function in coronary heart disease. *Am J Cardiol* 1988;**61**:1050–1055.

58 The ESVEM Investigators. Determinants of predicted efficacy of antiarrhythmic drugs in the Electrophysiologic Study Versus Electrocardographic Monitoring Study. *Circulation* 1993;**87**:323–329.

59 Swerdlow CD, Winkle RA, Mason JW. Determinants of survival in patients with ventricular tachyarrhythmias. *N Engl J Med* 1983; **308**:1436–1442.

60 Poole JE, Mathison TL, Kudenchuk PJ, et al. Long-term outcome in patients who survive out of hospital ventricular fibrillation and undergo electrophysiologic studies: evaluation by electrophysiologic subgroups. *J Am Coll Cardiol* 1990;**16**:657–665.

61 Packer M. Hemodynamic consequences of antiarrhythmic drug therapy in patients with chronic heart failure. *J Cardiovasc Electrophysiol* 1991;**2(suppl)**:S240–S247.

62 Podrid PJ, Schoenberger A, Lown B. Congestive heart failure caused by oral dysopyramide. *N Engl J Med* 1980;**302**:614–617.

63 Ravid S, Podrid P, Lampert S, Lown B. Congestive heart failure induced by six of the newer antiarrhythmic drugs. *J Am Coll Cardiol* 1989;**14**:1326–1330.

64 Echt DS, Liebson PR, Mitchell LB, et al. Mortality and morbidity in patients receiving encainide, flecainide, or placebo. *N Engl J Med* 1991;**324**:781–788.
65 Flaker GC, Blackshear JL, McBride R, et al. Antiarrhythmic drug therapy and cardiac mortality in atrial fibrillation. *J Am Coll Cardiol* 1992;**20**:527–532.
66 Pratt CM, Eaton T, Francis M, et al. The inverse relationship between baseline left ventricular ejection fraction and outcome of antiarrhythmic therapy: a dangerous imbalance in the risk-benefit ratio. *Am Heart J* 1989;**118**:433–440.
67 Sheldon RS, Mitchell LB, Duff HJ, Wyse DG, Manyari DE. Right and left ventricular function during chronic amiodarone therapy. *Am J Cardiol* 1988;**62**:736–740.
68 Cleland JGF, Dargie HJ, Findlay IN, Wilson JT. Clinical, haemodynamic, and antiarrhythmic effects of long-term treatment with amiodarone of patients in heart failure. *Br Heart J* 1987;**57**:436–445.
69 Nicklas JM, McKenna WJ, Stewart RA, et al. Prospective, double-blind, placebo-controlled trial of low-dose amiodarone in patients with severe heart failure and asymptomatic frequent ventricular ectopy. *Am Heart J* 1991;**122**: 1016–1021.
70 Hamer AWF, Arkles LB, Johns JA. Beneficial effects of low dose amiodarone in patients with congestive cardiac failure: a placebo-controlled trial. *J Am Coll Cardiol* 1989;**14**:1768–1774.
71 Doval HC, Grancelli HO, Perrone SV, et al. Randomised trial of low-dose amiodarone in severe heart failure. *Lancet* 1994;**334**:493–498.
72 Vrobel TR, Miller PE, Mostow ND, Rakita L. A general overview of amiodarone toxicity: its prevention, detection and management. *Prog Cardiovasc Dis* 1989;**31**:393–426.
73 Weinberg BA, Miles WM, Klein LS, et al. Five-year follow-up of 589 patients treated with amiodarone. *Am Heart J* 1993;**125**:109–120.
74 Fletcher RD, Singh S, the CHF-STAT Investigators. Amiodarone decreases ability of baseline ventricular arrhythmia severity to predict mortality. *J Am Coll Cardiol* 1995; **25(suppl)**:15A.
75 Nademanee K, Singh BN, Stevenson WG, Weiss JN. Amiodarone and post-MI patients. *Circulation* 1993;**88**:764–774.
76 Burkart F, Pfisterer M, Kiowski W, Follath F, Burckhardt D. Effect of antiarrhythmic therapy on mortality in survivors of myocardial infarction with asymptomatic complex ventricular arrhythmias: Basel Antiarrhythmic Study of Infarct Survival (BASIS). *J Am Coll Cardiol* 1990;**16**:1711–1718.
77 Pfisterer M, Kiowski W, Burckhardt, Follath F, Burkart F. Beneficial effect of amiodarone on cardiac mortality in patients with asymptomatic complex ventricular arrhythmias after acute myocardial infarction and preserved but not impaired left ventricular function. *Am J Cardiol* 1992;**69**:1399–1402.
78 Navarro-López F, Cosin J, Marrugat J, et al. Comparison of the effects of amiodarone versus metoprolol on the frequency of ventricular arrhythmias and on mortality after acute myocardial infarction. *Am J Cardiol* 1993;**72**:1243–1248.
79 Schwartz PJ, Camm AJ, Frangin G, et al. Does amiodarone reduce sudden death and cardiac mortality after myocardial infarction? The European Myocardial Infarct Amiodarone Trial (EMIAT). *Eur Heart J* 1994;**15**:620–624.
80 Cairns JA, Connolly SJ, Roberts R, et al. Canadian Amiodarone Myocardial Infarction Arrhythmia Trial (CAMIAT): rationale and protocol. *Am J Cardiol* 1993;**72**:87F–94F.
81 Waldo AL, Camm AJ, de Ruyter H, et al. Preliminary mortality results from the Survival with Oral D-Sotalol (SWORD) trial. *J Am Coll Cardiol* 1995;**25(suppl)**:15A.
82 Leclerq JF, Coumel P, Denjoy I, et al. Long-term follow-up after sustained monomorphic ventricular tachycardia: causes, pump failure, and empiric antiarrhythmic therapy that modify survival. *Am Heart J* 1991;**121**: 1685–1692.
83 Hallstrom AP, Cobb LA, Yu BH, Weaver WD, Fahrenbruch CE. An antiarrhythmic drug experience in 941 patients resuscitated from an initial cardiac arrest between 1970 and 1985. *Am J Cardiol* 1991;**68**:1025–1031.
84 Eichhorn EJ. The paradox of β-adrenergic blockade for the management of congestive heart failure. *Am J Med* 1992;**92**:527–538.

85 Ertl G, Neubauer S, Gaudron P, et al. Beta-blockers in cardiac failure. *Eur Heart J* 1994;**15(suppl C)**:16–24.
86 Waagstein F, Bristow MR, Swedberg K, et al. Beneficial effects of metoprolol in idiopathic dilated cardiomyopathy. *Lancet* 1993;**342**: 1441–1446.
87 CIBIS Investigators and committees. A randomized trial of β-blockade in heart failure. The Cardiac Insufficiency Bisoprolol Study (CIBIS). *Circulation* 1994;**90**:1765–1773.
88 Kelly PA, Cannom DS, Garan H, et al. The automatic implantable cardioverter–defibrillator: efficacy, complications and survival in patients with malignant ventricular arrhythmias. *J Am Coll Cardiol* 1988;**11**:1278–1286.
89 Winkle RA, Mead RH, Ruder MA, et al. Long-term outcome with the automatic implantable cardioverter-defibrillator. *J Am Coll Cardiol* 1989;**13**:1353–1361.
90 Bardy GH, Johnson G, Poole JE, et al. A simplified, single-lead unipolar transvenous cardioversion–defibrillation system. *Circulation* 1993;**88**:543–547.
91 Manolis AS. Transvenous endocardial cardioverter defibrillator systems. Is the future here? *Arch Intern Med* 1994;**154**:617–622.
92 Fogoros RN, Elson JJ, Bonnet CA, Fiedler SB, Burkholder JA. Efficacy of the automatic implantable cardioverter-defibrillator in prolonging survival in patients with severe underlying cardiac disease. *J Am Coll Cardiol* 1990;**16**:381–386.
93 Newman D, Sauve J, Herre J, et al. Survival after implantation of the cardioverter defibrillator. *Am J Cardiol* 1992;**69**:899–903.
94 Powell AC, Fuchs T, Finkelstein DM, et al. Influence of implantable cardioverter–defibrillator on the long-term prognosis of survivors of out-of-hospital cardiac arrest. *Circulation* 1993;**88**:1083–1092.
95 O'Nunain S, Ruskin J. Cardiac arrest. *Lancet* 1993;**341**:1641–1647.
96 Kim SG, Maloney JD, Pinski SL, et al. Influence of left ventricular function on survival and mode of death after implantable defibrillator therapy (Cleveland Clinic Foundation and Montefiore Medical Center experience). *Am J Cardiol* 1993;**72**:1263–1267.
97 Mehta D, Saksena S, Krol RB. Survival of implantable cardioverter–defibrillator recipients: role of left ventricular function and its relationship to device use. *Am Heart J* 1992;**124**:1608–1614.
98 Kim SG, Fisher JD, Choue CW, et al. Influence of left ventricular function on outcome of patients treated with implantable defibrillators. *Circulation* 1992;**85**:1304–1310.
99 Saksena S, Camm AJ. Implantable defibrillators for prevention of sudden death. Technology at a medical and economic crossroad. *Circulation* 1992;**85**:2316–2321.
100 Kolttis TM, Saksena S. Prophylactic implantable cardioverter defibrillator therapy in high-risk patients with coronary artery disease. *Am Heart J* 1994;**127**:2264–2270.
101 Zipes DP. Implantable cardioverter–defibrillator. Lifesaver or a device looking for a disease? *Circulation* 1994;**89**:2934–2936.
102 The Cardiomyopathy Trial Investigators. Cardiomyopathy Trial. *PACE Pacing Clin Electrophysiol* 1993;**16**:576–581.

14

Current perspective on beta-blockers in heart failure

Norman Sharpe, Robert Doughty, Stephen MacMahon

Introduction

The rationale for the use of beta-blockers in heart failure relates to several factors:

- the poor prognosis for heart failure patients, which remains despite modern treatment including angiotensin converting enzyme (ACE) inhibition;
- studies of neurohormonal alterations and their prognostic importance in heart failure;
- clinical trials of the effects of beta-blockers on left ventricular function and exercise capacity in patients with heart failure; and
- larger clinical trials of the effects of beta-blockers on mortality in patients with myocardial infarction and evidence of heart failure.

In considering the possible application of beta-blockers in heart failure as part of a combined treatment regimen, it is important to emphasize that the various aims of treatment for heart failure are met through a number of different mechanisms which are not necessarily associated. For example, congestive symptoms and signs are relieved through reduction of elevated ventricular filling pressures and diuresis. Exercise performance may improve through relief of congestion but more significantly through peripheral circulatory changes and muscular conditioning. Ventricular function is altered through changes in myocardial contractility or loading conditions. Finally, survival benefit may be mediated through functional improvement but also importantly through neurohormonal blockade.

Neurohormonal alterations in heart failure

Activation of neurohormonal systems causes excessive vasoconstriction and volume expansion and worsening symptoms and signs of congestive heart failure. The benefit of blockade of the renin–angiotensin–aldosterone system with angiotensin converting enzyme (ACE) inhibition is well established. There may also be benefits from blockade of the sympathetic nervous system with beta-blockade which are complementary to those provided by ACE inhibitors.

Neurohormonal activation and survival

Data from the Studies of Left Ventricular Dysfunction (SOLVD) registry[1] have shown that elevated plasma levels of noradrenaline, renin, arginine, vasopressin, and atrial natriuretic peptide (ANP) are associated with a poor prognosis. However, only ANP and renin were independent predictors of mortality by multivariate analysis. The Veterans Administration Cooperative Vasodilator Heart Failure Trial (VHeFT)[2] has shown that elevated plasma levels of noradrenaline and renin are independently related to mortality and that the most beneficial response to ACE inhibition occurred in those with the most neurohormonal activation. These findings emphasize the importance of the relationship between neurohormonal activity and mortality and the relevance of neurohormonal blockade to improved survival.

Plasma noradrenaline levels

The plasma concentration of noradrenaline provides an index of sympathetic activity. Several studies have shown that plasma norepinephrine levels are increased in heart failure.[3–5] As well as a predictor of survival,[2,5] the level of circulating noradrenaline is directly proportional to the degree of left ventricular dysfunction.[3] Measurements of noradrenaline may provide a better prognostic guide than haemodynamic measurements such as cardiac index, stroke work index, or pulmonary capillary wedge pressure.[5]

Substudy data from the SOLVD trial[6] have demonstrated that sympathetic activation occurs before the development of clinical heart failure and is present in patients with asymptomatic left ventricular dysfunction. Sympathetic activation is therefore not solely a consequence of clinical heart failure. Overactivity of the sympathetic nervous system may result from chronic changes in stroke volume, cardiac output, and mean arterial pressure that result in deactivation of arterial baroreceptors, which play an important role in negative feedback control of the sympathetic nervous system.[7,8] Prolonged excessive activation of the sympathetic nervous system has many potential adverse effects, including direct toxic effects on the myocardium,[9] arrhythmogenesis,[10] decreased coronary blood flow, and tissue anoxia from vasoconstriction.[7]

Cardiac noradrenaline stores

Despite increased plasma concentrations of noradrenaline, the myocardium is depleted of noradrenaline[11,12] at least partly because of a profound decrease in reuptake.[13,14] The reuptake mechanism is a major determinant of both the concentration of noradrenaline within the synaptic cleft and the stores of noradrenaline in the neurone.

In addition to abnormal reuptake of norepinephrine, it has been suggested that abnormalities occur in the synthesis of noradrenaline within the neurone,[15,16] although this has not been a consistent finding.[17] The exact mechanism of the depleted noradrenaline stores is still uncertain and may depend on the underlying cause of the heart failure.

Effect of beta-blockade on plasma noradrenaline levels

A randomized trial of the effects of bucindolol in patients with idiopathic dilated cardiomyopathy[18] has demonstrated a 50% reduction in plasma noradrenaline levels in the bucinodolol-treated patients after 3 months. These findings and those from uncontrolled studies[19,20] suggest that beta-blockade may reduce circulating noradrenaline levels both by reducing spillover to the plasma from the synpatic cleft and by increasing clearance of noradrenaline.

Beta-blockers are also able to block directly the toxic effects of catecholamines, as demonstrated *in vitro* by the prevention of noradrenaline-induced myocyte necrosis by propranolol[21] and *in vivo* by reversal of the cardiomyopathy associated with phaeochromocytoma.[22]

In addition to the increase in plasma noradrenaline, other alterations occur in the adrenergic pathway, including changes in the beta-receptor density and function, guanine nucleotide regulatory proteins (or G-proteins), and cyclic-AMP levels.

Beta-adrenergic receptors

The beta-adrenergic receptor complex and the interrelation between noradrenaline, beta-receptors, G-proteins, and cyclic-AMP is shown schematically in Fig. 14.1. In the normal myocardium there is a predominance of the $beta_1$-subgroup of receptors. In heart failure there is a decrease in the total beta-receptor density; this decrease is related to the degree of heart failure.[23] It is due to a selective reduction, or 'down-regulation', in the $beta_1$-receptor density of about 60–70%.[24] In a study of papillary muscle extracts obtained from patients with severe heart failure undergoing transplantation[25] it was shown that down-regulation of $beta_1$-receptors is accompanied by a reduction in the corresponding messenger RNA (mRNA) for the $beta_1$-receptor. No such changes were seen in $beta_2$-receptor density or in $beta_2$-receptor mRNA. These findings suggest that the $beta_1$-receptor down-regulation is, at least partly, the consequence of a reduction in the synthesis of the $beta_1$-receptors. However, it is also possible that the $beta_1$-receptor down-regulation reflects an increase in receptor degradation,[26] although this remains to be proven in failing human hearts.

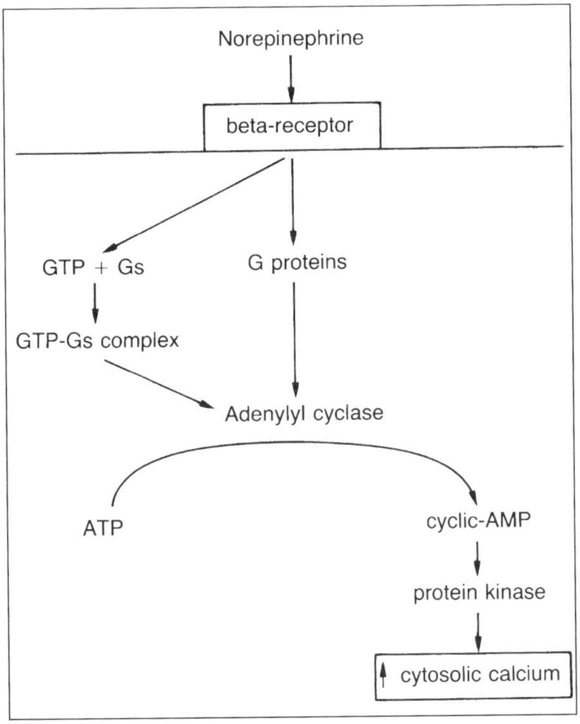

Fig. 14.1
The beta-adrenergic receptor complex and the interrelation between noradenaline receptors, G proteins and cyclic-AMP. G proteins – guanine nucleotide regulatory proteins; Gs – stimulatory proteins; cyclic AMP – cyclic adenosine monophosphate; ATP – adenosine triphosphate.

The absolute density of the $beta_2$-receptor is unchanged in heart failure, although the ratio of $beta_2$-receptors to $beta_1$-receptors is increased and their functional activity is reduced.[27] Several different mechanisms are involved in this receptor 'uncoupling'.[28] One important pathway involves initial phosphorylation of the agonist-occupied active receptors by beta-adrenergic receptor kinase.[29] Subsequently, an inhibitory protein, beta-arrestin,[30] binds to the phosphorylated receptor, resulting in uncoupling of the beta-receptor and the G-proteins and a reduction in their function.

Alterations in the beta-receptors may be a response to increased sympathetic activity or a result of progressive heart muscle damage, or both.[31] Thus, it is uncertain whether these alterations in beta-receptors are specific to heart failure or whether they merely reflect the marked sympathetic activation that occurs in this condition.[28] Down-regulation of the beta-receptors does not occur uniformly throughout the myocardium and is more marked in the sub-endocardial myocytes, which suggests that it is not simply related to the increase in sympathetic activity.[32]

Effect of beta-blockade on beta-receptor density

Uncontrolled studies of metoprolol in patients with idopathic dilated cardiomyopathy have suggested that chronic treatment with this agent increases beta-receptor density.[33,34] The patients in these series also showed significant haemodynamic improvement. A recent randomized trial with metoprolol has also demonstrated a significant increase in beta-receptor density after 6 months of treatment compared with placebo.[35] However, there were no significant changes in ejection fraction between the two groups.[36] Whereas the increase in $beta_1$-receptor density seen after treatment with beta-blockers appears to occur within days,[37] the clinical benefits of beta-blockade occur after longer-term therapy (more than 2 months),[18,38–54] and thus it is unlikely that this improvement is explained simply by beta-receptor up-regulation alone.

The underlying cause of the heart failure may influence the changes seen in the beta-receptor complex. Bristow et al[55] have shown that, compared with idiopathic dilated cardiomyopathy, cardiomyopathy due to ischaemic heart disease has less total beta-receptor down-regulation and greater uncoupling of left ventricular $beta_2$-receptors and right ventricular $beta_1$-receptors. These differences may explain why beta-blockade appears to produce greater effects on left ventricular function in idiopathic dilated cardiomyopathy than in ischaemic cardiomyopathy.[45] However, this apparent difference in response might also be attributable to a greater degree of spontaneous improvement in patients with idiopathic dilated cardiomyopathy.

G-proteins

The guanine nucleotide regulatory proteins, or G-proteins, exist on the inner surface of the cell membrane and provide the link between the beta-receptor and adenylate cyclase. Some G-proteins stimulate adenylate cyclase (Gs-proteins) and others are inhibitory (Gi-proteins). They share a common structure, each being composed of alpha, beta, and gamma subunits with the alpha subunit thought to be responsible for regulating the effector systems.[56,57] There are alterations in these proteins in the failing human myocardium, including an increase of as much as a third in the Gi-protein,[58,59] and a reduction in the Gs-protein.[60,61] These alterations in the G-proteins, as well as the receptor modifications mentioned above, probably account for the 'uncoupling' of the $beta_2$-receptors seen in heart failure.[31] The Gs-proteins interact directly with the catalytic unit of adenylate cyclase, and it appears that this subunit is not altered in heart failure.[31]

Clinical trials of beta-blockers in heart failure

Traditionally, beta-blockers have been considered contraindicated in heart failure because of their acute negative inotropic effect. The first report of their application in heart failure described seven patients with severe idiopathic dilated cardiomyopathy who appeared to have a favourable clinical response to beta-blockade with metoprolol.[62] The same workers later reported a further 24 patients (with 13 control subjects) who showed clinical improvement during beta-blockade.[63] It was suggested that, in comparison with historical controls, survival was prolonged with the beta-blocker treatment. A further report of patients with idiopathic dilated cardiomyopathy indicated improvement in haemodynamics and symptoms with beta-blockade,[64] and significant haemodynamic deterioration on withdrawal.[65]

The initial observations suggestive of benefit were all derived from non-randomized studies, but these have been followed by a number of randomized, placebo-controlled trials of beta-blockers in patients with heart failure of different types. Table 14.1 outlines the randomized controlled trials of beta-blockade in patients with heart failure that have been reported to date.[18,38–54] These trials have predominantly included patients with idiopathic dilated cardiomyopathy, although, some have involved patients with ischaemic cardiomyopathy. Most, but not all, have reported an improvement in symptoms and a reduction in NYHA functional class with longer-term treatment. Those studies that did not report improvement had, generally, a short treatment period and relatively small numbers of patients.

Haemodynamic effects of beta-blockade in heart failure

In patients with heart failure that is mainly due to idiopathic dilated cardiomyopathy, long-term beta-blockade has been shown to result in significant haemodynamic improvement with increased left ventricular stroke work index and left ventricular ejection fraction, and to decreased pulmonary capillary wedge pressure. In those studies that measured ejection fraction, the mean increase in the beta-blocker group relative to the control was 5.7% (see Table 14.1). (This increase is derived from the

Reference number	Number of patients	Beta-blocker	Follow-up (months)	Ejection fraction (%)	Exercise tolerance (treadmill)
38	17	acebutolol	1	not available	decrease
39	10	metoprolol	1	+3.0	no change
40	50	metoprolol	19	not available	no change
41	25	metoprolol	12	+2.0	increase
42	12	labetalol	2	not avilable	increase
43	20	bucindolol	3	0.0	increase
18	24	bucindolol	3	+8.0	no change
45	50	bucindolol	3	+0.5	no change
46	10	metoprolol	3	not available	increase
47	383	metoprolol	12–18	+6.0	no change
48	49	carvedilol	3.5	+5.5	not available
50	60	carvedilol	4	+10.0	not available
52	29	nebivolol	3	+8.0	no change
51	50	metoprolol	6	+5.0	not available
44	139	bucindolol	3	+4.1	decrease
49	40	carvedilol	6	+11	no change
53	25	metoprolol	3	+8	not available
54	641	bisoprolol	23	not available	not available
	1634 patients			**+5.7%**	

Table 14.1
Randomized, controlled trials of beta-blockers in congestive heart failure. (Mean difference in ejection fraction calculated as the difference between the mean change during active treatment and the mean change during control, and adjusted for number of patients.)

mean ejection fraction data from the published studies in which this was assessed.)

The mechanisms of haemodynamic improvement with long-term beta-blockade in heart failure are unclear. Acute intravenous beta-blockade has been demonstrated to have an adverse effect on left ventricular systolic function.[66] However, long-term oral therapy is well tolerated and can result in significant improvement. Most studies investigating the possible mechanisms of improvement have been uncontrolled and involved small numbers of patients and the data are conflicting.

Eichhorn et al,[67] in an uncontrolled study of the effects of 3 months' treatment with bucindolol in patients with heart failure, demonstrated an increase in left ventricular ejection fraction that was related to reductions in both end-systolic and end-diastolic volumes, which suggests an improvement in myocardial contractility. This was confirmed by improvements in the end-systolic pressure–volume relationship and peak dP/dt–end-diastolic volume relationship, both of which are relatively load-independent measures of contractility. Despite these improvements in contractility and mechanical work, there was no increase in myocardial oxygen consumption.

The finding of improved contractility following long-term beta-blockade has also been demonstrated in a placebo-controlled study of nebivolol, a $beta_1$-selective antagonist with vasodilating properties, in patients with dilated cardiomyopathy.[52] This study demonstrated no significant change in wall stress, suggesting that the significant increase in ejection fraction observed was due to improved contractility rather than ventricular unloading.

In addition to improvements in resting haemodynamics following beta-blockade, improvements have also been demonstrated in cardiac index, stroke volume index, stroke work index, and pulmonary capillary wedge pressure with exercise.[17,19] In association with these improvements there was no increase in myocardial oxygen consumption suggesting increased myocardial work load without higher metabolic costs.

Few data are available regarding the effects of beta-blockade on diastolic function in heart failure. Improvements have been demonstrated in isovolumic relaxation, with no change in chamber stiffness, following treatment with bucindolol.[67] Improved diastolic function may be an important component of the response to beta-blockade and requires further investigation.

Effects of beta-blockade on exercise tolerance in heart failure

The findings related to exercise capacity in these studies have been conflicting. Although some studies have reported statistically significant improvements in total exercise duration with beta-blockade, others have not (see Table 14.1). Long-term beta-blockade can attenuate maximum oxygen consumption[68] and, consequently, maximal exercise tolerance testing may not be the appropriate method for assessing improvement in functional capacity. In a randomized trial of the effects of the vasodilating beta-blocker carvedilol,[69] submaximal exercise time (determined by stressing patients at a workload fixed at 85% of their baseline maximal oxygen consumption) was significantly increased in the beta-blocker group compared with placebo, while maximal exercise time was not changed. A similar study[52] has recently shown a significant increase in the distance traversed during a 6-minute walk test in the group treated with beta-blockers compared with group treated with placebo. This method of assessing submaximal performance is often preferred by patients and may reflect improvement in their regular daily physical activity better than maximal exercise testing does.

Effects of beta-blockade on survival in heart failure

In the Metoprolol in Dilated Cardiomyopathy (MDC) study,[47] 383 patients with heart failure on standard treatment were randomized to receive either metoprolol or placebo and followed for 12–18 months. There were significant improvements in haemodynamics and symptoms as well as fewer hospital readmissions in the group treated with beta-blockers. There was no statistically significant effect on total mortality, but fewer metoprolol-treated patients were placed on the transplant list. In the Cardiac Insufficiency Bisoprolol Study (CIBIS),[54] 641 patients with heart failure of various aetiologies on standard treatment were randomized to bisoprolol or placebo for a mean period of 1.9 years. Significantly fewer patients in the beta-blocker group required hospitalization and significantly more showed improvement in functional class. There was no significant difference between the groups in mortality. Definitive larger scale mortality studies currently in progress should reliably assess the plausible survival benefit of beta-blocker treatment.

An overview of the likely survival benefit from beta-blockade in heart failure can be obtained from a meta-analysis of all randomized controlled trials. A total of 19 trials have been identified and included in the analysis.[18,38–54,70] In these trials, 74% of the patients had idiopathic dilated cardiomyopathy, the median ejection fraction was 23%, median NYHA class was 2.7, and average duration of follow-up was 15 months. The majority of the patients were from the MDC or CIBIS studies, and there were 17 smaller trials. None of the trials individually was large enough to detect reliably an effect of beta-blocker treatment on mortality. Mortality in patients assigned beta-blocker treatment was 10.5% versus 13% in controls (odds ratio 0.82, 95% confidence interval 0.6–1.1) (Fig. 14.2a). When the meta-analysis was repeated using the MDC study combined end-point of mortality and transplant listing, the mortality in treated patients was 10.8% versus 15.3% in controls (odds ratio 0.69, 95% confidence interval 0.51–0.92) (Fig. 14.2b). A large-scale trial with longer follow-up is required for reliable determination of a plausible effect of beta-blocker treatment on mortality in heart failure.

Currently available data indicating improvements in haemodynamics, clinical symptoms and exercise performance are not yet sufficient to justify the widespread use of beta-blockers in all patients with heart failure. In particular, further information is required about the effects of beta-blockade in heart failure of ischaemic aetiology, which is the most common aetiology, as there is some evidence to suggest that this may respond differently to beta-blockade.[45,54] Additional data, which are still preliminary and unpublished, suggest however a very favourable effect of treatment with carvedilol in patients with heart failure that is predominantly of ischaemic aetiology.

The experience with other agents in heart failure, such as milrinone,[71] that produce favourable acute haemodynamic and clinical effects but actually increase mortality in the long term, indicates the importance of mortality data in the consideration of general treatment recommendations. However, some mortality data from the numerous trials of beta-blockers following myocardial infarction are relevant and reassuring.

Beta-blockers following myocardial infarction

Observations from the placebo group of the Multicentre Diltiazem Post-infarction

Trial	Number of patients	% Events Study	% Events Control	Odds ratio (OR) and 95% confidence intervals (CI)
17 smaller trials	592	4.3%	7.0%	
Larger trials				
MDC	383	11.9%	10.1%	
CIBIS	641	16.6%	20.9%	
Subtotal	1024	14.8%	16.9%	
Total	1616	10.5%	13.0%	

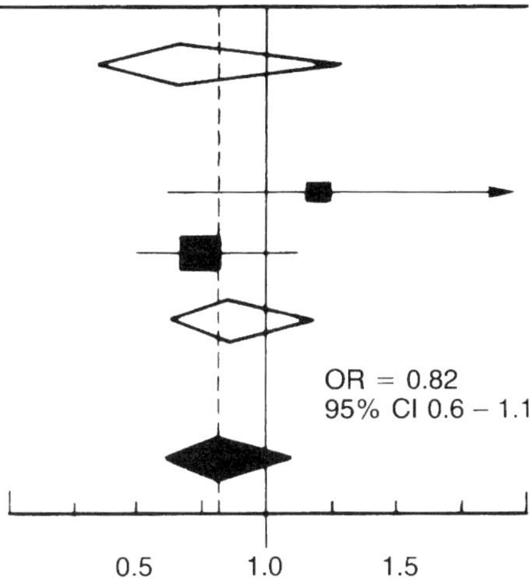

Treatment effect 2P=0.19
X^2 test for heterogeneity between subgroups = 0.42, 1df p=0.52
X^2 test for heterogeneity overall = 5.13, 9df p=0.82

Fig. 14.2
Beta-blockers in heart failure. A. Meta-analysis of mortality data.

Research Group[72] suggested that beta-blockers were less frequently used in patients with ejection fraction of less than 30%, râles, a third heart sound, or radiological pulmonary congestion. However, for each level of left ventricular function, the chance of developing heart failure requiring treatment was actually less if the patient was on a beta-blocker. Mortality was less if the patient was on a beta-blocker for every correlate of left ventricular function except a third heart sound.

Further evidence that beta-blockers may confer survival benefit in patients with heart failure has accrued from the Beta-Blocker Heart Attack Trial (BHAT).[73] In this trial, of the 3837 patients randomized, 710 had a history of heart failure. Among this heart failure group there was about one quarter fewer deaths in those assigned propranolol than in the placebo group. This difference, while of borderline statistical significance (p = 0.07), appeared to be of similar magnitude to the highly significant difference in mortality observed in the much larger group of patients without a history of heart failure. The lower mortality among patients with heart failure assigned propranolol primarily resulted from a reduction in sudden death of about a half (p = 0.02).

In the Beta-blocker Pooling Project,[74] results from nine trials involving a total of 13 679 patients were combined in order to allow greater power for the detection of treatment

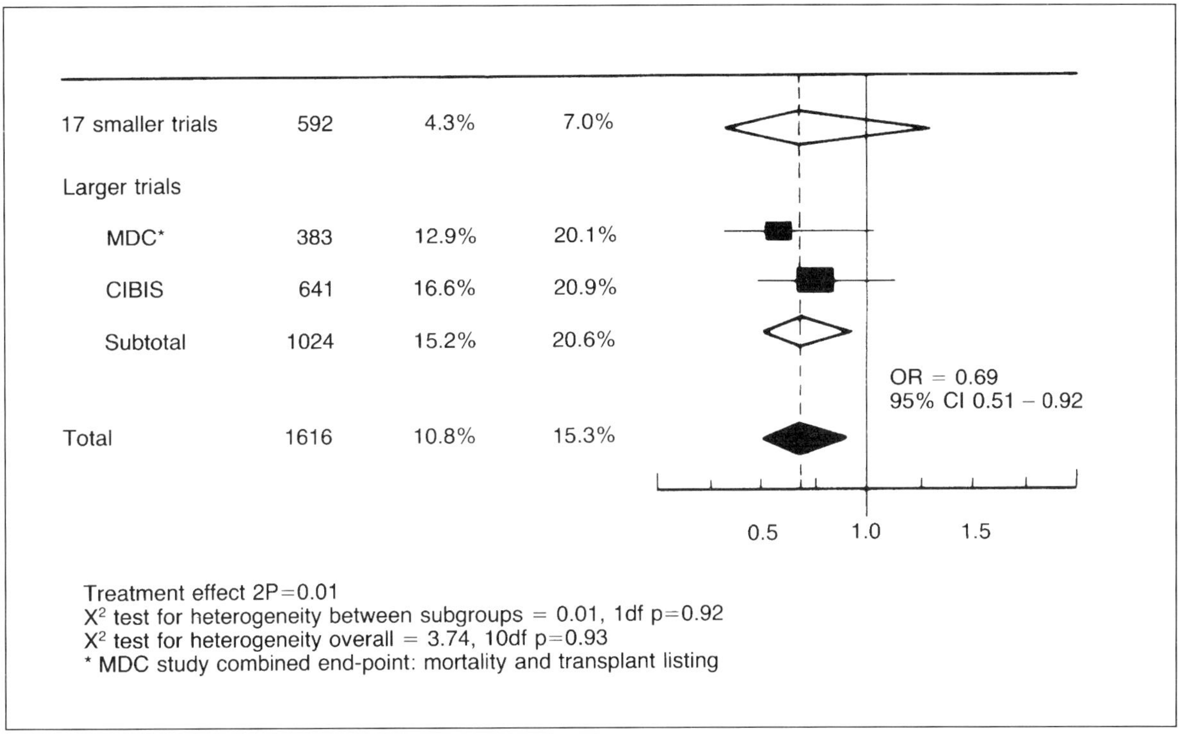

***Fig. 14.2** (cont.)*
Beta-blockers in heart failure. B. Meta-analysis using combined endpoint data from MDC study.

effects among subgroups of randomized patients. Although the subgroup with chronic heart failure was made up almost entirely of BHAT patients, there was additional information provided on the effects of treatment in a total of 3519 patients with prior heart failure (as indicated by pulmonary oedema, cardiogenic shock, persistent hypotension, basilar râles or other symptoms or signs of heart failure at the time of the acute infarction). Among these patients there was a significant reduction in total mortality of about one quarter in those assigned treatment with a beta-blocker ($p = 0.004$). Similarly among the 2625 patients with systolic blood pressure below 110 mmHg there was a significant reduction in total mortality of about one half ($p = 0.0002$) in those treated with a beta-blocker (a similar result was observed in those with diastolic blood pressure less than 70 mmHg). Finally, among the 957 patients receiving digitalis prior to randomization, mortality was reduced by about a third ($p = 0.01$) in those assigned a beta-blocker.

Thus, it is apparent that some patients with heart failure or left ventricular dysfunction following acute myocardial infarction may benefit from beta-blocker therapy. However, the general relevance of these results from the post-infarction trials is uncertain, given that the populations chosen for study were highly selected.

Potential benefits of beta-blockers in the context of current management

Studies with ACE inhibitors[75,76] have clearly demonstrated that these agents can reduce deaths caused by progressive heart failure, with a questionable effect on sudden death. The possibility that beta-blockade may provide further benefit through reducing the risk of sudden death is relevant since sudden death still accounts for one third to one half of all deaths in patients with heart failure.

The exact mechanism of action of beta-blockers in the prevention of sudden death following myocardial infarction is uncertain. A reduction in ventricular arrhythmias has been postulated from a retrospective analysis of subgroups of patients in BHAT.[77] Those with arrhythmias had the most pronounced effect from beta-blockade, with mortality being halved in the treatment group. Following myocardial infarction, metoprolol has been reported to have a pronounced effect on prevention of ventricular fibrillation.[78] Beta-blockers have an effect on the fibrillation threshold rather than on ventricular ectopics and this effect may confer protection from sudden death.[79]

Several other cardioprotective actions of beta-blockers have been proposed apart from anti-arrhythmic effects[80] including decreased myocardial oxygen demand,[65] antithrombotic effect,[81] and prevention of plaque rupture.[82] Beta-blockers are able to decrease the myocardial oxygen demand : supply ratio by decreasing heart rate, blood pressure, and myocardial contractility, and they thus may prevent ischaemia. In keeping with this, a four-fold reduction in the incidence of non-fatal reinfarction was observed in an overview of the long-term treatment trials.[83] A reduction in the rate of recurrent myocardial infarction has also been demonstrated with ACE-inhibition,[84,85] although the mechanisms of benefit are probably different. ACE inhibitors may have useful vascular-protective and possible anti-atherosclerotic effects,[86] thus extending the rationale for complementary benefits from beta-blockade following myocardial infarction and in heart failure with combined ACE inhibitor/beta-blocker treatment.

Conclusion

Congestive heart failure is a common problem and, despite recent improvements in treatment, mortality remains high. Complex neurohormonal alterations occur in heart failure which are deleterious in the long term and adversely affect survival. ACE inhibition has been shown to have beneficial effects on haemodynamics, symptoms, and survival. Beta-adrenergic antagonists are also able to modulate the neurohormonal activation of heart failure. Clinical trials of beta-blockers in ischaemic and idiopathic dilated cardiomyopathy have shown good tolerability and improved haemodynamics and symptoms. Following myocardial infarction, beta-blockers reduce mortality particularly in patients with heart failure. Further studies are required to determine whether beta-blockade can further reduce mortality in heart failure and provide a useful addition to existing therapy. Indeed, at least two large-scale, definitive mortality studies are planned with several thousand patients using bucindolol (the BEST study) and carvedilol (the CHOICE study). These studies, the outcomes of which should be known in the next few years, will be crucial in defining exactly the potentially considerable treatment benefit from beta-blockers in heart failure.

References

1 Nicklas JM, Benedict C, Johnstone ED, et al. Relationship between neurohormonal profile and one year mortaility in patients with congestive heart failure and/or left ventricular dysfunction [abstract]. *Circulation* 1991;**84(suppl II)**:II-468.

2 Cohn JN, Simon A, Johnson G, VHeFT Study Group. Relationship of plasma norepinephrine and plasma renin activity to mortality in heart failure: V-HeFT II [abstract]. *Circulation* 1991;**84(suppl II)**:II-310.

3 Thomas JA, Marks BH. Plasma norepinephrine in congestive heart failure. *Am J Cardiol* 1978;**41**:233–243.

4 Francis GS, Goldsmith SR, Cohn JN. The relationship of exercise capacity to resting left ventricular performance and basal plasma norepinephrine levels in patients with congestive heart failure. *Am Heart J* 1982;**104**:725–731.

5 Cohn JN, Levine B, Olivari MT, et al. Plasma norepinephrine as a guide to prognosis in patients with chronic congestive heart failure. *N Engl J Med* 1984;**311**:819–823.

6 Francis GS, Benedict C, Johnstone DE, et al, for the SOLVD Investigators. Comparison of neuroendocrine activation in patients with left ventricular dysfunction with and without congestive heart failure. A substudy of the Studies of Left Ventricular Dysfunction (SOLVD). *Circulation* 1990;**82**:1724–1729.

7 Mancia G. Sympathetic activation in congestive heart failure. *Eur Heart J* 1990:**11(suppl A)**:3–11.

8 Olivari MT, Levine TB, Cohn JN. Abnormal neurohumoral response to nitroprusside infusion in congestive heart failure. *J Am Coll Cardiol* 1983;**2**:411–417.

9 Szakacs JE, Cannon A. Norepinephrine myocarditis. *Am J Clin Pathol* 1958;**30**:425–435.

10 Bigger JT. Why patients with congestive heart failure die: arrhythmias and sudden cardiac death. *Circulation* 1987;**75(suppl IV)**:IV-28–IV-35.

11 Chidsey CA, Braunwald E, Morrow AG. Catecholamine excretion and cardiac stores of norepinephrine in congestive heart failure. *Am J Med* 1965;**39**:442–451.

12 Daly PA, Sole MJ. Myocardial catecholamines and the pathophysiology of heart failure. *Circulation* 1990;**82(suppl I)**:I-35–I-43.

13 Sandoval AB, Gilbert EM, Rose CP, Bristow MR. Cardiac norepinephrine uptake and release is decreased in dilated cardiomyopathy [abstract]. *Circulation* 1989;**80(suppl II)**:II-393.

14 Petch MC, Nayler WG. Uptake of catecholamines by human cardiac muscle *in vitro*. *Br Heart J* 1979;**41**:336–339.

15 Sole MJ, Helke CJ, Jacobowitz DM. Increased dopamine in the failing hamster heart: transvesicular transport of dopamine limits the rate of norepinephrine synthesis. *Am J Cardiol* 1982;**49**:1682–1690.

16 Pierpont GL, Francis GS, DeMaster EG, et al. Heterogenous myocardial catecholamine concentrations in patients with congestive heart failure. *Am J Cardiol* 1987;**60**:316–321.

17 Anderson FL, Port JD, Reid BB, Larrabee P, Hanson G, Bristow MR. Myocardial catecholamine and neuropeptide Y depletion in failing ventricles of patients with idiopathic dilated cardiomyopathy. Correlation with beta-adrenergic receptor down regulation. *Circulation* 1992;**85**:46–53.

18 Gilbert EM, Anderson JL, Deitchman D, et al. Long-term betablocker vasodilator therapy improves cardiac function in idiopathic dilated cardiomyopathy: a double-blind, randomised study of bucindolol versus placebo. *Am J Med* 1990;**88**:223–229.

19 Nemanich JW, Veith RC, Abrass IB, Stratton JR. Effects of metaprolol on rest and exercise cardiac function and plasma catecholamines in chronic congestive heart failure secondary to ischaemic or idiopathic cardiomyopathy. *Am J Cardiol* 1990;**66**:843–848.

20 Andersson B, Blomstrom-Lundqvist C, Hedner T, Waagstein F. Exercise haemodynamics and myocardial metabolism during long-term, beta-

adrenergic blockade in severe heart failure. *J Am Coll Cardiol* 1991;**18**:1059–1066.

21 Mann DL, Cooper G. Propranolol prevents the myopathic effects of catecholamines in vitro: implications for patients with congestive heart failure. *Circulation* 1988;**78(suppl II)**:II-576.

22 Imperato-McGinley J, Gautier T, Ehlers K, Zullo T, Goldstein DS, Vaughan ED. Reversibility of catecholamine-induced dilated cardiomyopathy in a child with a phaeochromocytoma. *N Engl J Med* 1987;316: 793–797.

23 Fowler MB, Laser JA, Hopkins GL, Minobe W, Bristow MR. Assessment of the beta-adrenergic receptor pathway in the intact failing human heart: progressive receptor down-regulation and subsensitivity to agonist response. *Circulation* 1986;**74**:1290–1302.

24 Bristow MR, Ginsburg R, Umans V, et al. $Beta_1$- and $beta_2$-adrenergic subpopulations in nonfailing and failing human ventricular myocardium: coupling of both receptor subtypes to muscle contraction and selective $beta_1$-receptor down-regulation in heart failure. *Circ Res* 1986;**59**:297–309.

25 Ungerer M, Bohm M, Elce JS, Erdmann E, Lohse MJ. Altered expression of beta-adrenergic receptor kinase and $beta_1$-adrenergic receptors in the failing human heart. *Circulation* 1993;87:454–463.

26 Mahan LM, Koachman AM, Insel PA. Genetic analysis of beta-adrenergic receptor internalisation and down regulation. *Proc Natl Acad Sci USA* 1985;**82**:129–133.

27 Bristow MR, Hershberger RE, Port JD, Minobe W, Rasmussen R. $Beta_1$- and $beta_2$-adrenergic receptor-mediated adenylate cyclase stimulation in non-failing and failing human ventricular myocardium. *Mol Pharmacol* 1989;**35**:295–303.

28 Hammond HK. Mechanisms for myocardial beta-adrenergic receptor densensitization in heart failure. *Circulation* 1993;**87**:652–654.

29 Lohse MJ, Benovic JL, Caron MG, Lefkowitz R. Multiple pathways of rapid $beta_2$-adrenergic receptor densensitisation. *J Biol Chem* 1990;**265**:3202–3209.

30 Lohse MJ, Benovic JL, Codina J, Caron MG, Lefkowitz RJ. Beta-arrestin: a protein that regulates beta-adrenergic receptor function. *Science* 1990;**248**:1547–1550.

31 Bristow MR, Hershberger RE, Port JD, et al. Beta-adrenergic pathways in nonfailing and failing human ventricular myocardium. *Circulation* 1990;**82(suppl I)**:I-12–I-25.

32 Murphee SS, Saffitz JE. Distribution of beta-adrenergic receptors in failing human ventricular myocardium. Implications for the mechanisms of down-regulation. *Circulation* 1989; **79**:1214–1225.

33 Heilbrunn SM, Shah P, Bristow MR, Valantine HA, Ginsburg R, Fowler MB. Increased beta-receptor density and improved haemodynamic response to catecholamine stimulation during long-term metoprolol therapy in heart failure from dilated cardiomyopathy. *Circulation* 1989;**79**:483–490.

34 Waagstein F, Caidahl K, Wallentin I, Bergh C, Hjalmarson A. Long term beta-blockade in dilated cardiomyopathy. Effects of short and long term metoprolol treatment followed by withdrawal and readministration of metoprolol. *Circulation* 1989;**80**:551–563.

35 Bristow MR, Gilbert EM, Olsen S, Larrabee P. Renlund DG, O'Connell JB. Long-term metoprolol therapy increases myocardial beta-adrenergic receptor density relative to placebo controls [abstract]. *J Am Coll Cardiol* 1993;**21(suppl A)**:101A.

36 Bristow MR, Port JD, Hershberger RE, Gilbert EM, Feldman AM. The beta-adrenergic receptor-adenylate cyclase complex as a target for therapeutic intervention in heart failure. *Eur Heart J* 1989;**10(suppl B)**:45–54.

37 Whyte K, Jones CR, Howie CA, Deighton N, Sumner DJ, Reid JL. Haemodynamic metabolic and lymphocyte beta2-adrenoceptor changes following chronic beta-adrenoceptor antagonism. *Eur J Clin Pharmacol* 1987;**32**: 237–243.

38 Ikram H, Fitzpatrick D. Double-blind trial of chronic oral betablockade in congestive cardiomyopathy. *Lancet* 1981;**ii**:490–493.

39 Currie PJ, Kelly MJ, McKenzie A, et al. Oral beta-adrenergic blockade with metaprolol in chronic severe dilated cardiomyopathy. *J Am Coll Cardiol* 1984;**3**:203–209.

40 Anderson JL, Lutz JR, Gilbert EM, et al. A randomized trial of low-dose beta-blockade

therapy for idiopathic dilated cardiomyopathy. *Am J Cardiol* 1985;**55**:471–475.

41 Engelmeier RS, O'Connell JB, Walsh R, Rad N, Scanlon PJ, Gunnar RM. Improvement in symptoms and exercise tolerance by metoprolol in patients with dilated cardiomypathy: a double-blind randomized, placebo-controlled trial. *Circulation* 1985;**72**:536–546.

42 Leung W, Lau C, Wong C, Cheng C, Tai Y, Lim S. A double-blind cross-over trial of labetalol in patients with dilated cardiomyopathy [abstract]. *Circulation* 1989;**80(suppl II)**:II-118.

43 Pollock SG, Lystash J, Tedesco C, Craddock G, Smucker ML. Usefulness of bucindolol in congestive heart failure. *Am J Cardiol* 1990;**66**:603–607.

44 Bristow MR, O'Connell JB, Gilbert EM, et al for the Bucindolol Investigators. Dose-reponse of chronic betablocker treatment in heart failure from either idiopathic dilated or ischaemic cardiomyopathy. *Circulation* 1994;**84**:1632–1642.

45 Woodley SL, Gilbert EM, Anderson JL, et al. Betablockade with bucindolol in heart failure caused by ischaemic versus idiopathic dilated cardiomyopathy. *Circulation* 1991;**84**:2426–2441.

46 Paolisso G, Gambardella A, Marrazzo G, et al. Metabolic and cardiovascular benefits deriving from β-adrenergic blockade in chronic congestive heart failure. *Am Heart J* 1992;**123**:1397–1404.

47 Waagstein F, Bristow MR, Swedberg K, et al, for the Metoprolol in Dilated Cardiomyopathy (MDC) Trial Study Group. Beneficial effects of metoprolol in idiopathic dilated cardiomyopathy. *Lancet* 1993;**342**: 1441–1446.

48 Krum H, Schwartz B, Sackner-Bernstein J, et al. Double-blind, placebo-controlled study of the long-term efficacy of carvedilol in patients with severe heart failure treated with converting-enzyme inhibitors [abstract]. *J Am Coll Cardiol* 1993;**21(suppl A)**: 114A.

49 Metra M, Nardi M, Giubbini R, Dei Cas L. Effects of short- and long-term carvedilol administration on rest and exercise haemodynamic variable, exercise capacity and clinical conditions in patients with idiopathic dilated cardiomyopathy. *J Am Coll Cardiol* 1994;**24**:1678–1687.

50 Olsen SL, Gilbert EM, Renlund DG, et al. Carvedilol improves symptoms and left ventricular function in patients with congestive heart failure due to ischaemic or idiopathic delated cardiomyopathy [abstract]. *J Am Coll Cardiol* 1993;**21(suppl A)**:114A.

51 Fisher ML, Gottlieb SS, Plotrick GD, et al. Beneficial effects of metoprolol in heart failure associated with coronary artery disease: a randomised trial. *J Am Coll Cardiol* 1994;**23**:943–950.

52 Wisenbaugh T, Katz I, Davis J, et al. Long-term (3 month) effects of a new beta-blocker (nebivolol) on cardiac performance in dilated cardiomyopathy. *J Am Coll Cardiol* 1993;**21**:1094–1100.

53 Eichhorn EJ, Heejch CM, Barnet JH, et al. Effect of metoprolol on myocardial function and energetics in patients with nonischaemic dilated cardiomyopathy: a randomized, double-blind, placebo-controlled study. *J Am Coll Cardiol* 1994;**24**:1310–1320.

54 CIBIS Investigators. A randomized trial of beta-blockade in heart failure. The Cardiac Insufficiency Bisoprolol Study. *Circulation* 1994;**90**:1765–1773.

55 Bristow MR, Anderson FL, Port D, et al. Differences in beta-adrenergic neuroeffector mechanisms in ischaemic versus dilated cardiomyopathy. *Circulation* 1991;**84**:1024–1039.

56 Insel PA, Ransnas LA. G proteins and cardiovascular disease. *Circulation* 1988;**78**:1511–1513.

57 Horn EM, Bilezikian JK. Mechanisms of abnormal transmembrane signalling of the beta-adrenergic receptor in congestive heart failure. *Circulation* 1990;**82(suppl I)**:I-26–34.

58 Feldman AM, Cates AE, Veazey WB, et al. Increase of the 40,000-mol wt pertussis toxin substrate (G protein) in the failing human heart. *J Clin Invest* 1988;**82**:189–197.

59 Neumann J, Schmitz W, Scholz H, von Meyerinck L, Doring V, Kalmar P. Increase in myocardial Gi-proteins in heart failure. *Lancet* 1988;**ii**:936–937.

60 Lau C, Pun K, Leung W. Reduced stimulatory guanine nucleotide binding regulatory protein

in idiopathic dilated cardiomyopathy. *Am Heart J* 1991;**122**:1787–1788.

61 Ransnas LA, Hjalmarson A, Insel PA. Dilated cardiomyopathy is associated with an impaired activation of the stimulatory G-protein, Gs by GTP in heart membranes [abstract]. *Circulation* 1988;**78(suppl II)**:II-178.

62 Waagstein F, Hjalmarson A, Varnauskas E, Wallentin I. Effect of chronic beta-adrenergic receptor blockade in congestive cardiomyopathy. *Br Heart J* 1975;**37**:1022–1036.

63 Swedberg K, Hjalmarson A, Waagstein F, Wallentin I. Prolongation of survival in congestive cardiomyopathy by beta-receptor blockade. *Lancet* 1979;**i**:1374–1377.

64 Swedberg K, Hjalmarson A, Waagstein F, Wallentin I. Beneficial effects of long term betablockade in congestive cardiomyopathy. *Br Heart J* 1989;**44**:117–133.

65 Swedberg K, Hjalmarson A, Waagstein F, Wallentin I. Adverse effects of betablockade withdrawal in patients with congestive cardiomyopathy. *Br Heart J* 1980;**44**:134–142.

66 Haber HL, Gimple LW, Simek CL, et al. Why do patients with congestive heart failure tolerate the initiation of betablocker therapy [abstract]? *Circulation* 1992;**86(suppl I)**:17.

67 Eichhorn EJ, Bedotto JB, Malloy CR, et al. Effect of beta-adrenergic blockade on myocardial function and energetics in congestive heart failure. Improvements in hemodynamic, contractile and diastolic performance with bucindolol. *Circulation* 1990;**82**:473–483.

68 Sweeney ME, Fletcher BJ, Fletcher GF. Exercise testing and training with beta-adrenergic blockade: role of drug washout period in 'unmasking' a training effect. *Am Heart J* 1989;**118**:941–946.

69 Olsen SL, Yanowitz FG, Gilbert EM, et al. Betablocker related improvement in submaximal exercise tolerance in heart failure from idiopathic dilated cardiomyopathy [abstract]. *J Am Coll Cardiol* 1992;**19(suppl A)**:146A.

70 Sano H, Kawabata N, Yonezawa K, Hirayama H, Sakuma I, Yasuda H. Metaprolol was more effective than captopril for dilated cardiomyopathy in Japanese patients. *Circulation* 1989;**80(suppl II)**:II-118.

71 Packer M, Carver JR, Rodeheffer RJ, et al. Effect of oral milrinone on mortality in severe chronic heart failure. *N Engl J Med* 1991;**325**:1468–1475.

72 Lichstein E, Hager D, Gregory JJ, Fleiss JL, Rolnitzky LM, Bigger JT for the Multicenter Diltiazem Post-infarction Research Group. Relation between beta-adrenergic blocker use, various correlates of left ventricular function and the chance of developing congestive heart failure. *J Am Coll Cardiol* 1990;**16**:1327–1332.

73 Chadda K, Goldstein S, Byington R, Curb JD. Effect of propranolol after acute myocardial infarction in patients with congestive heart failure. *Circulation* 1986;**73**:503–510.

74 The Beta-Blocker Pooling Project Research Group. The Beta-Blocker Pooling Project (BBPP); subgroup findings from randomised trials in post-infarction patients. *Eur Heart J* 1988;**9**:8–16.

75 The CONSENSUS Trial Study Group. Effects of enalapril on mortality in severe congestive heart failure. Results of the Cooperative North Scandinavian Enalapril Survival Study (CONSENSUS). *N Engl J Med* 1987; **316**:1429–1435.

76 The SOLVD Investigators. Effect of enalapril on survival in patients with reduced left ventricular ejection fractions and congestive heart failure. *N Engl J Med* 1991;**325**:293–302.

77 Furberg C, for the BHAT trial. Effect of propranolol in post-infarction patients with mechanical or electrical complications. *Circulation* 1984;**69**:761–765.

78 Ryden L, Ariniego R, Arnman K, et al. A double-blind trial metoprolol in acute myocardial infarction. Effects on ventricular arrythmias. *N Engl J Med* 1983;**308**:614–618.

79 Lichstein E. Why do beta-receptor blockers decrease mortality after myocardial infarction? *J Am Coll Cardiol* 1985;**6**:973–975.

80 Bigger JT, Coromilas J. How do beta-blockers protect after myocardial infarction? *Ann Intern Med* 1984;**101**:256–258.

81 Weksler BB, Gillick M, Pink J. Effects of propranolol on platelet function. *Blood* 1977;**49**:185–196.

82 Frishman WH, Lazar EJ. Reduction of mortality, sudden death and non-fatal reinfarction with beta-adrenergic blockers in survivors of acute myocardial infarction: a new hypothesis regarding the cardioprotective action of beta-

adrenergic blockade. *Am J Cardiol* 1990; **66**:66G–70G.

83 Yusuf S, Peto R, Lewis J, Collins R, Sleight P. Betablockade during and after myocardial infarction: an overview of the randomised trials. *Prog Cardiovasc Dis* 1985;**27**:335–371.

84 Pfeffer MA, Braunwald E, Moyé LA, et al. Effect of captopril on mortality and morbidity in patients with left ventricular dysfunction after myocardial infarction. Results of the Survival and Ventricular Enlargement Trial. *N Engl J Med* 1992;**327**:669–677.

85 Yusuf S, Pepine CJ, Garces C, et al. Effect of enalapril on myocardial infarction and unstable angina in patients with low ejection fractions. *Lancet* 1992;**340**:1173–1178.

86 Anon. From cardiac to vascular protection: the next chapter [editorial]. *Lancet* 1992; **340**:1197–1198.

15

What lessons should we learn from the negative trials?

Alan J Cowley

Introduction

In a relatively few years our understanding of heart failure has increased dramatically. We now realize that it is a major public health problem, we know more about its effects on patients' quality of life and life expectancy, and we have also learned much about its treatment, particularly with drugs. Our knowledge of the effects of drugs, beneficial or otherwise, is derived from the results of properly conducted clinical trials. However, each clinical trial is designed to answer a particular question, and if that original question is not of clinical relevance the results of the trial in guiding practice will be misleading. Therefore, we must be very clear about what we are trying to achieve in treating patients with heart failure, and then ask the appropriate questions about each new treatment.

What are we trying to achieve?

There are three main questions that are asked of treatments for heart failure:

- Does it improve symptoms?
- Does it improve survival?
- Does it delay progression?

Improve symptoms

Heart failure is an important cause of symptomatic impairment and disability. Once a patient has developed the syndrome it is unlikely that any drug treatment will return the exercise capability to normal and therefore there will always be, at the very least, mild symptoms. The measurement of symptomatic impairment is not easy, but a number of ways are used to try to quantify patients' incapacity. These include symptom-limited exercise tolerance measured in a laboratory on a treadmill or bicycle. Although this type of test allows close control, it involves an unusual form of exercise because it is performed to symptom-limited maximum and because the changes in workload are fixed. Patients need to learn the technique and some may not be capable of this. Furthermore, there are differences between the different types of exercise – bicycle compared with treadmill – and, even if the same type of exercise is used, between different protocols.[1] It is difficult to relate incapacity measured in this way to patients' symptomatic impairment during normal daily activities when they determine their own workloads. However, despite the disadvantages of this type of test it remains the mostly widely used measure of symptomatic impairment and is frequently used (and required by the licensing authorities) to assess the efficacy of treatment.

More relevant to patients are tests in which they choose their own work rate; such tests, including corridor walk tests, are gaining in popularity although they are not universally accepted. Probably the most relevant measure of the degree of patients' symptomatic impairment is an assessment of their daily activity which has been demonstrated to be markedly reduced compared to normal subjects. Studies measuring footfall with pedometers have shown that patients often walk less than 25% of the distance of healthy, age-matched normal subjects.[2] This clearly indicates a marked limitation in their wish or ability to exercise and indicates the considerable impact of heart failure on normal life. The effect of drug treatment on this type of assessment is not known but presumably effective therapy would improve these measures of customary activity.

Other methods of quantifying symptomatic severity include measurement of quality of life. Using quality-of-life questionnaires patients with heart failure have been shown to score their quality of life lower than virtually all other non-malignant chronic diseases, including chronic obstructive airways disease, angina, and diabetes (Table 15.1).[3] Again this indicates the enormous symptomatic burden of heart failure.

Although all of these methods of assessing symptomatic impairment have advantages and disadvantages, they all demonstrate considerable disability in heart failure. The extent of this disability has major implications for the social support and caring of the patients in the community and in hospital. For this reason alone the financial cost of heart failure is huge and places an enormous and increasing burden on health care systems.

Chronic condition	Score
Hypertension (n = 2595)	+0.8
Diabetes (n = 844)	−35.6
Arthritis (n = 2079)	−50.4
Chronic lung problems (n = 731)	−55.8
Angina (n = 532)	−60.6
CHF (n = 297)	−80.9

Table 15.1
Quality of life in common chronic illnesses. Average deviation from patients without chronic conditions (composite score). A more negative score represent greater impairment of quality of life.

Improve survival

Heart failure due to any cause is a lethal condition. In those with the most severe forms annual mortality rates are well in excess of 50%[4] and even in those whom we wrongly label as having mild heart failure it is still around 10%.[5] These survival figures compare unfavourably with many malignant diseases and, at worst, are only marginally better than patients with metastatic lung cancer. Clearly another aim of treatment must be to try to reduce mortality.

Delay progression

Heart failure is often thought of as the final result of a number of different processes including, most importantly, acute myocardial infarction. Infarct expansion and left ventricular remodelling and dilatation may in some patients precede the development of heart failure. If this is a true understanding of the pathophysiology of the development of heart failure, then it is possible that these processes can be interrupted and heart failure prevented or at least delayed. Prevention of the progression or development of heart failure is therefore a laudable aim. It may be achievable by reducing the incidence of coronary artery disease through education about smoking and weight, by better treatment of hypertension, by better treatment of acute myocardial infarction with thrombolytic agents, or by trying early in the pathophysiological process to prevent cardiac dilatation and hypertrophy.

Multiple combined endpoints in clinical trials?

It is fashionable to combine multiple endpoints in clinical trials to form one composite result on which to base a statistical analysis. This may have the advantage of reducing the number of patients who need to be included in the trial but is clearly a 'blunderbuss' approach which leaves the interpretation of the results, at best, cloudy. If we wish to know if a drug improves symptoms or survival we must have the scientific rigor to address each question separately. The lumping together of multiple endpoints, including mortality and measures of morbidity and symptoms, makes results difficult to interpret and they cannot be used as good guides to clinical practice. We must define precisely the aims of treatment.

Although much of the current interest in heart failure addresses the problem of mortality we must not lose sight of the impact heart failure has on quality of life and well-being, and to lessen this must remain the major aim of treatment. If an associated reduction in mortality and delayed progression of heart failure can also be achieved then this is the 'icing on the cake'. Additionally we need to address the question of the price we are willing to pay for improved well-being, particularly in severely ill, often elderly, patients. In this situation even a lack of adverse effect on survival may be over-optimistic and we may need to accept improved symptoms at the expense of a risk of reduced survival.

The established drugs

Loop diuretics

Loop diuretics have attracted a considerable amount of undeserved criticism because they activate the renin–angiotensin system. There is an established association between the degree of activation of neurohumoral mechanisms and mortality and further activation of the renin–angiotensin system by diuretics is belived to be detrimental. Although many of us have grown up in the world of powerful loop diuretics, their introduction a little over 20 years ago was an undoubted advance on sulphonylureas, thiazides and mercuryl diuretics.[6] The clinical trial proving efficacy was presumably like that of penicillin and needed only one patient, the advance being so dramatic. Despite theoretical disadvantages, a natriuretic agent will always be required in patients who have fluid retention, and no other treatment is capable of replacing diuretics in volume overloaded patients. They are currently, therefore, the keystone of treatment.

ACE inhibitors

ACE inhibitors have now been shown to improve symptomatic well-being,[7] to reduce the necessity for hospital admission, and to delay the progression and to improve survival in all grades of heart failure.[4,5] They represent a major advance in treatment but they are not the complete and final answer. Virtually all patients with heart failure have some degree of restricted exercise capability despite treatment with an ACE inhibitor and many remain severely incapacitated. There is therefore a need to investigate additional treatments. In patients with severe heart failure, mortality rates also remain high despite ACE inhibitors, and survival needs to be further improved, ideally with a cocomitant improvement in well-being.

Digoxin

The use of digoxin in patients in sinus rhythm is more dependent on culture than fact. The enthusiasts believe that the trials that show a reduction in exercise capability with withdrawal of diogoxin is evidence of efficacy. The sceptics believe that deterioration after withdrawal is not the same as benefit when adding the drug. The two are clearly not the same, particularly as the withdrawal studies already include highly selected patients (namely those who can tolerate digoxin).[8]

The real problem with digoxin is its narrow therapeutic window. It must be remembered that heart failure is a problem that affects predominantly middle and older age groups, who do not participate in the major trials that rely on laboratory-based symptom limited exercise capability as evidence of efficacy. In these patients the difference between acceptable efficacy and unacceptable toxicity is minimal and blurred.

The effect of digoxin on survival is not known but is currently being examined.

These then are the established drugs, and while they have brought about improvement in all areas of treatment they are not the total answer to the problem and other drugs still need to be evaluated.

Experimental drugs

The clinical investigation of a new drug involves a series of separate but contiguous stages. First, information has to be obtained about the drug's pharmacology and pharmacokinetics. Next a dose ranging study will need to be performed. Dose ranging is usually assessed with invasive haemodynamic monitoring; the dose of the drug is titrated upwards from a subtherapeutic amount to a dose that produces maximum haemodynamic effect or until the development of adverse events or side-effects. This type of investigation is usually undertaken with the patients resting and, as most patients develop symptoms only on exercise, it may not be entirely appropriate. Further dose ranging may be performed with other measures of efficacy, but whatever method is used the dose of the drug chosen for further evaluation tends to be at the top end of the therapeutic range rather than a minimum effective dose.

As the measurement of changes in central haemodynamics provide little information about changes in symptomatic well-being, formal exercise studies are believed to be required to assess efficacy and, ultimately, to assess whether appropriate survival studies will be performed. Formal, laboratory-based exercise tests, on a treadmill or bicycle, have advantages and disadvantages which have been discussed above. They are a highly artificial form of exercise and perhaps some type of self-paced test such as a corridor walk test is more representative of incapacity. Other studies of a more specialized nature, such as the effects on neurohumoral activation or regional haemodynamics, may additionally be performed.

Inotropic agents

Left ventricular systolic dysfunction is often thought to be the primary abnormality in heart failure, and a direct improvement in systolic performance is therefore believed to be a desirable aim. For this reason a number of inotropic agents that improve systolic function have been investigated. The most extensively investigated agents are those that increase intracellular levels of cyclic adenosine monophosphate (cAMP). This leads to an increase in calcium available to the contractile apparatus of the myocyte by enhancing release from the endoplasmic reticulum and to an influx of calcium into the cell. There are two ways of increasing cAMP levels: by stimulating its production, or by inhibiting its breakdown.

cAMP phosphodiesterase inhibitors

At least two cAMP phosphodiesterase inhibitors have now been shown to reduce survival. The PROMISE trial,[9] which was designed to investigate the effects of oral milrinone on survival (Fig. 15.1), and more recently a trial designed to investigate the effect of enoximone[10] (Fig. 15.2) were stopped prematurely by the ethical committees because of reduced survival in the actively treated groups. In the PROMISE trial, quality of life was not measured but data from different studies, which were also terminated prematurely by the sponsoring company because of the results of PROMISE, show improved exercise capability with milrinone in patients already taking diuretics and ACE inhibitors with or without digoxin.[11] However, in PROMISE, adverse events and side-effects were reported as being more common in the actively treated group. It must be remembered that the doses of milrinone used were high and the trial design was such that attempts were made to titrate up to the maximum tolerated dose. The excess mortality appeared to be due to sudden death, which could be predicted from Holter recordings; prolongation of runs of ventricular tachycardia or the development of new episodes of ventricular tachycardia were associated with subsequent death. A possible interaction with concomitant digoxin was also thought to be contributory to the excess deaths.

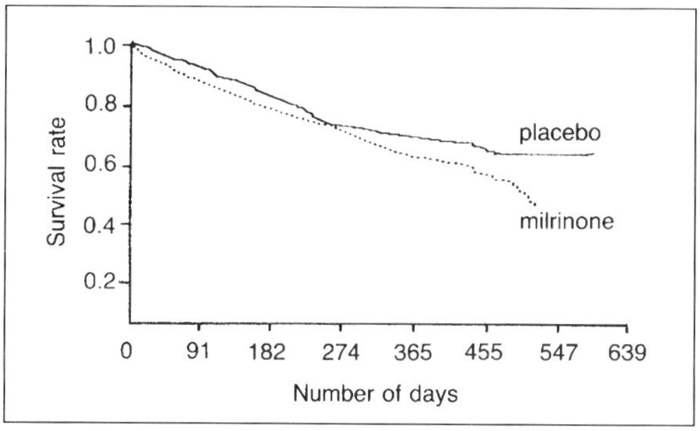

Figure 15.1
Kaplan–Meier analysis showing cumulative rates of survival in patients with chronic heart failure treated with milrinone of placebo.

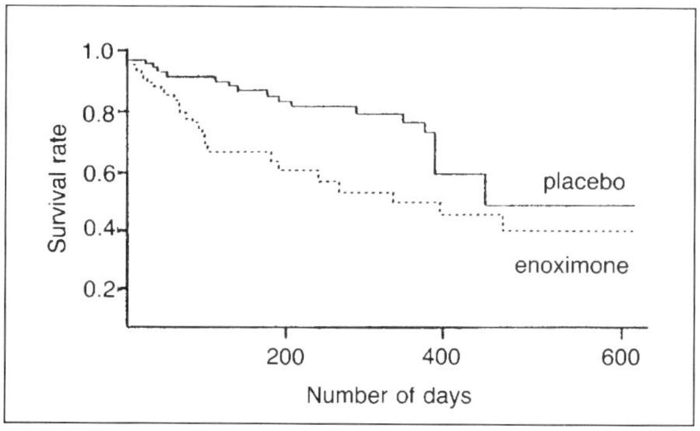

Figure 15.2
Kaplan–Meier survival curves. All patients: maximum follow-up.

In the enoximone trial,[10] which was conducted in severely ill patients already treated with maximum therapy including ACE inhibitors, quality of life was measured with two different questionnaires. One was disease-specific and the other was not; both demonstrated an improvement in quality of life in the actively treated group. The disease-specific questionnaire, which inquired about all aspects of the patients' life, showed a clinically significant improvement (Fig. 15.3) whereas the Nottingham Health Profile (a non-disease

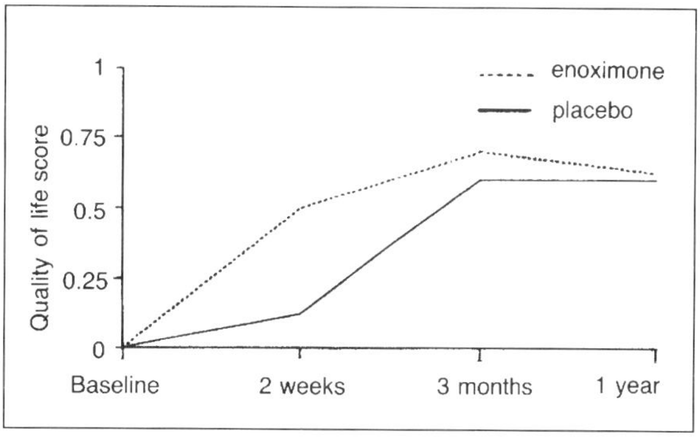

Figure 15.3
Effect of enoximone on quality of life.

specific questionnaire) showed an improvement in the index of mobility. In this study, as in PROMISE, the dose of enoximone was titrated upwards to the maximum tolerated. The number of patients included was not large enough to allow definite conclusions about mechanisms of death (sudden or due to deteriorating heart failure) or possible drug interactions, particularly with digoxin.

It would therefore appear that this class of drug improves well-being but at the expense of a reduction in survival. This does not necessarily mean that agents in this class should be abandoned because the reduction in survival is often small and patients with severe symptoms, particularly if they are elderly, may prefer an increased quality of life and independence at the risk of an increase in mortality.

Adenyl cyclase stimulators

Another way of increasing cAMP levels is by stimulation of adenyl cyclase. One agent that does this is prostacyclin, but it has the disadvantage of having to be administered by constant intravenous infusion. In an ambitious study, which was also terminated early by the safety committee, prostacyclin was compared with placebo.[12] Comparatively high doses were again used (40% of the maximum tolerated dose of 13 (2) ng/kg per minute). An excess mortality occurred in the actively treated group with no apparent beneficial effect of symptomatic well-being or exercise capability.

All agents which produce inotropic activity by increasing intracellular cAMP levels appear to reduce survival but the cAMP phosphodiesterase inhibitors may at least improve well-being.

Sympathomimetic agents

Sympathomimetic agents continue to play an important role in the treatment of acute or acutely decompensated heart failure. However, for use in patients with chronic heart failure (CHF), tachyphylaxis may occur and preclude long-term use, as does the parenteral route of administration of many of the agents. Although intermittent infusions have been used with either benefit[13] or harm,[14] this is still not wholly desirable and has never found an established place in routine practice. Furthermore, xamoterol, the partial beta-agonist which at high heart rates also acts as an antagonist, has been shown to cause a reduced survival in severely ill patients (Fig. 15.4).[15]

Dopaminergic agents are also extensively used to treat patients with acute heart failure. Ibopamine is an orally active dopamine agonist that may be much more suitable for the treatment of patients with CHF. It has been shown in some trials to improve symptomatic well-being in patients treated with diuretics and in patients also taking ACE inhibitors.[16,17] Although it causes selective vasodilatation in the renal vascular bed and despite its natriuretic properties, which are of obvious theoretical importance, it does not appear to be diuretic sparing (R Andrews, personal communication). Its effects on mortality are not known but there

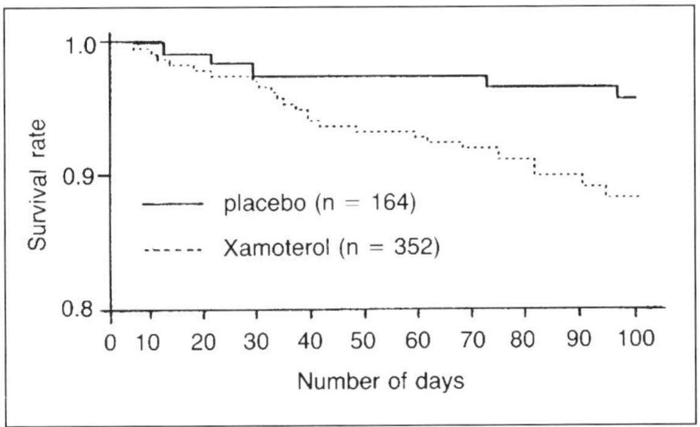

Figure 15.4
Three-month surival probalities for the placebo and xamoterol groups.

is a survival trial currently underway and this should report at the latest by the end of 1996.

Sympathomimetic blocking agents

As it has become apparent that complete and even partial beta-agonism is not beneficial and more likely deleterious in CHF, the emphasis has shifted to beta-blockade to attenuate the long-term effects of sympathetic activation. Following the original uncontrolled observations of possible benefit,[18] the early studies were inconsistent. Larger studies conducted more recently indicate modest benefits in exercise tolerance and symptoms.[19] Even more recently beta-blockers have been developed which cause peripheral vasodilatation by concomitant alpha-blockade, and initial results with these agents is encouraging.

The effect of beta-blockade on mortality is not fully resolved. There was thought to be a reduction in death in patients with dilated cardiomyopathy, but the Metoprolol Dilated Cardiomyopathy (MDC) trial does not confirm this.[20] The evidence for a similar effect in patients with ischaemic heart disease is even less compelling.

Because of the difficulty in initiating treatment and titrating dose, beta-blockade is not a routine treatment for chronic heart failure and in this context the harmful effect of xamoterol, which may have been a 'safe' beta-blocker, are disappointing.

Inotropic agents that act independently of cAMP

Vesnarinone is an inotropic agent whose precise mechanism of action is unclear. It has been shown to improve exercise tolerance and symptomatic well-being. In one study that has evaluated its effects on survival, high doses caused a worsening of survival but low doses had the opposite effect, prolonging life expectancy

	Deaths
60 mg daily	3
120 mg daily	16*
Placebo	6

*p = 0.01

Table 15.2
The effects of vesnarinone on survival. (253 patients randomly assigned to receive 60 mg daily, 120 mg daily, or placebo.)

(Table 15.2).[21] This result is even more curious in that the beneficial effect of vesnarinone occurs at doses that do not have any haemodynamic effects. A possible explanation for this rather implausible result is that vesnarinone has an antiarrhythmic effect similar to class III antiarrhythmic agents. However, the reduction in mortality was from both sudden death and progressive heart failure, and it therefore presumably cannot be due to the simple reduction in life-threatening arrhythmias. One potentially serious side-effect is that it causes reversible white cell depression.

Pimobendan is said, in addition to having cAMP phosphodiesterase properties, to sensitize the cellular contractile apparatus to calcium. This will also cause increased inotropic activity but more efficiently than by increasing cAMP levels. It has been shown to improve symptoms and exercise tolerance after short-term and long-term administration and interestingly appears more effective at low doses.[22]

Direct acting vasodilators

Flosequinan

Flosequinan, a direct acting vasodilator thought to produce smooth muscle relaxation by inhibition of the inositide trisphosphate pathway, has also recently been withdrawn because of an

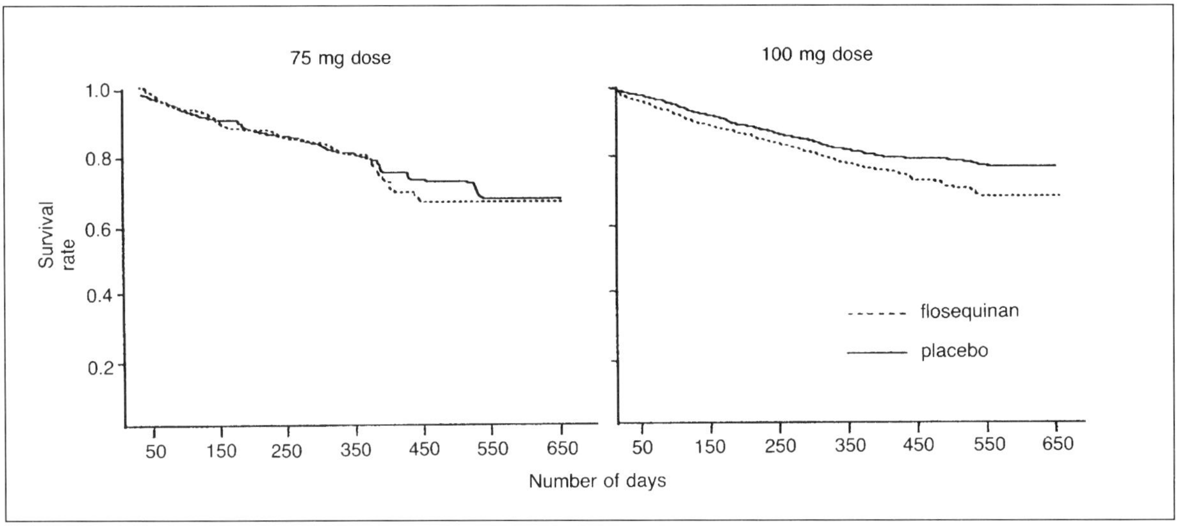

Figure 15.5
Profile – preliminary analysis (Boots Pharmaceuticals).

adverse effect on survival. Two doses of flosequinan were used in the trial, 100 mg and 75 mg daily, and the adverse effect was only apparent at the higher dose with no obvious harmful effect at the lower dose (Fig. 15.5) (unpublished data, Boots Pharmaceuticals). This is similar to other studies that have shown harm at the top end of the therapeutic dose range but not at lower doses. In view of the long pharmacological half-life of flosequinan (approximately 36 hours), it is possible that accumulation of the drug occurred during long-term administration. At high doses, flosequinan inhibits cAMP phosphodiesterase and therefore may have similar effects to milrinone and enoximone. Preliminary reports suggest that the adverse effect was confined to those patients with impaired renal function, which would support the idea of drug accumulation as being responsible.

Unlike the PROMISE trial[10] the reduced survival appeared to be due to progression of heart failure and not sudden death. This suggests that the mechanism was different from that of milrinone, and that inhibition of cAMP phophodiesterase may not be the cause of the reduced survival. The differentiation between sudden death and death due to progressive heart failure can be difficult but, if this difference is real, the precise cause of the excess mortality is not and probably will not be known.

Despite the detrimental effect of flosequinan on survival, there is considerable evidence that it leads to an improvement in symptomatic well-being. Initial studies showed a consistent and sustained improvement in central haemodynamic variables. Furthermore, the improved cardiac output seems, at least in part, to be directed to the limb and therefore to skeletal muscle.[23] As skeletal muscle blood flow is a major determinant of exercise capability, flosequinan should increase treadmill exercise capability.

A number of placebo-controlled, blinded studies have evaluated the effects of flosequinan in patients taking diuretics only. It has been shown to improve various measures of symptomatic well-being, including treadmill exercise capability.[24] Compared with placebo it has also been shown to improve corridor walk tests and New York Heart Association (NYHA) classification.

Several studies have also directly compared it with ACE inhibitors in patients taking diuretics and shown comparability if not superiority. One study compared its effects with enalapril over a comparatively short time and showed a greater improvement in exercise capability and other measures of symptomatic well-being than with the ACE inhibitor.[25]

Another study compared it with captopril over a much longer 12-month period. At the end of the study, there was a similar improvement in exercise capacity with both drugs but during the trial there was a higher withdrawal rate in those patients who received flosequinan.[26] The doses of flosequinan used in the study were again high and most of the withdrawals were due to side-effects that were probably caused by smooth muscle relaxation. In particular these were headache caused by dilatation of the cerebral vessels and nausea, which occurred either because of a central effect or because of relaxation of the smooth muscle of the gut. In terms of symptomatic well-being, flosequinan seems to be as effective as ACE inhibitors both in the short term and over longer periods, and it does not seem to induce tolerance.

Other clinical trials have also evaluated the effects of flosequinan in patients already established on ACE inhibitors. In one study, exercise capability improved in the actively treated group whereas there was little change in those patients treated with placebo.[27] In another study there was a clear trend to improved symptom limited exercise time and a significant improvement in NYHA class in those who received active therapy. Quality of life or other measures of symptomatic well-being were not measured.

Flosequinan would therefore appear to improve exercise tolerance, if not other measures of symptomatic well-being, in patients taking conventional therapy including ACE inhibitors. At high doses it has an adverse effect on survival which is not obvious at lower doses.

Calcium antagonists

The role of calcium antagonists in heart failure remains to be clearly defined. The first generation of calcium antagonists, verapamil, nifedipine and diltiazem, are harmful and cause a deterioration in symptoms and probably a reduction in survival, most likely due to the negative inotropic action of the agents.

The newer calcium antagonists, amlodipine and felodipine, have less negative inotropy and do not stimulate neurohumoral mechanisms.[28,29] Their effects on symptoms and exercise tolerance remain inconsistent, and small uncontrolled studies of felodipine show apparent benefit not observed in the controlled trials.[30] One large study with amlodipine has shown an improvement in exercise tolerance in patients taking diuretics, digoxin, and ACE inhibitors. Another somewhat smaller study has failed to show any benefit with a number of different exercise tests, or in changes in central and regional haemodynamics, or in skeletal muscle metabolism (J Walsh, personal communication). Although calcium antagonists may not necessarily improve symptomatic well-being, they do not appear to cause harm and may be useful in patients with concomitant angina.

Their effect on mortality is currently being investigated.

New innovative compounds

A number of new innovative compounds are in the process of being developed. The most advanced and exciting of these are the angiotensin II receptor antagonists and neutral endopeptidase inhibitors.

What lessons should we learn?

So what does all this mean and what should we learn from the trials that showed reduction in survival? The starting point is to decide what we are trying to achieve in treating patients with heart failure. Do we want the only goal to be improvement in survival or are there equally or more important aims? We must remember that heart failure is a disease predominantly of the elderly. Data from Framingham suggest an annual incidence of 1 in 100 in 75-year-olds and 1 in a little under 10 in 85-year-olds.[31] The majority of patients with heart failure, therefore, are not those who were included in the clinical trials. The wishes of these patients and their expectations from treatment may not be for longer survival but they may prefer to maintain their independence, avoid long-term hospitalization and experience reduced symptoms and improved quality of life at the expense of reduced survival. These expectations may be entirely different from those of a young person with comparatively mild symptoms whose major desire is a prolongation of life.

Symptoms or survival?

Effective drug treatment may improve either of these two endpoints and may even do so at the expense of the other. Until recently, our belief has been that there are so many drugs available that we need only accept those which have a favourable effect on both quality and duration of life. With the aid of hindsight this is no longer the case and we must be quite clear what our aims are in any individual patient. Having established this, it becomes obvious that some of the agents that have been discarded still have an important place in the treatment of some patients. Although these drugs cannot be resurrected we must be sure not to make the same mistake again. There is a very important place for a drug that improves well-being at the possible expense of reduced survival, particularly in severely symptomatic elderly patients.

Assessment of benefit

We must then address the question of whether there are better ways of assessing new treatments as they become available. A decade ago the major, if not only, aim of treatment was to improve central haemodynamic variables. We now believe, however, that these tell us little about symptomatic impairment or improvement in response to treatment. The reason for this is that there is no correlation with symptom-limited exercise tolerance or changes in symptom-limited exercise tolerance measured in the laboratory. This type of exercise test seems to be much more dependent on local skeletal muscle blood flow than on central haemodynamics.[32] But in view of what we know about the epidemiology of heart failure, is this the best way of measuring symptomatic impairment? Many elderly patients will be incapable of this type of exercise and even in younger patients, exercising in the tightly controlled environment of the laboratory may not tell us anything about symptoms during daily life. Other ways of assessing exercise capability are needed which are more applicable to all patients and are more indicative of exercise intolerance during normal daily activities.

Corridor walk tests and measures of daily customary activity are likely to be much better indicators of symptomatic impairment and should be used more frequently. If this type of activity is measured, there are correlations with cardiac output, which suggests that it is more important in determining normal activity than it is in influencing laboratory-based symptom-limited tests.[33] Presumably cardiac output may have subtle and yet undetermined effects on motivation and depression, which are important in determining self-paced tests and customary activity.

Measurement of quality of life includes all aspects of patients' life styles and is of obvious importance. The measurement of quality of life has not attracted much attention in trials. There may be a number of reasons for this, including lack of objectivity (quality of life is by definition subjective) and difficulties in identifying the best questionnaire. A number of questionnaires have now been used and are capable of showing changes in response to treatment. It is to be hoped that measurement of quality of life will receive much more attention in the future.

How to choose the dose?

Having questioned the methods used to assess treatments, should we also question the methods used to arrive at the therapeutic doses of treatment? Neurohumoral activation is believed to be harmful. Inhibition or blockade of these systems should be as complete as the patient can tolerate. The doses of ACE inhibitors and beta-blocking agents should therefore be high and the doses titrated up to the maximum. Conversely the doses of drugs that do not block the neurohumoral systems – inotropic agents and direct acting vasodilators – should be lower to produce an effect but not cause further neurohumoral activation. This may be the minimum effective dose. Using this type of approach the trials of milrinone, enoximone, and flosequinan may have produced different results. It is also possible that low doses of two different agents (e.g. an inotrope and a calcium antagonist) may have additive effects.

Do all drugs need to be subjected to a mortality trial?

The last question is whether all drugs for heart failure need to be subjected to a mortality trial? The sensible answer is an emphatic 'no'. The phamaceutical industry cannot and should not be expected to make the huge investment, both in terms of money and the loss of patents, that conducting such studies before a drug is licensed would entail. If companies are expected or even compelled to do so then interest in heart failure will clearly decline. Efficacy must remain the major aim of treatment for the majority of patients and drugs should be granted a licence on the basis of improvement in symptoms. Some data on mortality might then be reasonably expected after a period of, say, 5 years from licensing. We have already 'lost' too many potentially useful drugs and we must not let this happen again.

References

1 Cowley AJ, Fullwood L, Stainer K, Hampton JR. Exercise tolerance in patients with heart failure: how should it be measured? *Eur Heart J* 1991;**12**:50–54.

2 Hoodless DJ, Stainer K, Savic N, Batin P, Hawkins M, Cowley AJ. Reduced customary activity in chronic heart failure: assessment with a new shoe-mounted pedometer. *Int J Cardiol* 1994;**43**:39–42.

3 Stewart AL, Greenfield S, Hays R, et al. Functional status and well being of patients with chronic conditions. *JAMA* 1989; **262**:907–913.

4 The CONSENSUS Trial Study Group. Effects of enalapril on mortality in severe congestive heart failure; results of the Cooperative North Scandinavian Enalapril Survival Study (CONSENSUS). *N Engl J Med* 1987; **316**:1429–1435.

5 The SOLVD Investigators. Effect of enalapril on survival in patients with reduced left ventricular ejection fraction and congestive heart failure. *N Engl J Med* 1991;**325**:293–302.

6 Verel D, Stantiford NH, Rahman F, Saynor R. A clinical trial of frusemide. *Lancet* 1964;**ii**:1088–1092.

7 Cowley AJ, Rowley JM, Stainer K, Hampton JR. Captopril for heart failure: a placebo controlled trial. *Lancet* 1982:**ii**:730–732.

8 Packer M, Gheorghiade M, Siegrist J, Just H, et al, for the RADIANCE Study Group. Withdrawal of digoxin from patients with chronic heart failure treated with angiotensin converting enzyme inhibitors. *N Engl J Med* 1993;**329**:1–7.

9 Packer M, Carver JR, Rodeheffer RJ, et al. Effect of oral milrinone on mortality in severe chronic heart failure. *N Engl J Med* 1991;**325**:1468–1475.

10 Cowley AJ, Skene A. The treatment of severe heart failure: quantity or quality of life? A trial of enoximone. *Br Heart J* 1994;**72**:226–230.

11 Colucci WS, Sonnenblick WH, Adams KF, et al. Chronic efficacy trials of milrinone in combination with converting enzyme inhibitors in patients with moderate congestive heart failure. *J Am Coll Cardiol* 1993;**22**:113–118.

12 McKenna WJ, Swedberg K, Zannad F, et al, on behalf of the FIRST Investigators. Experience of chronic intravenous epoprostenolinfusion in end stage cardiac failure: results of FIRST. *Eur Heart J* 1994;**15**:36S.

13 Liang CS, Sherman LG, Doherty JU, Wellington K, Lee VW, Hood WB. Sustained improvement of cardiac function in patients with congestive heart failure after short term infusion of dobutamine. *Circulation* 1984;**69**:113–119.

14 Dies F, Krell MJ, Whitlow P, et al. Intermittent dobutamine in ambulatory outpatients with chronic heart failure. *Circulation* 1985;**74(suppl II)**:38.

15 1990 Xamoterol in Severe Heart Failure Group. Xamoterol in severe heart failure. *Lancet* 1990;**336**:1–6.

16 Roland E, Sabino F, Cantoni V, Ghirardhi P, Marcketti GV, Cichetti V. Long-term therapy of chronic congestive heart failure with ibopamine: a multicentre trial. *J Cardiovasc Pharmacol* 1989;**14**:S93–S103.

17 Van Veldhuisen DJ, Man in't Veld AJ, Dunselman PHJM, et al. Double-blind placebo-controlled study of ibopamine and digoxin in patients with mild to moderate heart failure: results of the Dutch Ibopamine Multicentre Trial (DIMT). *J Am Coll Cardiol* 1993;**22**:1564–1573.

18 Waagstein F, Hjalmarson A, Varnauskas E, Wallentin I. Effects of chronic beta-adrenergic receptor blockade in congestive cardiomyopathy. *Br Heart J* 1975;**37**:1022–1036.

19 Engeimeier RS, O'Connell JB, Walsh R, Rad N, Scanlon PF, Gunnar RM. Improvement in symptoms and exercise tolerance by metoprolol in patients with dilated cardiomyopathy; a double-blind, randomised, placebo controlled trial. *Circulation* 1985;**72**:536–546.

20 Waagstein F, Bristow MR, Swedberg K, et al. Beneficial effects of metoprolol in idiopathic dilated cardiomyopathy. *Lancet* 1993;**342**: 1441–1446.

21 Feldman MA, Bristow MR, Parmley WW, et al. Effects of vesnarinone on morbidity and mortality in patients with heart failure. *N Engl J Med* 1993;**329**:149–155.

22 Kubo SH, Gollub S, Bourge R, et al. Beneficial effects of pimobendan on exercise tolerance and quality of life in patients with heart failure: results of a multicenter trial. *Circulation* 1992;**85**:942–949.

23 Cowley AJ, Wynne RD, Stainer K, Fullwood L, Rowley JM, Hampton JR. Flosequinan in heart failure: acute haemodynamic and longer term symptomatic effects. *BMJ* 1988;**297**:169–173.

24 Cowley AJ, McEntegart DJ. Placebo-controlled trial of flosequinan in moderate heart failure. The possible importance of aetiology and method of analysis in the interpretation of the results of heart failure trials. *Int J Cardiol* 1993;**38**:167–175.

25 Silke B, Tennet H, Fisher-Hansen N, Keller N, Heikkila J, Salminen K. A double blind, parallel group comparison of flosequinan and enalapril in the treatment of chronic heart failure. *Eur Heart J* 1992;**13**:1092–1100.

26 Cowley AJ, McEntegart DJ, Hampton JR, et al. The long term evaluation of treatment for chronic heart failure: a one year comparative trial of flosequinan and captopril. *Cardiovasc Drugs Ther* 1994;**8**:829–836.

27 Massie BM, Berk MR, Brozena SC, et al. Can further benefit be achieved by adding flosequinan to patients with congestive heart failure who remain symptomatic on diuretic, digoxin and an angiotensin converting enzyme inhibitor? Results of the flosequinan ACE inhibitor trial (FACET). *Circulation* 1993;**88**:492–501.

28 Packer M, Nicod P, Khanderia BR, et al. Randomized, multicenter, double blind, placebo controlled evaluation of amlodipine in patients with mild to moderate heart failure. *J Am Coll Cardiol* 1991;**17**:274A.

29 Timmis AD, Smyth P, Kenny JF, et al. Effects of vasodilator treatment with felodipine on haemodynamic response to treadmill exercise in congestive heart failure. *Br Heart J* 1994;**52**:314–320.

30 Littler WA, Sheridan DJ, on behalf of the UK Study Group. Placebo controlled trial of felodipine in patients with mild to moderate heart failure. *Br Heart J* 1995;**73**:428–433.

31 Kannel WB, Belanger AJ. Epidemiology of heart failure. *Am Heart J* 1991;121:951–957.

32 Cowley AJ, Stainer K, Rowley JM, Hampton JR. Abnormalities of the peripheral circulation and respiratory function in patients with severe heart failure. *Br Heart J* 1986;**55**:75–80.

33 Cowley AJ, Fullwood L, Muller AF, Stainer K, Skene AM, Hampton JR. Exercise capability in heart failure: is cardiac output important after all? *Lancet* 1991;**337**:771–773.

16

Digitalis in the 21st century

Inder S Anand

Introduction

Digitalis has been used in the treatment of heart failure for thousands of years, and even the ancient Indian Ayurvedic texts referred to its usefulness.[1] Around 1000 BC the famous Indian physician Sushruta Chikitsa wrote 'After purification procedures, the patient should be administered aqueous decoction of the roots of yellow oleander (Ashwa Maraka), ratti and kakadani' and 'This medicine either cures patients or kills them'.[2] There is evidence that the Romans also used this drug.[3] It is, therefore, amazing that, having been in use for nearly 3000 years the efficacy of digitalis is still debated despite the fact that scientific investigation into this question began over 200 years ago.[4]

Most clinicians agree that digitalis has a definite role in the management of patients with heart failure complicated by supraventricular tachyarrhythmias such as atrial fibrillation or flutter, where it acts mainly by slowing heart rate.[5,6] However, the role of digitalis in the management of chronic heart failure in patients with sinus rhythm has been seriously questioned. This controversy started at the turn of the century when Sir James Mackenzie, on the basis of his considerable clinical experience in Britain, advocated the use of digoxin only in patients with heart failure in atrial fibrillation.[7] However, his equally experienced counterpart in the United States, Thomas Christian, held the view that digoxin was effective in heart failure irrespective of the rhythm.[8] The views of these stalwarts prevailed in their respective countries for years.

With the introduction of cardiac catheterization, studies from both sides of the Atlantic in the early 1940s showed that digoxin improved hemodynamics of patients with chronic heart failure even in sinus rhythm.[9,10] Later, it was confirmed that the acute positive inotropic effects of digoxin[11] persist chronically without tachyphylaxis.[12] Yet the clinical efficacy of chronic digoxin therapy remained less clear. During the 1970s a number of reports showed that discontinuation or withdrawal of digoxin from patients with chronic heart failure and sinus rhythm did not produce any adverse effects.[13–19] While most of these studies were small and uncontrolled and had serious flaws such as inadequately documented heart failure, they did help to renew interest in the controversy and led to the development of several randomized controlled trials.

An important aspect of these early uncontrolled studies, often not appreciated, is that most patients in these studies were receiving diuretics and or vasodilators. Optimal treatment with diuretics is very effective in normalizing body fluid compartments[20] and this might have confounded any beneficial effects of digoxin that were seen in the earlier studies. Since digoxin has a narrow therapeutic-to-toxic window, it is important to question whether the addition of a potentially toxic drug to patients optimally treated with diuretics and angiotensin converting enzyme (ACE) inhibitors confers any advantage. This is all the more important now, since ACE inhibitors are not only effective in the treatment of chronic heart failure but also prevent the development and progression of heart failure and improve survival.[21–23] In contrast, all the inotropic agents tested so far increase mortality.[24–27]

A proper reassessment of the role of digoxin must take into account the present-day objectives in the management of heart failure:

- to prevent the occurrence of heart failure following the initial myocardial injury;
- to delay progression of the disease;
- to alleviate signs and symptoms and to improve quality of life; and
- to prolong survival.

There is no evidence that digoxin, unlike the ACE inhibitors, has any effect on ventricular remodelling following myocardial infarction[28] – a process that leads to the development of heart failure. On the other hand, there are studies that have shown digoxin to be harmful in the year following myocardial infarction.[29–31] There are also no data to show that digoxin has any effect on the progression of the disease. However, a number of trials have tried to address the question of long-term clinical benefits of digoxin therapy in patients with chronic heart failure. One meta-analysis and several reviews have tried to analyze these trials.[32–35]

This chapter analyzes all the randomized trials that have used a double-blind, placebo-controlled design in patients with well-defined chronic heart failure, systolic dysfunction, and sinus rhythm. A special effort will be made to see whether the two most recent trials (PROVED[36] and RADIANCE[37]) have been able to end the digoxin controversy and to redefine its role for the 21st century.

Randomized placebo-controlled trials

During the last 15 years there have been eight small single-center and seven large multicenter randomized, double-blind, placebo-controlled trials of digoxin in chronic heart failure (Table 16.1). These trials enrolled patients with mild to moderate heart failure with systolic dysfunction who were in sinus rhythm. Most patients tested were being treated with diuretics, some were receiving vasodilators (ACE inhibitors in only one study) but many had received digoxin before being randomized. Therefore, most of these are drug withdrawal studies.

Small single center trials

Dobbs et al[38] were the first to report the results of a placebo-controlled, double-blind, crossover trial with digoxin. They investigated 46 patients receiving long-term digoxin therapy. Patients were randomly allocated to receive either digoxin or placebo, and after 6 weeks they were crossed over to the alternate treatment. Sixteen of the 46 patients deteriorated on placebo but only eight of these improved when digoxin was reintroduced. In the remainder, additional diuretics were required to control heart failure. Unfortunately, there are a number of problems with this study: 10 patients had cor pulmonale and only 60% of the patients were receiving diuretics. Moreover, 13 patients were in atrial fibrillation and it is not made clear whether only those patients with atrial fibrillation deteriorated. The authors concluded that digoxin was an effective drug.

In 1982, Lee et al[39] studied 25 patients using a crossover design. During the lead-in period the dose of diuretics was adjusted until the weight, symptoms and signs were stable. All but three patients were receiving diuretics; six patients were also receiving a vasodilator but

Trials	No. of patients	Design	Duration (wk)	NYHA class	EF (%)	Digoxin level (ng/ml)	Concomitant therapy (% patients) Diur	Vaso	ACE	Ex capacity	% Change in EF from baseline	Worsening HF. (%) P	D	Overall clinical benefit
Small single center trials														
Dobbs et al[38]	46	CO/DW	6	NA	Not done	0.9	60	0	0	Not done	Not done	34	0*	Yes but flawed study
Lee et al[39]	25	CO/DW	9	II to III	29	1.15	88	24	0	Not done	No change	56	24*	Yes in selected patients
Fleg et al[40]	30	CO/DW	12	II to III	23(FS)	1.4	76	16	0	No change	↓9%(V_{cf})P*	10	10	No
Taggart et al[41]	22	CO/DW	12	I to II	Not done	1.2	95	35	0	Not done	↓5%(STI)P*	18	10	No
Guyatt et al[42]	20	CO/DW	7	II to III	19(FS)	1.75	90	55	0	↑5% D*	↓19%(FS)P*	35	0*	Yes
Pugh et al[43]	44	CO/DW	8	NA	28(FS)	0.8	75	9	0	Not done	↓(STI)P*	25	11*	Yes
Fleg et al[45]	10	CO/DW	4	II to III	33	1.4	100	41	0	No change	↓16%P* on ex	0	0	No
Haerer et al[46]	28	PA/DI	3	II to III	25(FS)	1.8	0	0	0	Not done	↓(FS)D*	–	–	Not evaluated
Large multicenter trials														
Captopril-Digoxin[47]	196	PA/DW	24	II to III	25	0.7	84	0	0	No change	↑16%D*	29	15*	Yes
Xamoterol[48]	213	PA	12	II to III	Not done	0.9	25	10	0	No change	Not done	6	4	No
DiBianco et al[49]	111	PA/DW	12	II to III	25	1.1	100	48	0	↑14% D*	↑3.4%D*	47	15*	Yes but flawed study
Just et al[50]	133	PA	52	II	50	NA	0	0	0	No change	Not done	NA	NA	Yes even with good EF
DIMT[51]	108	PA	26	II to III	28	0.9	0	0	0	↓12% P*	Not done	4	0	No
PROVED[36]	88	PA/DW	12	II to III	27	1.2	100	0	0	↓18% P*	↓10%P*	39	19*	Yes
RADIANCE[37]	178	PA/DW	12	II to III	26	1.2	100	0	100	↓7.5% P*	↓13%P*	25	5*	Yes

Table 16.1

*Randomized, double-blind, placebo-controlled trials of digoxin in heart failure. Diur – diuretics; Vaso – vasodilators; ACE – angiotensin converting enzyme inhibitors; D – digoxin; P – placebo; CO – crossover; DW – digoxin withdrawal; NA – not available; PA – parallel design; DI – digoxin introduction; FS – fraction shortening by echocardiography; V_{cf} – velocity of circumferential fiber shortening; STI – systolic time intervals; ex – exercise; HF – heart failure; * – $p < 0.05$ placebo vs digoxin.)*

ACE inhibitors were not used. Although the mean ejection fraction was 29%, six patients had ejection fractions over 50%. Using a scoring system that evaluated symptoms, signs, cardiac dimension on chest X-ray and echocardiogram, the study showed that 14 of the 19 patients with ejection fractions under 50% improved with digoxin therapy. All 14 patients who improved had a third heart sound, compared with only one of the 11 patients who did not improve. Six patients underwent right heart catheterization during both placebo and digoxin phases. Four of these six patients responded to digoxin and all had high pulmonary wedge pressures. Digoxin did not improve the ejection fraction but it did decrease the cardiac size on chest X-ray and reduce left ventricular diastolic dimension on echocardiography. The authors concluded that, although digoxin was useful, only those patients who have a third heart sound or raised pulmonary wedge pressures respond to it. Another interpretation of this study might be that patients who responded to digoxin were inadequately treated and that optimal treatment with diuretics and vasodilators might have improved them to an extent where digoxin would have had no effect.

Fleg et al[40] reported their observations on 30 patients with NYHA class II to class III heart failure in a double-blind digoxin withdrawal protocol. Only 76% of the patients were taking diuretics, 16% received vasodilators, and none received an ACE inhibitor. Digoxin withdrawal caused only a small increase in left ventricular end-diastolic diameter and a small decrease in velocity of circumferential shortening by echocardiography, but there was no change in exercise capacity or clinical status over a 3-month period. In 17 of the 30 patients, digoxin was not given for the next 18 months and no deterioration in heart failure was noted.

In a similarly designed trial, Taggart et al[41] also found that digoxin withdrawal had no significant effect on the clinical end points in the majority of 22 patients with mild heart failure (NYHA class I to class II, all except one patient on diuretics) although there was a small but significant improvement in the non-invasive indices of left ventricular performance on digoxin. The authors concluded that, although digoxin had a sustained positive inotropic effect during maintenance therapy, no clinical benefit was seen.

Guyatt et al[42] studied 20 patients with chronic mild to moderate heart failure in a placebo-controlled crossover trial. All patients had digoxin dose titrated to attain serum levels between 1.54 and 2.56 nmol/l during the prerandomization phase. Ninety per cent of the patients were taking diuretics and 55% were receiving a vasodilator other than an ACE inhibitor. Seven out of 20 patients required premature termination of the study because of progressive symptoms during the placebo phase, but none deteriorated while taking digoxin. In addition, dyspnoea, clinical heart failure score, 6-minute walk test, heart size on chest X-ray, and echocardiographic fractional shortening were significantly better during the digoxin phase.

In 1989, Pugh et al[43] reported the results of a double-blind placebo-controlled, crossover study of digoxin withdrawal and reintroduction in 44 patients with mild to moderate heart failure. Over a period of 2 months, digoxin withdrawal caused clinical deterioration in a significantly greater number of patients (25%) than digoxin treatment (11%). However, worsening heart failure could be controlled by increasing diuretics in all but two (5%) of these patients. Deterioration during digoxin withdrawal was accompanied by decrease in some indices of contractility (systolic time intervals) but not in others (echocardiographic).

Importantly, administration of diuretics during deterioration was also able to reverse these indices. Moreover, reintroduction of digitalis after increasing diuretic therapy did not further improve contractility. The authors concluded that diuretics are often successful in relieving symptoms in patients who deteriorate following digoxin withdrawal, and digitalis has little to offer in way of additional inotropic support in these patients. There was another interesting finding in this study: patients who did not deteriorate when digoxin was withdrawn showed no change in their digoxin (Na^+–K^+ ATPase) binding sites on erythrocytes or in rubidium-86 uptake (a measure of Na^+ ion transport) and the intracellular Na^+ in red cells did not change. However, 1 week after reintroduction of digoxin the number of binding sites and the rubidium-86 uptake first fell and then rose again after 8 weeks of continuous therapy, suggesting pharmacological tolerance. In contrast, patients who deteriorated after digoxin withdrawal showed an increase in both the number of digoxin binding sites and rubidium-86 transport, which returned to pre-withdrawal values after 8 weeks of digoxin withdrawal. These findings suggest that patients who do not deteriorate on digoxin withdrawal may be the ones who develop tolerance to digoxin, a finding also reported in an earlier study.[44] Thus, the effects of digoxin may vary from patient to patient, and more needs to be learned about the different ways by which the myocardium adapts to long-term treatment with digoxin.

Fleg et al[45] in another randomized placebo-controlled crossover trial studied 10 patients with heart failure having ejection fractions of 32 ± 12%. The study was carried out over a short period of only 4 weeks in patients with relatively mild heart failure. Digoxin had no effect on exercise capacity, peak oxygen consumption or any other indices of gas exchange. There was no change in ejection fraction at rest but ejection fraction at peak exercise was less on placebo than digoxin.

The above studies used the drug withdrawal design and, as will be seen later, these protocols have considerable problems with interpretation. Haerer et al[46] in 1988 reported the first trial ever to study the effect of introducing digoxin (28 patients, NYHA class II to class III), who were not taking any other cardiac medication and were randomized to digoxin, diuretics, or placebo. Unfortunately, complete details of this study are not available and it has only appeared in abstract form. Nevertheless, the data show that 3 weeks of treatment with digoxin decreased pulmonary capillary wedge pressure, reduced ventricular diameter, and increased the echocardiographic indices of myocardial contractility, whereas placebo treatment increased wedge pressure and did not change cardiac dimensions or contractility.

Large multicenter trials

Since 1988 there have been seven large multicenter randomized placebo-controlled digoxin trials. The captopril–digoxin trial[47] compared captopril, digoxin, and placebo in 300 patients, 84% of whom were on diuretics and 65% of whom had been on long-term digoxin. During the pre-randomization period digoxin and vasodilators were stopped but diuretics were continued. Digoxin increased ejection fraction (4.4 percentage points), but had no effect on exercise capacity or NYHA class. Worsening heart failure (hospitalization, emergency room visits, or increased diuretic requirement) occurred more often in the placebo-treated patients (29%) than in the digoxin group (15%, $p < 0.05$). This occurred despite considerable bias against digoxin, because 30 patients could not tolerate withdrawal of digoxin during the pre-randomization phase and so were not randomized.

In the German–Austrian Xamoterol trial[48] 433 patients with mild to moderate symptoms of heart failure but without any objective documentation of left ventricular systolic dysfunction were randomized to digoxin, xamoterol, or placebo. After 3 months, as compared to placebo, patients on digoxin therapy had improvement in some symptoms and signs of heart failure using the Likert scale, but there was no effect on exercise capacity. The study was seriously flawed because the extent of left ventricular dysfunction was not defined, 25% of the patients were in NYHA class I, and an equal number were not taking diuretics.

DiBianco et al[49] reported the results of the Milrinone Multicenter trial in 1989. In this trial, 230 patients with an average ejection fraction of 25% were stabilized on diuretics and digitalis for 4–8 weeks and then randomized to digoxin, placebo, milrinone alone, or digoxin and milrinone combination. The digoxin group remained on an uninterrupted regimen of digoxin and diuretics. The placebo group was treated with diuretics alone. Milrinone was substituted for digoxin in the milrinone group and was added to digoxin in the combination group. It is interesting that in the digoxin continuation group, the ejection fraction and exercise capacity increased significantly during the 12-week follow-up period, whereas exercise capacity remained unchanged in the placebo group. This unexpected increase in ejection fraction and exercise capacity in the digoxin group despite there being no change in therapy is difficult to explain. The ejection fraction fell, however, and there were more treatment failures in the placebo group (18%) than in the digoxin group (3%).

The Captopril and Digoxin Study (CADS)[50] evaluated the effects of captopril (25 mg twice a day), digoxin (0.25 mg/day), and placebo in 222 patients in a multicenter double-blind placebo-controlled trial. This study included patients, at least 2 months following myocardial infarction, who had regional wall motion abnormalities but well-preserved global ejection fraction (about 50% or more). They had symptoms of mild heart failure (NYHA class IIA and class IIB) when taken off all medication but were asymptomatic otherwise. Patients were randomized to digoxin, captopril, or placebo after all drugs had been discontinued for a 14-day run-in period. After 1 year, digoxin improved the NYHA class in 45% of the patients compared to 25% of the patients on placebo. The symptoms and quality of life also improved with digoxin compared to placebo ($p < 0.05$), but exercise tolerance did not change in either group.

In the Dutch Ibopamine Multicenter Trial (DIMT),[51] 161 patients with mild to moderate heart failure, treated with diuretics alone, were randomized to digoxin, ibopamine (dopamine agonist), or placebo. After 6 months, the exercise capacity in the digoxin group was significantly higher than in the placebo group only by intention-to-treat analysis. The incidence of worsening heart failure was no different from the placebo group.

Although many of the above trials were well performed, there were wide variations in study design. Many were of short duration or small sample size, lacked objective criteria of left ventricular systolic dysfunction, and lacked optimization of medical therapy before randomization, especially with ACE inhibitors. This left doubts about the role of digitalis in the present day management of patients with chronic heart failure. Nevertheless, the data from these withdrawal studies make it clear that digitalis has long-term inotropic effects. The non-invasive indices of contractility were better in those treated with digoxin than in placebo groups in all studies where these indices were measured. However, clear beneficial *clinical* effects of positive inotropy were seen in only half the studies.

Moreover, these effects appeared to be small and were seen only in a selected group of patients, particularly those who had cardiomegaly, third heart sound, and signs of fluid retention (i.e. probably those not optimally treated with diuretics). A convincing increase in exercise capacity was seen in only three of the eight trials in which it was measured.

PROVED and RADIANCE trials

In order to address some of the abovementioned deficiencies and also to answer the important question as to whether digoxin confers an additional benefit in patients optimally treated with diuretics and ACE inhibitors, two model clinical trials – PROVED[36] and RADIANCE[37] – were recently completed. These companion trials had an identical design, except that in the PROVED trial the effect of digoxin withdrawal was tested on patients receiving a background therapy with diuretics alone, whereas in the RADIANCE trial the effect of digoxin withdrawal was tested on patients receiving optimal treatment with both diuretics and ACE inhibitors. Both trials were randomized, double-blind, placebo-controlled, withdrawal studies in patients with chronic heart failure (NYHA class II and class III). Only patients with systolic dysfunction in sinus rhythm with ejection fractions less than 35%, echocardiographic left ventricular end-diastolic dimension greater than 60 mm, and reduced exercise capacity on treadmill test were randomized (Table 16.2). Eligible patients underwent an 8-week single blind phase during which digoxin dose was adjusted to achieve serum digoxin levels of 0.9–2.0 ng/ml. Patients were required to remain stable on their medication for at least 4 weeks before randomization. After 8 weeks of single blind phase, patients were randomized to continue digoxin (digoxin group) or to discontinue digoxin (placebo group). All patients in the PROVED trial were maintained on constant doses of diuretics whereas patients in the RADIANCE trial were on a constant dose of diuretic and ACE inhibitors. Treatment lasted 12 weeks and patients were seen every 2 weeks. Clinical evaluation by a physician, evaluation by the patient of his own progress, a maximal treadmill exercise test, a 6-minute walk test, quality of life assessment by the Minnesota Living with Heart Failure questionnaire,[52] left ventricular dimensions by echocardiography, ejection fraction by radionuclide gated blood pool imaging and a clinico-radiological heart failure score were assessed at intervals. Primary end points for both studies were:

1. incidence of treatment failure (increase or change in medical therapy, emergency room visits, hospitalization for heart failure or death);
2. time to treatment failure;
3. maximal treadmill exercise time; and
4. distance covered in the 6-minute walk test. Secondary end points included change in signs and symptoms, response to the quality of life questionnaire, heart failure score, evaluation of progress by the patient, left ventricular ejection fraction and dimensions, heart rate, blood pressure, and body weight (Table 16.3).

The PROVED trial was stopped prematurely after only 88 patients were randomized because of difficulty in finding patients who were not taking ACE inhibitors. There were 46 patients in the placebo group and 42 patients in the digoxin group. The RADIANCE trial randomized 178 patients, 93 to placebo and 85 to digoxin. The demographic variables of patients in both trials are shown in

	PROVED		RADIANCE	
	Placebo (n=46)	Digoxin (n=42)	Placebo (n=93)	Digoxin (n=85)
Age (years)	64 ± 2	64 ± 2	59 ± 1	61 ± 1
Sex (males %)	77	90	81	70
Etiology (ICM/non-ICM, %)	67/33	60/40	56/44	65/35
Duration of heart failure (years)	3.1 ± 0.5	3.6 ± 0.5	–	–
NYHA class II/III (%)	83/17	83/17	75/25	71/29
Heart rate (beats/min)	73 ± 1	73 ± 2	78 ± 1	77 ± 1
JVD (% patients)	22	45	–	
CTR (%)	50 ± 0.01	50 ± 0.01	53 ± 0.01	54 ± 0.01
LVEF (%)	29 ± 2	27 ± 1	28 ± 1	26 ± 1
LVEDD (mm)	67 ± 1	67 ± 1	67 ± 1	69 ± 1
Median treadmill time (sec)	540	494	571	510
Average digoxin dose (mg)	0.375	0.375	0.4	0.37
Digoxin level (ng/ml)	1.1 ± 0.05	1.2 ± 0.05	1.1 ± 0.03	1.2 ± 0.03
Average daily captopril dose (mg)	–	–	73	77
Average daily enalapril dose (mg)	–	–	13	17

Table 16.2
Comparison of patient characteristics in PROVED and RADIANCE trials. (ICM – ischemic cardiomyopathy; non-ICM – dilated cardiomyopathy, hypertension and end stage valve disease; JVD – jugular venous distension; CTR – cardiothoracic ratio; LVEF – left ventricular ejection fraction; LVEDD – left ventricular dimension in diastole.)

Table 16.2. While pretreatment characteristics in the placebo and digoxin groups were well matched in the RADIANCE trial, there was a higher incidence of jugular venous distention in the digoxin (45%) than in the placebo group (22%, $p = 0.02$) in the PROVED trial. Although a statistical comparison of patient characteristics between the two trials cannot be made, they appear to be fairly similar except perhaps for a greater percentage of NYHA class III patients in the RADIANCE trial. The RADIANCE patients, as shown in Table 16.2, were on adequate doses of ACE inhibitors. Unfortunately, the dose of diuretics used was not reported in either trial, making it difficult to assess whether PROVED patients had to be stabilized on higher doses of diuretics than the RADIANCE patients.

In the RADIANCE trial, significant deterioration in all four primary end points was seen more in the placebo group than the digoxin group (see Table 16.3). The most striking difference was in the incidence of treatment failure (placebo 25% *vs* digoxin 5%). Deterioration of NYHA class, quality of life, chronic heart failure score and patients own evaluation of progress was also significantly worse in the placebo group. In addition, left ventricular ejection fraction decreased more and left ventricular dimensions, heart rate, and body weight increased by

	PROVED		RADIANCE	
	Placebo (n=46)	Digoxin (n=42)	Placebo (n=93)	Digoxin (n=85)
Primary endpoints				
Treadmill time	↓18%	↑1%‡	↓7.5%	No change†
6-minute walk distance	No difference		↓11%	No change*
Incidence of treatment failure	39%	19%†	25%	5%*
Time to treatment failure	Significantly less in placebo		Significantly less in placebo	
Secondary endpoints				
Increase in signs and symptoms of CHF	No difference		38%	18%†
Quality of life	No difference		↓48%, ↑33%	↓41%, ↑47%†
CHF score (increase in NYHA class)	No difference		27%	10%†
Global evaluation (assessed by patient)	No difference		↓31%	↓9%*
LVEF	↓10%	↑7%†	↓13%	↓4.0%*
LVEDD	No change	No change	↑3%	↓1.5%†
Heart rate	↑15%	No change‡	↑9%	No change*
Body weight	↑0.6%	↓1%†	↑1%	↓1%*

Table 16.3
*Comparison of primary and secondary end points in PROVED and RADIANCE trials. (LVEF – left ventricular ejection fraction; LVEDD – left ventricular dimension in diastole; * – $p < 0.001$ placebo vs. digoxin group; ‡ – $p < 0.01$ placebo vs digoxin group; † – $p < 0.05$ placebo vs. digoxin group.)*

a greater extent in the placebo group. In the PROVED trial, all four primary end points except for the 6-minute walk test showed significant differences between placebo and digoxin. There was also a significant decrease in ejection fraction, increase in heart rate, and increase in body weight in placebo compared to digoxin. However, no significant differences were seen in the NYHA class, quality of life, chronic heart failure score or patient's own evaluation of progress. There was only one episode of digoxin toxicity in the RADIANCE and none in the PROVED trial, despite use of relatively high doses of digoxin (0.375 mg/day in PROVED and 0.370 mg/day in RADIANCE).

It is interesting to compare the results of these two trials in an attempt at better defining the role of digoxin during background treatment with ACE inhibitors (see Table 16.3). Although the incidence of treatment failure was significantly higher in the placebo group than in the digoxin group for both trials, a far greater number of patients in both the placebo and digoxin groups had treatment failure in the PROVED trial (39% and 19%) compared to the RADIANCE trial (25% and 5%). It is likely that this difference was due to the additional beneficial effect of ACE inhibitors in the RADIANCE patients. The fact that significant clinical deterioration in heart failure occurred on withdrawal of digoxin in the RADIANCE trial suggests that ACE inhibitor therapy, in moderate doses, is unable to prevent worsening heart failure when digoxin is withdrawn. Alternatively, it could be argued that these patients were not treated with optimal doses of ACE inhibitors and diuretics.

Another interesting observation in these trials was that the curves relating the incidence of treatment failure continued to diverge throughout the 12-week study period. The reason for this is not clear since tissue stores of digoxin are known to clear from the body much earlier than the duration of this study.[53] This finding also underscores the importance of performing trials with a long duration of follow-up because trials of shorter duration may miss clinical deterioration seen with withdrawal of digoxin.

In summary, these two well-designed companion trials were able to overcome many of the problems of previous studies. They demonstrate that patients with mild to moderate chronic heart failure due to left ventricular systolic dysfunction who are clinically stable on either maintenance therapy of digoxin and diuretics (PROVED), or with additional background therapy with ACE inhibitors (RADIANCE), are at considerable risk of clinical deterioration if digoxin is withdrawn. The problem remains, however, that because these were withdrawal studies, they did not answer the important clinical question of whether or not initiation of digitalis therapy in patients optimally treated with maximally tolerated doses of diuretics and ACE ihibitors further improves clinical state, functional capacity, and survival.

Comparison of digoxin with ACE inhibitors

ACE inhibitors are clearly indicated in the treatment of all stages of chronic heart failure, making it most important to compare digoxin with ACE inhibitors. There are six randomized trials that have compared digoxin with an ACE inhibitor using either a placebo or non-placebo protocol (Table 16.4). Some of the placebo-controlled trials have been described above.

Alicandri et al[54] compared captopril with digoxin in 16 patients with NYHA class II to class III heart failure in a single-blind, crossover trial. All patients were receiving diuretics and digoxin when admitted to the trial. During a 5–10 day lead-in period, digoxin was stopped but diuretics were continued. Patients were then randomized to captopril or digoxin for 30 days. At the end of this period, a 5–10 day washout period was allowed before starting the alternate therapy for another 30 days. Both drugs increased exercise duration, non-invasive indices of contractility, and plasma neurohormones to the same extent.

In the previously described captopril–digoxin trial,[47] digoxin produced a significant increase in ejection fraction while captopril did not. Captopril, on the other hand, significantly increased exercise time whereas digoxin did not. The number of patients who either improved or deteriorated clinically was not significantly different in either group.

Beaune[55] reported the results of the French enalapril versus digoxin trial in 1989. This multicenter, double-blind, parallel group trial compared the effects of enalapril and digoxin on clinical signs, symptoms and exercise capacity in 142 patients with moderately severe congestive heart failure. Patients were stabilized on optimal doses of digoxin and diuretics for 2–4 weeks and then randomly assigned either to continue treatment with digoxin and diuretics or to switch to enalapril and diuretics. After 8 weeks, both groups showed significant and similar improvement in NYHA class and exercise capacity. The reason for improvement in patients who continued to receive digoxin (also seen in the digoxin–milrinone trial) is not clear and raises the question of a training effect. There are other flaws in this trial. About 15–20% patients in this trial had atrial fibrillation. The

Trials	No. of patients	Design	Duration (week)	NYHA Class	Baseline EF (%)	% patients with improvement in heart failure		% patients with worsening heart failure		% increase in ex capacity from baseline		Increase in EF from baseline (percentage points)	
						Digoxin	ACE	Digoxin	ACE	Digoxin	ACE	Digoxin	ACE
Allicandri et al[54]	16	CO/DW	4	II to III	NM	–	–	–	–	27*	36*	↑(STI)*	↑(STI)*
Captopril-Digoxin[47]	200	PA/DW	24	II to III	25	31	41	16	16	9.6	14.3*	4.4*†	1.8
Beaune[55]	142	PA/DW	8	II to IV	NM	28*	35*	–	–	9.4	8.4*	NM	NM
Kromer et al[56]	19	CO‡	6	II	24(FS)	NM	NM	NM	NM	3.8	6.3*	1(FS)	1(FS)
Davies et al[57]	145	PA‡	14	II to III	30	19	18	30	13	12*	8*	5(FS)*	5(FS)*
Herlitz[76]	217	PA¶	12	II to III	<45	16	17	2	5	6.2	11.4*	NM	NM
CADS[50]	129	PA	52	II	50	–	–	NA	NA	3.7	4.1	NM	NM

Table 16.4

*Randomized trials comparing ACE inhibitors with digoxin in heart failure. (EF – ejection fraction; ACE – angiotensin converting enzyme inhibitors; CO – crossover; DW – digoxin withdrawal; PA – parallel design; NM – not measured; STI – systolic time intervals; FS – fraction shortening by echocardiography; Ex – exercise; * – $p < 0.05$ from baseline; † – $p < 0.05$ digoxin vs ACE; ‡ – digoxin withdrawn before randomization in those using it; ¶ – Digoxin naive patients.)*

design of the trial was also unusual, which makes it difficult to separate the effect of initiation of enalapril from the effect of digoxin withdrawal in the enalapril group.

Kromer et al[56] compared digoxin with the ACE inhibitor quinapril in 19 patients with mild (NYHA class II) chronic heart failure using a single-blind crossover protocol. Randomization to active drug was preceded by an 8-week period of fixed treatment with 25 mg hydrochlorothiazide while all other cardiac medication was stopped. Active treatment for 6 weeks was followed by 4 weeks of placebo washout phase and then crossover to the other drug. Six weeks of digoxin therapy had no effect on exercise duration, heart size, plasma norepinephrine or plasma aldosterone levels, while all these parameters improved with quinapril when compared to baseline.

Davies et al[57] reported data from the Canadian enalapril versus digoxin study, which compared the effects of enalapril and digoxin in 145 patients with NYHA class II and class III chronic heart failure. In this trial digoxin was withdrawn from all patients who were receiving it (60%) and these patients were stabilized on frusemide for at least 2 weeks before they were randomized in a double-blind, parallel design to receive digoxin or enalapril for a period of 14 weeks. Exercise capacity and left ventricular fractional shortening improved with both drugs to a similar extent. After 14 weeks, improvement in functional class was similar for both enalapril and digoxin. However, more patients in the digoxin group were withdrawn because of an adverse clinical event.

Herlitz[58] reported the results of the Multicenter Lisinopril–Digoxin study in 1992. They used a double-blind, parallel-group, randomized design to compare lisinopril and digoxin in 217 patients with NYHA class II and class III heart failure with ejection fraction less than 45% who were maintained on diuretics. After 6 weeks, exercise capacity increased significantly with both drugs but by 12 weeks the increase in exercise capacity was no longer significant in the digoxin group. However, the difference in the increase in exercise capacity between lisinopril and digoxin groups was not significant at 12 weeks. Both drugs also showed similar improvement in NYHA class and symptoms of heart failure. Digoxin appeared to be better for improving symptoms and signs of fluid overload.

In the Captopril and Digoxin Study (CADS)[50] described previously, patients with well-preserved ejection fractions (50%) showed greater improvement in symptoms and quality of life with digoxin than captopril, but exercise capacity did not change with either drug after 1 year of treatment.

Taken together, these trials showed that both digoxin and ACE inhibitors confer comparable symptomatic benefit in patients with mild to moderate chronic heart failure and mildly reduced ejection fraction. While captopril increased exercise capacity in all except the CADS trial, digoxin increased exercise capacity in only three of the seven trials. However, digoxin improved ejection fraction in two of the three trials and captopril increased it in only one.

Neurohormonal effects of digoxin

There is increasing evidence that neurohormonal activation seen in congestive heart failure is an important mechanism for progression of the disease.[59] Therefore, agents that reduce neurohormones may be beneficial in heart failure. The high- and low-pressure baroreceptors modulate sympathetic and neurohormonal activity and help to maintain arterial blood pressure.

Whenever systemic blood pressure falls, baroreceptor nerve activity decreases, leading to a reflex increase in sympathetic activity. The result is an increase in the release of renin and arginine vasopressin and a decrease in parasympathetic activity. In chronic heart failure, baroreceptor activity is attenuated because of resetting of baroreceptors, and this contributes to the increase in sympathetic and neurohormonal activation seen in patients with chronic heart failure.[60] It was believed that the inotropic effects of digoxin improve the hemodynamics of patients with heart failure, leading to reflex reduction in sympathetic activity. However, recent evidence from direct recording of baroreceptor[61] and sympathetic neural activity has shown that digitalis can directly stimulate baroreceptor endings, restoring a more normal sympathetic tone.[62]

It is possible that digitalis may have both hemodynamic and direct autonomic modulating effects. Which of these effects is more important in clinical congestive heart failure is under active investigation. At least three studies have recently shown that digitalis decreases the levels of neurohormones in patients with congestive heart failure (Table 16.5). Alicandri et al[54] were the first to show that long-term digoxin treatment decreased plasma norepinephrine in patients with mild to moderate chronic heart failure. In the Dutch Ibopamine Multicenter Trial,[51] digoxin caused a marginal increase in exercise duration at 6 months' follow-up and this was associated with decreased plasma norepinephrine and renin activity. Digoxin also increased heart rate variability at 3 months in these patients, suggesting an improvement in autonomic function.[63] More recently, Krum et al[64] measured plasma norepinephrine and parasympathetic activity from heart rate variability in 27 patients with mild to moderate chronic heart failure before and after 4–8 weeks of digoxin therapy. Digoxin caused a significant decrease in plasma norepinephrine and substantial improvement in parasympathetic activity. However, a number of studies have not confirmed these findings. Kromer et al[56] found that plasma norepinephrine did not change significantly after treatment with digoxin. Gheorghiade et al[65] found that in

Trials	No. of patients	Change in plasma norepinephrine (pg/ml)	
		Placebo	Digoxin
Alicandri et al[54]	16	–	↓113*
Kromer et al[56]	19	–	↑50
DIMT[51]	84	↑62	↓106*
Gheorghiade et al[65]	16	–	↓36
Gheorghiade et al[66]	20	↑127	↓209
Krum et al[64]	27	–	↓162*

Table 16.5
Effect of digoxin on plasma norepinephrine. (– $p < 0.05$ digoxin vs placebo or baseline.)*

optimally treated patients, when the dose of digoxin was increased from 0.2 to 0.4 mg/day, digoxin levels (0.7–1.2 ng/ml) and ejection fraction increased significantly after 6 weeks but that there was no effect on any of the neurohormones. Similarly, digoxin withdrawal did not increase neurohormones significantly in a subset of 11 patients in the RADIANCE trial despite a significant decrease in the ejection fraction.[66] Therefore, firm conclusions about potential direct neurohormonal modulating effects of digoxin cannot be drawn from these studies, and further research in this area is clearly required.

Digitalis dosage

The optimal serum level of digoxin and the need to titrate the dose of digoxin in patients with chronic heart failure has never been adequately addressed. Limited clinical evidence suggests that digitalis augments myocardial contractility in a dose-dependent manner but that there is little additional therapeutic benefit (and a dramatic increase in toxic effects) when digoxin levels are increased beyond 1.5–2.0 ng/ml.[67] Hence, serum digoxin levels of 1.0–2.0 ng/ml have generally been considered optimal. A recent retrospective analysis of the PROVED and RADIANCE trials, however, did not find any significant difference in exercise duration between patients with low (0.5–0.9 ng/ml) or high (over 1.2 ng/ml) serum digoxin levels.[68] Most recent trials have used an average digoxin dose of 0.375 mg/day to achieve serum digoxin levels of 1–2 ng/ml.[36,37] These doses, considered high by usual clinical practice, were not associated with clinical digitalis toxicity. It must be remembered, however, that most of these patients were relatively young and had normal renal function. Lower doses of digoxin may well be adequate to produce comparable levels in older patients with impaired renal function.

Problems with withdrawal trials

A major concern, common to most trials discussed in this chapter, is the problem inherent with the interpretation of withdrawal studies.[69] Such studies address only the question of whether a drug once started should or should not be stopped; they do not answer the question of whether adding a drug to the treatment in the first place confers additional advantage to the patient. In this context it is important to remember that, unlike digoxin trials, all other studies that have tested new inotropic agents have used drug introduction protocols in patients who have never received that experimental drug previously.[26,48,49] These studies have shown that, although most inotropic drugs have short-term beneficial clinical effects, their prolonged use increases mortality.[24–27] Even more interesting is the observation that some patients develop marked clinical deterioration when inotropic drugs like amrinone[70] or flosequinan (M Packer, personal communication) are withdrawn.

One explanation of these findings might be that prolonged administration of these drugs somehow damages the myocardium but that their inotropic effects are sufficiently efficacious to conceal any clinical deterioration while the patient receives the drug. Clinical deterioration seen after cessation may, under such circumstances, provide a measure of harm caused by the drug. A number of inotropic drugs have been shown to hasten myocyte death.[71–73] It is, therefore, entirely possible that deterioration after digoxin withdrawal has a similar mechanism. Another limitation of withdrawal studies is the inherent bias in patient selection. These patients are at least known to tolerate the drug and are, therefore, more likely not only to have a low incidence of adverse reaction but also more likely to benefit from the drug.

Conclusion

This review has summarized most of the randomized, double-blind, placebo-controlled trials of digoxin in patients with chronic heart failure and sinus rhythm. Analysis of these trials leads to two important conclusions:

- digoxin has important long-term inotropic effects which ever way they are measured; and
- the clinical effects of digoxin are not dramatic.

Withdrawal of digoxin causes clinical deterioration in only about a quarter of the patients who have been clinically stable on digoxin and diuretics with or without ACE inhibitors. Patients with more severe heart failure and with evidence of fluid overload fare worse.[39,74] The problem, however, is that these data come mainly from digoxin withdrawal studies. As discussed above, the clinical effect of adding digoxin to patients with chronic heart failure is not necessarily the opposite of withdrawing it. Therefore, two key questions remain unanswered: first, whether introduction of digoxin confers any further benefit to patients who have never received digoxin and who are optimally treated with diuretics and ACE inhibitors; second and perhaps more important, is whether treatment with digoxin prolongs survival as it does with the ACE inhibitors. It is clear from PROVED, RADIANCE, and other trials that treatment failure on placebo could easily be managed by increasing diuretic therapy. A more aggressive diuretic and ACE inhibitor regimen could achieve the same results as digoxin. Addition of a potentially toxic drug like digoxin to therapy in chronic heart failure would, therefore, make sense only if it were also to prolong survival.

It is possible that we may have satisfactory answers to both these questions from the Digitalis Investigators Group (DIG) trial.[75] This mortality trial, sponsored by the National Institutes of Health and Department of Veterans Affairs Cooperative Studies Program, enrolled 7788 patients when randomization ended in August 1994. Of these, 3365 patients were taking digoxin while 4423 patients had never received maintenance digoxin at the time of randomization. We eagerly await the outcome on 3784 of the 4423 patients who had never received digoxin, who had ejection fractions less than 45%, and who were randomized to digoxin or placebo (R Garg, personal communication). The results are scheduled to be announced at the American College of Cardiology Annual Scientific Sessions in March, 1996. Until these results are available it would be prudent to continue using digoxin in all patients with severe chronic heart failure and in those with mild to moderate heart failure who either remain symptomatic on maximally tolerated doses of diuretics and ACE inhibitors or are unable to tolerate these drugs.

References

1 Sharma J. Cardiovascular system and its diseases in the ancient Indian literature. *Indian J Dis* 1986;**9**:32.

2 Yusuf S. Clinical experience in protecting the failing heart. *Clin Cardiol* 1993;**16**:1127–1129.

3 Moore D. William Withering and digitalis. *BMJ* 1985;**290**: 324.

4 Withering W. An account of the foxglove, and some of its medical uses: with practical remarks on dropsy, and other diseases. M Swinney, London, 1785.

5 Shapiro W. Digitalis update. *Arch Intern Med* 1981;**141**:17–18.

6 Anon. A reappraisal of digoxin usage [editorial]. *Drug Ther Bull* 1979;**13**:49–51.

7 MacKenzie J. *Diseases of the Heart*, 3rd edition. Oxford University Press, London, 1913.

8 Christian H. Digitalis effects in chronic cardiac cases with regular rhythm in contrast to auricular fibrillation. *Med Clin North Am* 1922; **5**:1173–1190.

9 Harvey R, Ferrer M, Cathcart R, et al. Some effects of digoxin upon the heart and circulation in man: digoxin in left ventricular failure. *Am J Med* 1949;**7**:439–453.

10 McMichael J, Sharpey-Schafer E. The action of intravenous digoxin in man. *Q J Med* 1944; **13**:123–135.

11 Gheorghiade M, Hall V, Lekier J, et al. Comparative hemodynamic and neurohormonal effects of intravenous captopril and digoxin and their combinations in patients with severe heart failure. *J Am Coll Cardiol* 1989;**13**:134–142.

12 Arnold S, Bird R, Meister W, et al. Long-term digitalis therapy improves left ventricular function in heart failure. *N Engl J Med* 1980; **303**:1443–1448.

13 Starr I, Luchi R. Blind study of the action of digitoxin on elderly women. *Am Heart J* 1969;**78**:740–751.

14 Johnston G, McDevitt D. Is maintenance digoxin necessary in patients with sinus rhythm? *Lancet* 1979;**i**:567–570.

15 Dall J. Maintenance digoxin in elderly patients. *BMJ* 1970;**2**:705–706.

16 Krakauer R, Petersen B. The effects of discontinuing maintenance digoxin therapy. *Dan Med Bull* 1979;**26**:10–13.

17 Hull S, Mackintosh A. Discontinuation of maintenance digoxin therapy in general practice. *Lancet* 1977;**ii**:1054–1055.

18 Gheorghiade M, Beller G. Effects of discontinuing maintenance digoxin therapy in patients with ischemic heart disease and congestive heart failure in sinus rhythm. *Am J Cardiol* 1983;**51**:1243–1250.

19 McHaffie D, Purcell H, Mitchell-Hegs P, et al. The clinical value of digoxin in patients with heart failure and sinus rhythm. *Q J Med* 1978;**47**:401–419.

20 Anand I, Veall N, Kalra G, Ferrari R, Sutton G, et al. Treatment of heart failure with diuretics: body compartments, renal function and plasma hormones. *Eur Heart J* 1989;**10**:445–450.

21 The CONSENSUS Trial Study Group. Effect of enalapril on mortality in severe congestive heart failure: results of the Cooperative North Scandinavian Enalapril Survival Study (CONSENSUS). *N Engl J Med* 1987; **316**:1429–1435.

22 The SOLVD Investigators. Effect of enalapril on survival in patients with reduced left ventricular ejection fractions and congestive heart failure. *N Engl J Med* 1991;**325**:293–302.

23 Pfeffer MA, Moye LA, Basta L, et al. Effect of captopril on mortality and morbidity in patients with left ventricular dysfunction after myocardial infarction. Results of the survival and ventricular enlargement trial. The SAVE Investigators. *N Engl J Med* 1992;**327**:669–677.

24 Krell M, Kline E, Bates E, et al. Intermittent, ambulatory dobutamine infusions in patients with severe congestive heart failure. *Am Heart J* 1986;**112**:787–791.

25 Dies F, Krell M, Whitlow P, et al. Intermittent dobutamine in ambulatory outpatients with

chronic cardiac failure [abstract]. *Circulation* 1986;**74**:II38.

26 Packer MCJ, Rodeheffer RJ, et al. Effect of oral milrinone on mortality in severe chronic heart failure. *N Engl J Med* 1991;**325**:1468–1475.

27 Curfman G. Inotropic therapy for heart failure – an unfulfilled promise. *N Engl J Med* 1991; **325**:1509–1510.

28 Sabbah H, Shimoyama H, Kono T, et al. Effects of long-term monotherapy with enalapril, metoprolol, and digoxin on the progression of left ventricular dysfunction and dilation in dogs with reduced ejection fraction. *Circulation* 1994;**89**:2852–2859.

29 Bigger J, Fleiss J, Rolnitzky L, Merab J, Ferrick K. Effect of digitalis treatment on survival after acute myocardial infarction? *Am J Cardiol* 1985;**55**:623–630.

30 Moss A, Davis H, Conrad D, DeCamilla J, Odoroff C. Digitalis-associated cardiac mortality after myocardial infarction. *Circulation* 1981;**64**:1150–1156.

31 The Digitalis Subcommittee of the Multicenter Post-infarction Research Group. The mortality risk associated with digitalis treatment after myocardial infarction. *Cardiovasc Drugs Ther* 1987;**1**:125–132.

32 Poole-Wilson P, Robinson K. Digoxin: a redundant drug in congestive heart failure. *Cardiovasc Drugs Ther* 1989;**2**:733–741.

33 Jaeschke R, Oxman AD, Guyatt GH. To what extent do congestive heart failure patients in sinus rhythm benefit from digoxin therapy? A systematic overview and meta-analysis. *Am J Med* 1990;**88**:279–286.

34 Kelly RA, Smith TW. Digoxin in heart failure: implications of recent trials. *J Am Coll Cardiol* 1993;**22(suppl A)**:107A–112A.

35 Tauke J, Goldstein S, Gheorghiade M. Digoxin for chronic heart failure: a review of the randomized controlled trials with special attention to the PROVED (Prospective Randomized Study of Ventricular Failure and the Efficacy of Digoxin) and RADIANCE (Randomized Assessment of Digoxin on Inhibitors of the Angiotensin Converting Enzyme) trials. *Prog Cardiovasc Dis* 1994;**37**:49–58.

36 Uretsky BF, Young JB, Shahidi FE, Yellen LG, Harrison MC, Jolly MK. Randomized study assessing the effect of digoxin withdrawal in patients with mild to moderate chronic congestive heart failure: results of the PROVED trial. PROVED Investigative Group. *J Am Coll Cardiol* 1993;**22**:955–962.

37 Packer M, Gheorghiade M, Young JB, et al, for the RADIANCE Study. Withdrawal of digoxin from patients with chronic heart failure treated with angiotensin-converting enzyme inhibitors. *N Engl J Med* 1993;**329**:1–7.

38 Dobbs S, Kenyon W, Dobbs R. Maintenance digoxin after an episode of heart failure: placebo-controlled trial in outpatients. *BMJ* 1977;**i**:749–752.

39 Lee D, Johnson R, Bingham J, et al. Heart failure in outpatients: a randomized trial of digoxin versus placebo. *N Engl J Med* 1982; **306**:699–705.

40 Fleg L, Gottlieb S, Lakalta E. Is digoxin really important in compensated heart failure? *Am J Med* 1982;**73**:244–250.

41 Taggart A, Johnston G, McDevitt D. Digoxin withdrawal after cardiac failure in patients with sinus rhythm. *J Cardiovasc Pharmacol* 1983; **5**:229–234.

42 Guyatt G, Sullivan M, Fallen E, et al. A controlled trial of digoxin in congestive heart failure. *Am J Cardiol* 1988;**61**:371–375.

43 Pugh S, White N, Aronson J, et al. Clinical, hemodynamic, and pharmacological effects of withdrawal and reintroduction of digoxin in patients with heart failure in sinus rhythm after long-term treatment. *Br Heart J* 1989; **61**:529–539.

44 Ford A, Aronson J, Grahame-Smith D, Carver J. The acute changes seen in cardiac glycoside receptor sites, ^{86}rubidium uptake and intracellular sodium concentrations during early phases of digoxin therapy and after chronic therapy. *Br J Clin Pharmacol* 1979;**8**:135–142.

45 Fleg J, Rothfeld B, Gottlieb S. Effect of maintenance digoxin therapy on aerobic performance and exercise left ventricular function in mild to moderate heart failure due to coronary artery disease: a randomized placebo-controlled crossover trial. *J Am Coll Cardiol* 1991; **17**:743–751.

46 Haerer W, Bauer U, Hetzel M, Fehske J. Long-term effects of digoxin and diuretics in congestive heart failure – results of a placebo-con-

trolled randomized double blind study. *Circulation* 1988;**78**:53.
47 The Captopril-Digoxin Multicenter Research Group. Comparative effects of therapy with captopril and digoxin in patients with mild to moderate heart failure. *JAMA* 1988;**259**:539–544.
48 German and Austrian Xamoterol Study Group. Double-blind placebo-controlled comparison of digoxin and xamoterol in chronic heart failure. *Lancet* 1988;**i**:489–493.
49 DiBianco R, Shabetai R, Kostuk W, et al for the Milrinone Multicenter Trial Group. A comparison of oral milrinone digoxin, and their combination in the treatment of patients with chronic heart failure. *N Engl J Med* 1989; **320**:677–683.
50 Just H, Drexler H, Taylor SH, Siegrist J, Schulgen G, Schumacher M. Captopril versus digoxin in patients with coronary artery disease and mild heart failure. A prospective, double-blind, placebo-controlled multicenter study. The CADS Study Group. *Herz* 1993;**18(suppl 1)**:436–443.
51 van Veldhuisen DJ, Man in't Veld AJ, Dunselman PH, et al. Double-blind placebo-controlled study of ibopamine and digoxin in patients with mild to moderate heart failure: results of the Dutch Ibopamine Multicenter Trial (DIMT). *J Am Coll Cardiol* 1993; **22**:1564–1573.
52 Rector T, Kubo S, Cohn J. Patients' self-assessment of their congestive heart failure. II. Content, reliability, and validity of a new measure, the Minnesota Living with Heart Failure Questionnaire. *Heart Failure* 1987;**3**:198–209.
53 Lewis RP. Clinical use of serum digoxin concentrations. *Am J Cardiol* 1992;**69**:97G–106G.
54 Alicandri C, Fariello R, Boni E, et al. Captopril versus digoxin in mild-moderate chronic heart failure: a crossover study. *J Cardiovasc Pharmacol* 1987;**9**:S61–S67.
55 Beaune J, for the Enalapril Versus Digoxin French Multicenter Study Group. Comparison of enalapril versus digoxin for congestive heart failure. *Am J Cardiol* 1989;**63**:22D–25D.
56 Kromer E, Elsner D, Riegger G. Digoxin, converting-enzyme inhibition (quinapril), and the combination in patients with congestive heart failure functional class II and sinus rhythm. *J Cardiovasc Pharmacol* 1990;**16**:9–14.
57 Davies RF, Beanlands DS, Nadeau C, et al. Enalapril versus digoxin in patients with congestive heart failure: a multicenter study. Canadian Enalapril Versus Digoxin Study Group. *J Am Coll Cardiol* 1991;**18**:1602–1609.
58 Herlitz J, on behalf of the Lisinopril-Digoxin Study Group. Comparison of lisinopril versus digoxin for congestive heart failure during maintenance diuretic therapy. *Am J Cardiol* 1992;**70**:84C–90C.
59 Packer M. The neurohormonal hypothesis: a theory to explain the mechanism of disease progression in heart failure. *J Am Coll Cardiol* 1992;**20**:248–254.
60 Eckberg D, Drabinsky M, Braunwald E. Defective cardiac parasympathetic control in patients with heart disease. *N Engl J Med* 1971;**285**:877–883.
61 Gillis R, Quest J. The role of the nervous system in the cardiovascular effects of digoxin. *Pharmacol Rev* 1980;**31**:19–97.
62 Ferguson D, Berg W, Sanders J, Roach P, Kempf J, Kienzle M. Sympathoinhibitory responses to digitalis in heart failure patients. Direct evidence from sympathetic neural recordings. *Circulation* 1989;**80**:65–77.
63 Brouwer J, van Veldhuisen D, Man in't Veld A, et al, for the DIMT Study Group. Relation between heart rate variability and neurohumoral status in patients with heart failure. Effects of neurohumoral modulation by digoxin and ibopamine. *Circulation* 1993;**88**:I108.
64 Krum H, Bigger J Jr, Goldsmith R, Packer M. Effect of long-term digoxin therapy on autonomic function in patients with chronic heart failure. *J Am Coll Cardiol* 1995;**25**:289–294.
65 Gheorghiade M, Hall V, Alam M, et al. The effects of increasing digoxin dose on rest and exercise ejection fraction, exercise tolerance, and neurohormones in patients with heart failure on maintenance therapy with digoxin. *Circulation* 1992;**4**:I515.
66 Gheorghiade M, Hall V, Fenn N, et al. Chronic effects of digoxin withdrawal on neurohormones in patients with stable heart failure treated with converting-enzyme inhibitors. *Eur Heart J* 1993;**14**:131.

67 Lewis R. Digitalis. In: Leier C, ed. *Cardiotonic Drugs: A Clinical Survey*. Marcel Dekker, New York, 1987:85–150.
68 Young J, Gheorghiade M, Packer M, et al. on behalf of the PROVED and RADIANCE Investigators. Are low serum levels of digoxin effective in chronic heart failure? Evidence challenging the accepted guidelines for a therapueutic serum level of the drug. *J Am Coll Cardiol* 1993;**21**:378A.
69 Poole-Wilson PA. Digoxin withdrawal in patients with heart failure [letter]. *J Am Coll Cardiol* 1994;**24**:578–579.
70 Packer M, Medina N, Yushak M. Hemodynamic and clinical limitations of long-term inotropic therapy with amrinone in patients with severe chronic heart failure. *Circulation* 1984;**70**:1038–1047.
71 Rona G. Catecholamine cardiotoxicity. *J Mol Cell Cardiol* 1985;**17**:291–306.
72 Tan L, Jalil J, Pick R, Janicki J, Weber K. Cardiac myocyte necrosis induced by angiotensin II. *Circ Res* 1991;**69**:1185–1195.
73 Mann D, Kent R, Parsons B, Cooper G. Adrenergic effects on the biology of the adult mammalian cardiocytes. *Circulation* 1992; **85**:790–804.
74 Gheorghiade M, Young J, Uretsky B, et al. on behalf of the PROVED and RADIANCE Investigators. Predicting clinical deterioration after digoxin withdrawal in heart failure. *Circulation* 1993;**88**:I604.
75 Yusuf S, Garg R, Held P, et al. Need for a large randomized trial to evaluate the effects of digitalis on morbidity and mortality in congestive heart failure. Am J Cardiol 1992;**69**:64G–70G.

17

Inotropic agents: dead and buried?

Iain Squire, David Barnett

Introduction

Over the past decade or so, significant improvements have been made in the treatment of chronic congestive heart failure (CHF). Such improvements can be attributed in large part to the demonstration of the efficacy of vasodilator drugs, in particular the angiotensin converting enzyme (ACE) inhibitors.

Such therapy does not, however, address the fundamental physiological disturbance in the majority of CHF patients, namely impaired left ventricular function. The most direct theoretical approach to improving systolic function would appear to be the administration of therapy that improves the contractile state of the failing heart. The 1980s and early 1990s have seen much effort go into the development of agents designed to improve myocardial contractility. It is perhaps somewhat surprising that, as we approach the end of the 20th century, little progress appears to have been made and no new inotrope has an established place in therapy. No evidence exists of sustained benefit from any such agent either in terms of functional capacity or in terms of morbidity and mortality of the heart failure population. William Withering described the beneficial effects of digitalis glycosides in 'dropsy' in 1785, and for the intervening 200 years cardiac glycosides have been used in the treatment of heart failure. The positive inotrope digoxin improves functional capacity in at least a proportion of heart failure patients. Even for digoxin there is little evidence of any beneficial effect on mortality, and there is some evidence to suggest increased mortality in CHF. As for the other inotropic agents developed over recent years, the evidence is almost invariably that they have a detrimental effect on mortality. Does this mean that as far as the treatment of heart failure is concerned inotropic agents are dead and buried, or is resuscitation still possible?

All inotropes so far identified exert their effect by increasing the availability of intracellular free calcium, upon which myocardial contractility depends. Since the concentration of calcium and its availability for activation of the contractile proteins within the cell can be altered in a number of ways, there are several potential sites of drug action (Fig. 17.1). The ion channels that control calcium influx are voltage dependent, and the amount of calcium entering the cell can be increased by prolonging membrane depolarization. This may be the mechanism of action of some of the new inotropic drugs such as pimobendan. Alternatively, calcium may enter the cell in exchange for sodium; inhibition of the sodium-potassium ATPase (Na/K ATPase) is the accepted mechanism by which the digitalis glycosides increase intracellular calcium. Two of the major classes of inotropic agent, the phosphodiesterase inhibitors and the beta-adrenoceptor agonists, act to increase availability of the nucleotide cyclic AMP (cAMP), higher levels of which increase calcium influx at any

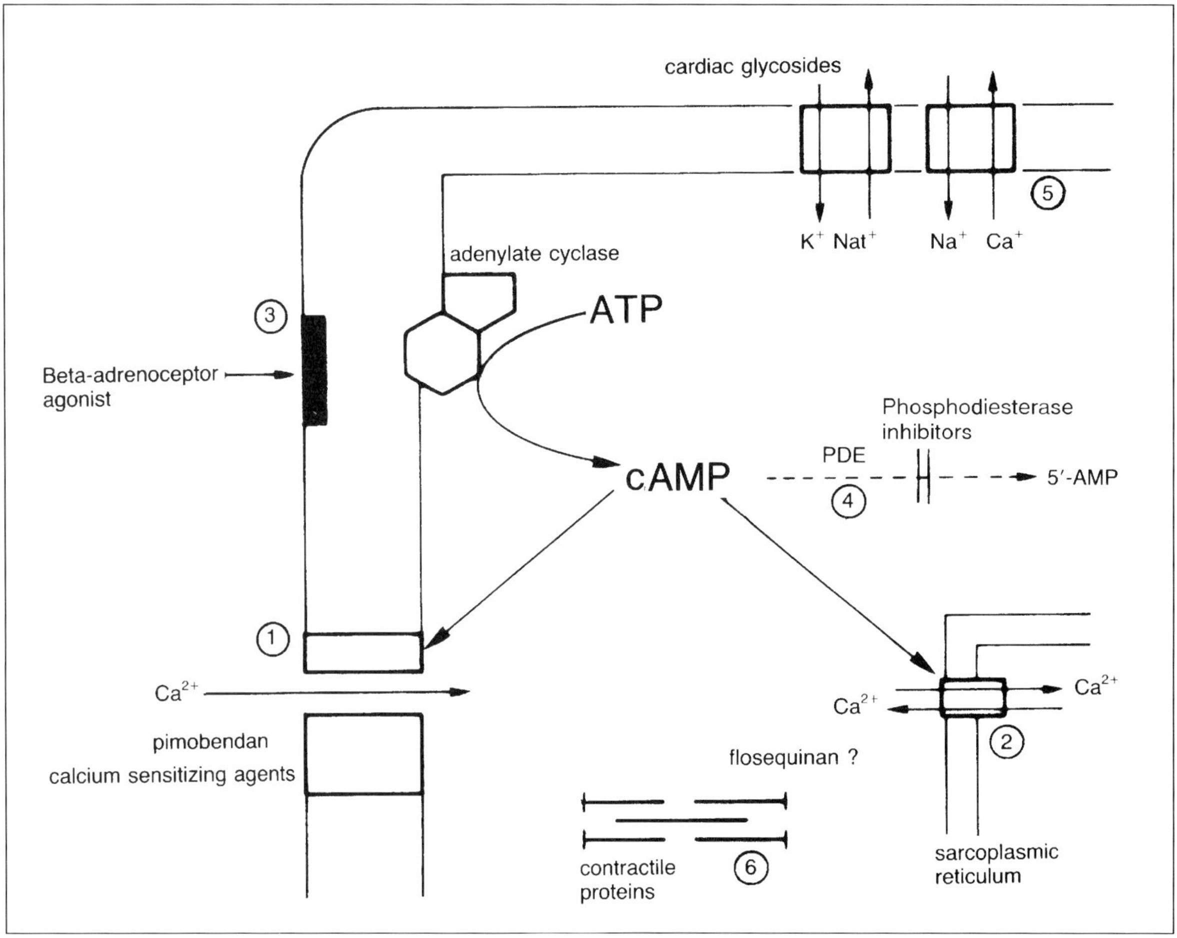

Fig. 17.1
Potential sites of action of positive inotropic agents. The nucleotide cAMP is intimately concerned with the modulation of intracellular free calcium concentration. cAMP influences both calcium flux across the voltage-dependent cell membrane calcium channel (1) and calcium release from the sarcoplasmic reticulum (2). Levels of cAMP can be increased by agents stimulating the cell-membrane beta-adrenoceptor (3) or by agents inhibiting its breadown (4). Enhancement of sodium–calcium exchange following inhibition of Na/K ATPase (5) increases intracellular free calcium independent of cAMP concentration. Sensitizing the contractile proteins to calcium (6) would increase contractility without the need for increased calcium influx. Calcium flux across the voltage-dependent channel may be influenced by calcium channel agonists without effect on cAMP (1). The release of calcium from the sarcoplasmic reticulum may be under the influence of inotropic agents such as flosequinan and digoxin.

level of cell membrane depolarization. Unlike the cardiac beta-adrenoceptor, the alpha-receptor is not linked to cAMP, and its inotropic response is dependent upon second messenger pathways associated with cell membrane inositol phosphates. The dependence or otherwise of a given agent on cAMP forms a convenient means of classifying inotropic drugs.

cAMP-dependent inotropic agents

Catecholamines

Adrenoceptors of beta-1 and beta-2 subtypes are found in human myocardium; the beta-1 subtypes predominate in ventricular tissue. Stimulation of either receptor subtype leads to increased cAMP levels via activation of adenylate cyclase. The catecholamines are unique among inotropic agents in having a direct chronotropic as well as an inotropic effect. In addition, beta-receptor agonists have a positive lusitropic effect, i.e., they increase the rate of relaxation of the cell. While activation of the sympathetic nervous system is a compensatory measure in early heart failure, progressive sympathetic activity appears to have deleterious effects in the long term. In spite of the fact that elevated plasma catecholamine levels are associated with increased mortality in CHF, much effort has gone into the development of orally active catecholamines as potential treatments for the condition. Initial interest was stimulated by the haemodynamic and clinical improvements from intermittent administration of intravenous dobutamine in CHF[1] and there is no doubt that treatment with oral catecholamines results in short-term improvements in both left ventricular filling pressure and cardiac output.[2–4] Although there is little information on the effects of oral catecholamines on mortality in CHF, the information that is available suggests an adverse effect. For example a much higher than expected mortality of 32% over 3 months was observed in a cohort of CHF patients treated with pirbuterol.[5] Experience with more recently introduced sympathomimetic agents has been no more encouraging. Xamoterol, a beta1-selective partial agonist, was developed as a treatment for heart failure in the 1980s. Xamoterol produced beneficial haemodynamic and symptomatic changes in patients with mild to moderate[6] or severe[7] heart failure.

However, a study of the safety and efficacy of xamoterol in severe heart failure[8] was terminated early, because active therapy was associated with a marked increase in mortality. Of the xamoterol group 9.1% died within 100 days of randomization compared to 3.7% of the placebo group. The beta-blocking effects of xamoterol were suggested by the study group to be a possible explanation. However this theory would appear to be at odds with evidence from studies of beta-receptor antagonism in heart failure. Following myocardial infarction, treatment with beta-blockers results in improved mortality.[9] The evidence suggests that in this setting, the benefit accrued from beta-blockade is greater among those patients with heart failure.[10] When beta-blockers with intrinsic sympathomimetic activity (ISA) are studied, the beneficial effects on mortality after myocardial infarction are no longer apparent.[9] Similarly, although beta-blockade results in improved haemodynamics in CHF,[11] no such beneficial effect is seen when the agent possesses ISA.[12] A causal effect of beta-blockade thus seems to be too simplistic an explanation for the increased mortality associated with xamoterol. Although sympathomimetic agents are undoubtedly potentially arrhythmogenic, there is no direct evidence from the study for this effect as an explanation for the observed findings.

It is accepted that plasma catecholamine level at the time of presentation is a strong predictor of mortality in CHF. Left ventricular dysfunction leads to a situation of chronic adrenergic stimulation, possibly due to deactivation of the normal neural reflexes controlling sympathetic nervous system activity. The end result of continuous receptor stimulation is a reduction in the number (down-regulation) of cell-surface beta-receptors, the extent of reduction depending on the severity of the heart failure.[13] The physiological result of this is an elevation in resting heart rate and an inability to mount an adequate heart rate response to exercise.[14] It is of interest that in the myocardium there is preferential down-regulation of beta-1 adrenoceptors compared to beta-2 adrenoceptors although there appears to be some uncoupling of the latter from adenylate cyclase.

The effect of CHF on adrenoceptor numbers is less clear. Animal models of heart failure have demonstrated that intermittent sympathomimetic stimulation improves exercise capacity, reduces resting heart rate, and improves heart rate during exercise. In addition, and perhaps significantly, plasma noradrenaline concentration and renin activity are reduced.[15]

Unfortunately, to date it has not been possible to translate encouraging animal experiments into beneficial effects in human heart failure. Initial studies of the effects of intermittent infusion of dobutamine in CHF patients resulted in improved haemodynamics, symptoms, and exercise tolerance. However a multicentre trial comparing intermittent inotropic therapy via weekly infusion of dobutamine (48 hours per week) to placebo was halted prematurely because of a dramatic increase in mortality with active therapy.[16] Can the regimen of inotropic stimulation employed explain the disparity between animal and patient studies? Recent evidence suggests this may be the case. In animal studies, dobutamine was infused over 1–2 hours whereas periods of 4–72 hours have been used in humans. Down-regulation of beta-receptors occurs only with continuous receptor stimulation for periods over 4 hours.[17] Adamopoulos et al have recently studied the effects of intermittent dobutamine infusion in a small number of patients with moderate to severe CHF. The regime used was infusion (20–25 mg/kg/min) of 30 minutes duration on 4 days a week for 3 weeks.[18] They found that this regime resulted in significant improvements in exercise capacity, reduction in peripheral vascular resistance and increases in lymphocyte beta-receptor density, indicating receptor up-regulation. As in animal studies, plasma noradrenaline concentration fell. The observed changes mimic those seen in response to exercise. This small, uncontrolled study, while in no way establishing a role for dobutamine or other inotropic therapy, will perhaps rekindle interest in the use of sympathomimetic agents in CHF.

Why should adrenergic stimulation in CHF be associated with progression of the condition and in the case of sympathomimetic agents, result in increased mortality for the patient with heart failure? The answer is not clear but it may be postulated that beta-receptor down-regulation is an adaptive measure to excessive receptor stimulation rather than a pathological consequence of CHF. The reduction in the number of receptors may therefore limit the myocardium's ability to respond to chronically elevated catecholamine levels and thereby reduce the rate of cardiac decompensation. Intermittent receptor stimulation or administration of a beta-adrenoceptor antagonist may interrupt the pathological cycle of receptor stimulation and down-regulation. Novel beta-adrenoceptor antagonists with vasodilator properties are now available and may hold significant therapeutic potential in CHF. These are discussed in chapter 18.

Phosphodiesterase inhibitors

Among the inotropic drugs, the phosphodiesterase inhibitors (PDIs) have undergone the most extensive clinical investigation, reflecting the enthusiasm with which the development of these agents was greeted. That such high hopes existed is understandable: inhibition of phosphodiesterase results in increased intracellular cAMP concentrations and thus in increased availability of calcium to cellular contractile elements. Inhibition of the enzyme in vascular smooth muscle cells results in balanced venous and arteriolar vasodilatation, a potentially beneficial effect in heart failure. As levels of myocardial cAMP are reduced in CHF,[19] treatments that increase its level in this condition would theoretically be of potential benefit.

These hopes have so far, however, proved to be unjustified. Experience in controlled clinical trials with phosphodiesterase inhibitors has been unfavourable, and in spite of beneficial haemodynamic effects, these agents have shown a detrimental effect on mortality in patients with heart failure. A number of PDIs have been evaluated in the treatment of CHF. All of the agents studied produce substantial short- and long-term haemodynamic improvement at rest and during exercise; this is true for amrinone,[20] milrinone,[21] piroximone,[22] enoximone,[23] flosequinan,[24] and vesnarinone.[25] Pharmacodynamic tolerance has been noted in only a few studies.[26,27] The laboratory and symptomatic improvements have not been paralleled by changes in mortality; with the possible exception of vesnarinone, the experience with all of these agents has been of detrimental effect in this regard. The clinical significance of the PDI properties of both flosequinan and vesnarinone is doubtful, and these agents lie at the interface between cAMP-dependent and -independent inotropes.

Initial experience with PDIs in heart failure was in the setting of uncontrolled trials. On the whole these demonstrated sustained haemodynamic improvement, but the incidence of undesirable side-effects was often high and apparently dose related. The use of lower, better tolerated doses seems to result in loss of therapeutic efficacy,[28] but this may not be the case for all PDIs.[29] Reported 1-year mortality varied widely in these studies, but was on average around 75%, which compares unfavourably with trials of standard vasodilator therapy in heart failure.[30]

It would of course not be reasonable to condemn PDIs on the basis of uncontrolled trials or those that were not designed to study the effects on mortality. One of the first controlled trials to report was the Enoximone Multicenter Trial Group,[31] although this too was not initially designed to evaluate mortality. This study, conducted in seven centres, randomly allocated 102 patients with CHF (NYHA classes II–III) to receive enoximone or placebo. In addition to failing to show any sustained benefit in terms of symptoms, there was a 20% mortality rate in the enoximone-treated patients compared to 5.8% in those receiving placebo. The finding of an increased mortality in patients with CHF treated with enoximone was confirmed in a placebo-controlled study whose purposes were to look at the effects of this agent on mortality and quality of life.[32] This study was terminated prematurely after 151 of an intended 200 patients with NYHA class III or IV symptoms had been recruited. The trial was terminated, owing to the finding of a significantly greater mortality in the patients treated with enoximone. Twenty-seven of 75 enoximone-treated patients and 18 of 76 placebo-treated patients died during the study period. However, quality of life was improved by active therapy.

When the PDI milrinone was compared to digoxin alone and to the combination of milrinone plus digoxin, no benefit was seen with the addition of the PDI, which was also seen to be less effective than digoxin alone in preventing decompensation of CHF.[33] In addition, there was a tendency for treatment with milrinone to be associated with aggravation of ventricular arrhythmias.

The definitive study of the effects of milrinone on mortality in CHF was published soon after this.[34] This study randomized 1088 patients to receive either milrinone 40 mg daily or placebo in addition to standard therapy, including digoxin and an ACE inhibitor. The study was terminated prematurely on the advice of the safety committee, based on the finding of increased mortality associated with active therapy. Milrinone therapy was associated with a 28% increase in all-cause mortality, and a 34% increase in cardiovascular mortality.

cAMP-independent inotropic agents

Calcium-sensitizing agents – vesnarinone and pimobendan

A number of agents has been identified which, in addition to inhibiting the phosphodiesterase enzyme, have a variety of other effects that may potentially explain their inotropic properties. Among these, several agents increase the sensitivity of cellular contractile elements to calcium. Two such agents, vesnarinone (OPC-8212) and pimobendan (UDCG-115) have reached the stage of clinical trials in heart failure. Pimobendan has both inotropic and direct vasodilator effects. *In vitro*, the drug increases the sensitivity of the contractile apparatus to calcium.[35] Administration of the drug in heart failure is associated with decreased systemic vascular resistance and mean arterial blood pressure, and increases in stroke volume, cardiac index, and heart rate.[36] Although no mortality studies have been published, pimobendan has been reported to improve both exercise duration and quality of life scores in CHF.[37]

Nony and colleagues have performed a meta-analysis of the effects on mortality of PDIs in CHF.[38] Using strict criteria for inclusion of a study in the analysis, the results of a total of 13 randomized, placebo-controlled trials were analysed. The conclusion was that treatment with PDIs was associated with a non-significant increase in mortality of 16% compared to placebo. However, the investigators found a heterogeneity in the results, a finding that disappeared when the three trials involving the agent vesnarinone were removed from the analysis. Subsequent analysis of the studies involving agents other than vesnarinone suggested that treatment with the other PDIs significantly increase (odds ratio [OR] 1.41) and vesnarinone significantly reduces (OR 0.3) mortality. This is a surprising and (if confirmed) an important finding for the treatment of CHF.

Two of the studies,[39,40] while reporting 'significant' improvements in mortality with vesnarinone compared to placebo, involved a total of 138 patients with one vesnarinone and eight placebo deaths. Such studies are unlikely to have had sufficient power to detect a meaningful difference in mortality. The third study[29] alone was responsible for the heterogeneity observed in the results of the analysis mentioned above. This study initially set out to compare vesnarinone at two dose levels, 60 or 120 mg daily, with placebo. However the trial design was altered after 253 patients had been enrolled, owing to the finding of a significantly higher mortality in the patients receiving 120 mg daily. Thereafter vesnarinone 60 mg was compared to placebo, 239 patients being randomized to active therapy and 238 patients to receive placebo therapy. Thirteen of the patients receiving 60 mg vesnarinone died, compared to 26 of those randomized to placebo, a 62% reduction in all-cause mortality. There was, in addition, a reduction in the rate of progression of heart failure and improvement in quality of life associated with active therapy, as assessed by the Sickness Impact Profile score. The beneficial effect was seen in spite of treatment of the patients in both groups with ACE inhibitors. The authors speculated that the apparently unique beneficial effects of vesnarinone in this setting may be due to its having a different mechanism of action from other PDIs. The drug has multiple effects on ion channels: inhibition of the delayed outward potassium current,[41] prolongation of the action potential duration,[42] increase in the fast inward sodium current,[43] and weak inhibition of phosphodiesterase.[44] Like all PDIs, vesnarinone causes a degree of vasodilatation due to inhibition of phosphodiesterase in vascular smooth muscle. Any one of the actions mentioned above would increase intracellular calcium concentration, and the relative contribution of each to the physiological response to vesnarinone is unclear.

Flosequinan

Although the positive inotropic properties of vesnarinone have been shown in both animal and human studies, in the study mentioned above no increase in ejection fraction was observed in the patients receiving 60 mg of vesnarinone and in whom the beneficial effects on mortality were seen. Flosequinan, like vesnarinone a quinolone derivative and a weak PDI, was marketed for the treatment of CHF but withdrawn by the manufacturers following an increase in mortality associated with its use.[45] Increased mortality was again seen only at higher doses of the drug. Flosequinan is primarily a vasodilator, the importance of its positive inotropic properties being questionable.[46] Animal and isolated tissue experiments have shown dose-dependent inotropic activity, but inotropic effect is not observed in the accepted therapeutic range.[47] Recent work with isolated cardiomyocytes from animals shows that at these concentrations, flosequinan is chronotropic and that PDI activity and positive inotropism are seen only at higher levels.[48]

The mechanism of the vasodilator action of flosequinan is not fully understood. The drug acts on the phosphatidylinositol pathway and may additionally influence release of calcium from the sarcoplasmic reticulum.[48] While flosequinan at low doses is primarily a vasodilator, higher doses selectively inhibit the PDE III isoenzyme. It is tempting to suggest that it is this property of the drug (and by implication other PDIs) which is responsible for its deleterious effect on mortality at higher dose levels, and that a therapeutic range potentially exists at which benefit may accrue.

Digoxin

In spite of its use for over 200 years the role of digoxin in the treatment of CHF remains to some extent controversial. This lack of consensus is reflected in the opposing views of its efficacy in the heart failure population as a whole – generally favourable in the USA and unfavourable in the UK. Such differences are nothing new and can be traced back to the early part of the century.[49] Marked differences in patterns of its use in CHF are also seen within the same country, including the USA. For example, in the SOLVD treatment trial, only 60% of CHF patients with ejection fraction less than 35% were receiving digoxin at entry to the study.[50]

There is evidence for both short-term and sustained haemodynamic benefits of digoxin in heart failure.[51] However, while it is clear that the drug is of benefit in atrial fibrillation, efficacy in patients in sinus rhythm has been questioned. Uncontrolled clinical trials have shown that withdrawal of digoxin from patients with stable CHF does not lead to adverse clinical effects.[52–54] More recently, a number of randomized, placebo-controlled trials have come to the opposite conclusion. A meta-analysis of seven such trials, involving 617 CHF patients with normal sinus rhythm, found a statistically significant benefit from continuation of digoxin compared to its withdrawal.[55] These studies were all limited by a number of factors, in particular by the fact that they studied the effects of the withdrawal of digoxin rather than its commencement in patients on maintenance diuretic therapy. In addition the applicability of these results to present clinical practice is unclear in that the patients were on the whole not receiving an ACE inhibitor.

The effects of digoxin withdrawal in patients whose regime included an ACE inhibitor were studied in the RADIANCE trial,[56] which again found that clinical deterioration was more likely in those patients in whom the drug was withdrawn. None of these trials was designed to examine the effect of digoxin on mortality in CHF, about which concerns have been expressed.[57] The results of a trial randomizing approximately 8000 patients with heart failure to placebo or digoxin in addition to standard therapy will be available within the next year or so and should answer more fully the questions surrounding the efficacy and mortality of digoxin in CHF. It should be pointed out that in terms of the symptomatic improvement elicited by digoxin in CHF, positive inotropism may be of secondary importance to other properties of the drug. Digoxin has a number of effects on autonomic function, causing vagal enhancement and impairment of sympathetic outflow, and there is enhanced sensitivity of baroreflexes. Acute inhibition of the activity of the renin–angiotensin–aldosterone axis is also seen. The net result is vasodilatation, which is of course in itself likely to be of benefit in CHF.

Why do inotropic agents worsen mortality in CHF?

Can the adverse effects of milrinone and other PDIs in CHF be explained on the basis of these or other known effects of the drugs? The excess mortality associated with PDIs appears to be dose related. It is difficult to establish, for any given agent, the relative contribution of positive inotropism compared to vasodilatation on the overall haemodynamic effect. It is even more difficult to establish which property of such a drug is responsible for effects on mortality. Angiotensin converting enzyme inhibitors and other vasodilators that have no inotropic effects improve mortality in patients with CHF. The increased mortality associated with PDIs is unlikely to be secondary to the vasodilatation which they elicit.

The theoretical reason for the use of PDIs in CHF is to increase myocardial levels of cAMP, known to be low in this condition. It is now suggested that this, like beta-receptor down-regulation, represents an adaptive change to, rather than a pathological consequence of, the process. Increased cAMP levels are toxic to the myocardium of experimental animals.[58] Inotropic drugs (PDIs and sympathomimetics) may increase myocardial energy consumption via stimulation of a number of metabolic pathways, leading to anaerobic metabolism and cellular ischaemia. This appears to be the case in CHF patients.[59,60] Increased intracellular calcium stimulates delayed depolarizations, suggested to be important in the genesis of arrhythmias, and the agents may be directly arrhythmogenic.[61] Many inotropic agents cause heart rate to increase. Thus, the increase in myocardial energy consumption and the acceleration of cell death that results from administration of PDI or sympathomimetic agents may explain the increased mortality. Receptor down-regulation and reduction in cAMP levels may simply represent energy saving adaptations to myocardial insufficiency. The evidence from clinical trials appears to support the assertion that PDIs hasten cell death and promote arrhythmia. Clinical progression of left ventricular dysfunction has been observed in patients treated with PDIs over periods of a few weeks.[26] This is in contrast to the observations in placebo-treated patients with heart failure observed over periods of up to a few months in various treatment trials.

The contrast between experience of the use of PDIs in heart failure and the results of animal studies is striking. For example, in a rat model of heart failure, milrinone (the agent for which the best human mortality data exist) has a beneficial effect on mortality comparable to that of ACE inhibitors.[62] However, there is a fundamental difference between the actions of milrinone in humans (particularly in patients with heart failure) and the actions in rats, in that the drug does not inhibit phosphodiesterase in rats, nor does it exhibit positive inotropic activity.[62]

At a cellular level, phosphodiesterase inhibitors and beta-adrenoceptor agonists act via increased intracellular concentrations of the second messenger cAMP. There is no doubt that beta-agonists and other agents that increase intracellular cAMP have arrhythmogenic potential. Why should the PDI group of drugs be different? On this matter the evidence from clinical trials is inconclusive. While a high frequency of ventricular ectopic activity has been noted in a number of trials of PDIs,[26,32,63] it is difficult to ascertain the true contribution of PDI therapy to this phenomenon in a group of patients with a high background incidence of arrhythmias. A high frequency of clinical ischaemic events in CHF patients with coronary artery disease was noted after starting amrinone therapy.[26] This same study recorded haemodynamically significant ventricular tachycardia in four of 29 patients treated with amrinone, in three cases within 24 hours of commencement. In the UK enoximone survival study,[32] sudden death occurred in 11 patients receiving enoximone and five receiving placebo. In this same study, the increase in mortality in patients treated with enoximone was seen in those individuals receiving over 120 mg frusemide daily. Milrinone therapy was associated with increased mortality in three particular groups of patients: those with the greatest cardiothoracic ratio; those with serum sodium concentration $\leqslant 137$ mmol/l; and those with the most severe symptoms (i.e. NYHA functional class IV).

The clinical features associated with the largest increase in mortality in each of these trials would suggest that those at greatest risk are those with severe CHF. Can we speculate that an agent hastening cell death would have a relatively greater effect on cell function in an already severely diseased myocardium? Symptoms suggestive of arrythmias were more common in the active treatment groups in placebo-controlled trials of amrinone,[26] enoximone,[31] and milrinone.[33]

Future developments

Where then do the inotropic agents stand in terms of future developments? Much work has yet to be done on aspects of PDI pharmacology and in particular on the relevance of animal studies to patients. The single clinical study showing improved mortality with vesnarinone 60 mg daily in CHF suggests that perhaps a therapeutic range may exist. A number of agents with multiple effects on ion channels are being developed. The door is not yet completely closed on modulation of the sympathetic nervous system in the treatment of CHF. A recent study suggests that a specific treatment regimen of dobutamine is of symptomatic value, although no data on mortality are yet available. The dopamine receptor agonists merit further attention. Clarification of the relative importance of myocardial as opposed to peripheral effects, and dopaminergic receptor as opposed to adrenergic receptor effects, with this class of agent may allow us to identify the mechanisms underlying the beneficial haemodynamic response. The effect on mortality of ibopamine, an orally active dopamine receptor agonist, is presently undergoing evaluation in a multicentre study, and the newer beta-receptor antagonists with vasodilator properties show promise as effective therapeutic agents. However, all of these agents have haemodynamic effects other than positive inotropism. It may be these other properties that result in clinical benefit. If it is the vasodilatory properties of phosphodiesterase inhibition that are responsible for their beneficial effects on symptoms in CHF then the future is indeed bleak for inotropic agents. Failing a beneficial effect on mortality, unless significant improvements in other parameters (such as quality of life) can be obtained, there can be no justification for using a vasodilator with a proven high incidence of adverse effects when alternative, safer and effective options are available.

References

1 Liang CS, Sherman LG, Doherty JU, Wellington K, Lee VW, Hood WB. Sustained improvement in patients with congestive heart failure after short-term infusion of dobutamine. *Circulation* 1984;**69**:113–119.

2 Sharma B, Hoback J, Francis GS, et al. Pirbuterol: a new oral sympathomimetic amine for the treatment of congestive heart failure. *Am Heart J* 1981;**102**:533–551.

3 Sharma B, Goodwin JF. Beneficial effect of salbutamol on cardiac function in severe congestive cardiomyopathy. *Circulation* 1978;**58**: 449–460.

4 Tweddel AC, Murray RG, Pearson D, Martin W, Hutton I. Cardiovascular effects of prenalterolon rest and exercise haemodynamics in patients with chronic congestive heart failure. *Br Heart J* 1982;**47**:375–380.

5 Dawson JR, Canepa-Anson R, Kuan P, Reuben SR, Poole-Wilson PA, Sutton GC. Symptoms, haemodynamics, and exercise capacity during long term treatment of chronic heart failure: experience with pirbuterol. *Br Heart J* 1983;**50**:282–289.

6 Pouleur H, Rousseau MF, Mengeot P, Veriter C, Brasseur LA. Improvement of global and regional left ventricular function in patients with previous myocardial infarction by a new beta-1 adrenoceptor partial agonist ICI 118, 587. *Eur Heart J* 1982;**3(suppl D)**:123–127.

7 McAlpine HM, Henderson F, Dargie H. Addition of xamoterol to captopril in severe chronic heart failure. *Eur J Clin Pharmacol* 1989;**36**:A71.

8 The Xamoterol in Severe Heart Failure Study Group. Xamoterol in Severe Heart Failure. *Lancet* 1990;**336**:1–6.

9 Yusuf S, Peto R, Lewis J, Collins R, Sleight P. Beta blockade during and after myocardial infarction: an overview of the randomized trials. *Prog Cardiovasc Dis* 1985;**27**:335–371.

10 Chadda K, Goldstein S, Byington R, Curb JD. Effect of propranolol after acute myocardial infarction in patients with congestive heart failure. *Circulation* 1986;**73**:503–510.

11 Eichhorn EJ, Bedotto BJ, Malloy CR, et al. Effect of β-adrenergic blockade on myocardial function and energetics in congestive heart failure. *Circulation* 1990;**82**:473–483.

12 Choong CYP, Roubin GS, Harris PJ, et al. A comparison of the effects of β-blockers with and without sympathomimetic activity on haemodynamics and left ventricular function at rest and during exercise in patients with coronary artery disease. *J Cardiovasc Pharmacol* 1986;**8**:441–448.

13 Fowler MB, Laser JA, Hopkins GL, Minobe W, Bristow MR. Assessment of the beta adrenergic pathway in the intact failing human heart: progressive receptor down regulation and subsensitivity to agonist response. *Circulation* 1986;**74**:1290–1302.

14 Colucci WS, Ribeiro JP, Rocco MB, et al. Impaired chronotropic response to exercise in patients with congestive heart failure: role of postsynaptic β-adrenergic desensitization. *Circulation* 1989;**80**:314–323.

15 Liang CS, Tuttle RR, Wood WB, Gavras H. Conditioning effects of chronic infusions of dobutamine: comparisons with exercise training. *J Clin Invest* 1979;**64**:2119–2131.

16 Dies F, Knell MJ, Whitlow P, et al. Intermittent dobutamine in ambulatory outpatients with chronic cardiac failure. *Circulation* 1984; **74(suppl II)**:II-39.

17 Tohmeh JF, Cryer PE. Biphasic adrenergic modulation of β-adrenergic receptors in man: agonist-induced early increment and late decrement of β-adrenergic receptor number. *J Clin Invest* 1980;**65**:836–840.

18 Adamopoulos S, Piepoli M, Qiang F, et al. Effects of pulsed β-stimulant therapy on β-adrenoceptors and chronotropic responsiveness in chronic heart failure. *Lancet* 1995;**345**:344–349.

19 Feldman MD, Copelas L, Gwanthmey JK, et al. Deficient production of cyclic AMP: pharmaco-

logic evidence of an important cause of contractile dysfunction in patients with end-stage heart failure. *Circulation* 1987;**75**:331–339.

20 Maskin CS, Forman R, Klein NA, Sonnenblick EH, LeJemtel TH. Long-term amrinone therapy in patients with severe heart failure: drug-dependent haemodynamic benefits despite progression of the disease. *Am J Med* 1982;**72**:113–118.

21 Baim DS, McDowell AV, Cherniles J, et al. Evaluation of a new bipyridine inotropic agent – milrinone – in patients with severe congestive heart failure. *N Engl J Med* 1983;**309**:748–756.

22 Petein M, Levine TB, Cohn JN. Persistent haemodynamic effects without long-term clinical benefits in response to oral piroximone (MDL 19205) in patients with congestive heart failure. *Circulation* 1986;**73(suppl III)**:III-230.

23 Herrmann HC, Ruddy TD, Dec GW, Strausse HW, Boucher CA, Fifer MA. Inotropic effect of enoximone in patients with severe heart failure. Demonstration by left ventricular end-systolic pressure-volume analysis. *J Am Coll Cardiol* 1987;**9**:1117–1123.

24 Packer M, Narahara KA, Elkayam U, et al. Double-blind, placebo-controlled study of the efficacy of flosequinan in patients with chronic heart failure. *J Am Coll Cardiol* 1993;**22**:65–72.

25 Asanoi H, Sassayama S, Kameyama T, Ishizaka S, Iuchi K. Sustained inotropic effects of a new cardiotonic agent OPC-8212 in patients with chronic heart failure. *Clin Cardiol* 1989;**12**:133–138.

26 Packer M, Medina N, Yushak M. Haemodynamic and clinical limitations of long-term inotropic therapy with amrinone in patients with severe chronic heart failure. *Circulation* 1984;**70**:1038–1047.

27 Shah PK, Amin DK, Hilse S, Shellock F, Swan HJC. Inotropic therapy for refractory congestive heart failure with oral fenoximone (MDL 17,043): poor long-term results despite early haemodynamic and clinical improvement. *Circulation* 1985;**71**:326–331.

28 Massie B, Bourassa M, Di Bianco R, et al, for the Amrinone Multicenter Trial Group. Long-term oral administration of amrinone for congestive heart failure: lack of efficacy in a multicenter controlled trial. *Circulation* 1985; **71**:963–971.

29 Feldman AM, Bristow MR, Parmley WW, et al. Effects of vesnarinone on morbidity and mortality in patients with heart failure. *N Engl J Med* 1993;**329**:149–155.

30 Packer M, Leier CV. Survival in congestive heart failure during treatment with drugs with positive inotropic actions. *Circulation* 1987;**75(suppl IV)**:IV-55–IV-63.

31 Uretsky BF, Jessup M, Konstam MA, et al. Multicenter trial of oral enoximone in patients with moderate to moderately severe congestive heart failure. Lack of benefit compared with placebo. *Circulation* 1990;**82**:774–780.

32 Cowley AJ, Skene AM. Treatment of severe heart failure: quantity or quality of life? A trial of enoximone. *Br Heart J* 1994;**72**:226–230.

33 Di Bianco R, Shabetai R, Kostuk W, Moran J, Schlant RC, Wright R. A comparison of oral milrinone, digoxin, and their combination in the treatment of patients with chronic heart failure. *N Engl J Med* 1989;**320**:677–683.

34 Packer M, Carver JR, Rodeheffer RJ, et al. Effect of oral milrinone on mortality in severe chronic heart failure. *N Engl J Med* 1991;**325**:1468–1475.

35 Fujino K, Sperelakis N, Solaro RJ. Sensitization of dog and guinea-pig heart myofilaments to Ca^{2+} activation and the inotropic effect of pimobendan: comparison with milrinone. *Circ Res* 1988;**63**:911–922.

36 Hasenfuss G, Holubarsch C, Heiss HW, Rattert B, Just HJ. Influence of the calcium sensitizer UDCG-115 on haemodynamics and myocardial energetics in patients with idiopathic dilated cardiomyopathy. Comparison with nitroprusside. In: Just HJ, Holubarsch CH, Scholz H, eds. *Inotropic Stimulation and Myocardial Energetics.* Springer, New York, 1989:225–233.

37 Kubo SH, Gollub S, Bourge R, et al. Beneficial effects of pimobendan on exercise tolerance and quality of life in patients with heart failure: results of a multicenter trial. *Circulation* 1992;**85**:942–949.

38 Nony P, Boissel JP, Leizorovic A, Haugh MC, Fareh S, de Breyne B. Evaluation of the effect of phosphodiesterase inhibitors in mortality in

chronic heart failure patients. *Eur J Clin Pharmacol* 1994;**46**:191–196.
39 OPC-8212 Multicenter Research Group. A placebo-controlled, randomized, double-blind study of in patients with mild chronic heart failure. *Cardiovasc Drugs Ther* 1990;**4**:419–426.
40 Feldman AM, Baughman KL, Lee WK, et al. Usefulness of OPC-8212, a quinolone derivative, for chronic congestive heart failure in patients with ischemic heart disease or idiopathic dilated cardiomyopathy. *Am J Cardiol* 1991;**68**:1203–1210.
41 Iijima T, Taira N. Membrane current changes responsible for the positive inotropic effect of OPC-1812, a new positive inotropic agent, in single ventricular cells of guinea pig heart. *J Pharmacol Exp Ther* 1987;**240**:60–62.
42 Lathrop DA, Varro A, Schwartz A. Rate-dependent electrophysiological effects of OPC 8212: comparison to sotalol. *Eur J Pharmacol* 1989;**164**:487–496.
43 Lathrop DA, Schwartz A. Evidence for possible increase in sodium channel open time and involvement of Na/Ca exchange by a new positive inotropic drug: OPC-8212. *Eur J Pharmacol* 1985;**117F**:391–392.
44 Yatani A, Imoto Y, Schwartz A, Brown AM. New positive inotropic agent OPC-8212 modulates Ca^{2+} channels in ventricular myocytes of guinea-pig. *J Cardiovasc Pharmacol* 1989;**13**:812–819.
45 Boots Company. Warning on flosequinan. *Lancet* 1993;**341**:1146.
46 Weishaar RE, Kirker ML, Wallace AM, Ferraris VA, Britton LW, Sim MF. Relationship between inotropic activity and phosphodiesterase activity inhibition for flosequinan and milrinone. *Eur J Pharmacol* 1993;**236**:363–366.
47 Yates DB. Pharmacology of flosequinan. *Am Heart J* 1991;**121**:974–983.
48 Kelso EJ, McDermott BJ, Silke B. Actions of the novel vasodilator, flosequinan, in isolated ventricular cardiomyocytes. *J Cardiovasc Pharmacol* 1995;**25**:376–386.
49 Christian HA. Digitalis effects in chronic cardiac cases with regular rhythm in contrast to auricular fibrillation. *Med Clin North Am* 1922;**5**:1173–1190.
50 SOLVD Investigators. Effect of enalapril on survival in patients with reduced left ventricular ejection fraction and congestive heart failure. *N Engl J Med* 1991;**295**:293–302.
51 Arnold SB, Byrd RC, Meister W, et al. Long-term digitalis therapy improves left ventricular function in heart failure. *N Engl J Med* 1980;**303**:1443–1447.
52 Dall JLC. Maintenance digoxin in elderly patients. *BMJ* 1970;**ii**:705–706.
53 Fonrose HA, Ahlbaum N, Bugatch E, Cohen M, Genovese C, Kelly J. The efficacy of digitalis withdrawal in an institutional aged population. *J Am Geriatr Soc* 1974;**22**:208–211.
54 Hull SM, Mackintosh A. Discontinuation of maintenance digoxin therapy in general practice. *Lancet* 1977;**ii**:1054–1055.
55 Jaeschke RJ, Oxman AD, Guyatt GH. To what extent do congestive heart failure patients in sinus rhythm benefit from digoxin therapy? A systematic overview and meta-analysis. *Am J Med* 1990:88:279–286.
56 Packer M, Gheorghiade M, Young JB, et al. Withdrawal of digoxin from patients with chronic heart failure treated with angiotensin-converting-enzyme inhibitors. *N Engl J Med* 1993;**329**:1–7.
57 Yusuf S, Garg R, Held P. Need for a large randomized trial to evaluate the effects of digitalis on morbidity and mortality in congestive heart failure. *Am J Cardiol* 1992;**69**:64G–70G.
58 Martorana PA. The role of cyclic AMP in isoprenaline induced cardiac necroses in the rat. *J Pharm Pharmacol* 1971;**23**:200–203.
59 Pozen RG, Di Bianco R, Katz RJ, Bortz R, Myerburg RJ, Fletcher RD. Myocardial metabolic and hemodynamic effects of dobutamine in heart failure complicating coronary artery disease. *Circulation* 1981;**63**:1279–1285.
60 Leier CV, Heban PT, Huss P, Bush CA, Lewis RP. Comparative systemic and regional hemodynamic effects of dopamine and dobutamine in patients with cardiomyopathic heart failure. *Circulation* 1978;**58**:466–475.
61 Katz AM. Potential deleterious effects of inotropic agents in the therapy of chronic heart failure. *Circulation* 1986;**73(suppl III)**:III-184–III-190.
62 Weishaar RE, Kobylarz-Singer DC, Steffen RP,

Kaplan HR. Subclasses of cyclic AMP-specific phosphodiesterase activity in left ventricular muscle and their involvement in regulating myocardial contractility. *Circ Res* 1987; **61**:539–547.

63 Naccarelli GV, Gray EL, Dougherty AM, Hanna JE, Goldstein RA. Amrinone: electrophysiologic and haemodynamic effects in patients with congestive heart failure. *Am J Cardiol* 1984;**54**:600–604.

18

Angiotensin II receptor antagonists for heart failure: do we need them?

John GF Cleland

Introduction

ACE inhibitors have revolutionized our understanding and treatment of heart failure. The first angiotensin receptor-1 (AT_1) antagonist has been licensed recently for use in hypertension, and clinical trials in heart failure are well underway.

What does this new class of agent have to offer? AT_1 receptor antagonists will undoubtedly help in the understanding of how the renin–angiotensin–aldosterone system operates in heart failure, and will give important insights into how ACE inhibitors work, but do they have anything to add to ACE inhibitors therapeutically? It is certainly likely that they will occupy a small niche for the management of patients who develop angioneurotic oedema or severe cough with ACE inhibitors, but this will hardly repay the efforts put into their development. The hope is that most of the benefits of ACE inhibition are mediated through the reduction of angiotensin II, and that AT_1 receptor antagonists will be rather better at preventing the adverse effects of angiotensin II. This chapter examines these assumptions and reviews the properties of AT_1 receptor antagonists.

The renin–angiotensin–aldosterone system

The organization of the renin–angiotensin–aldosterone system is outlined in Fig. 18.1. This section concentrates on the sites of action of ACE inhibitors and AT_1 receptor antagonists.

Angiotensin converting enzyme (ACE) is responsible not only for the production of angiotensin II but also the degradation of bradykinin. Other substrates for ACE include erythropoeitin and the enkephalins. Angiotensin II has numerous actions, which may be divided into acute and chronic effects. The acute effects of angiotensin II include regulation of vascular tone, autonomic function, and salt and water metabolism; the chronic effects include cardiac and vascular remodelling and a potential role in the genesis of atheroma (Table 18.1).

Less is known about bradykinin, firstly because it is difficult to measure (though it probably acts close to its site of synthesis with little spill-over into the circulation) and secondly because pharmacological tools for manipulating its actions have only recently become available. Current evidence suggests that, like angiotensin II, it may also have distinctly different acute and chronic effects (Table 18.2). In general, the actions of bradykinin are opposite to those of angiotensin II. Bradykinin may also be important in inhibiting the development of atheroma.

Alternative pathways for the generation of angiotensin II

Chymase or other endopeptidases can convert angiotensin I to II and are not inhibited by ACE

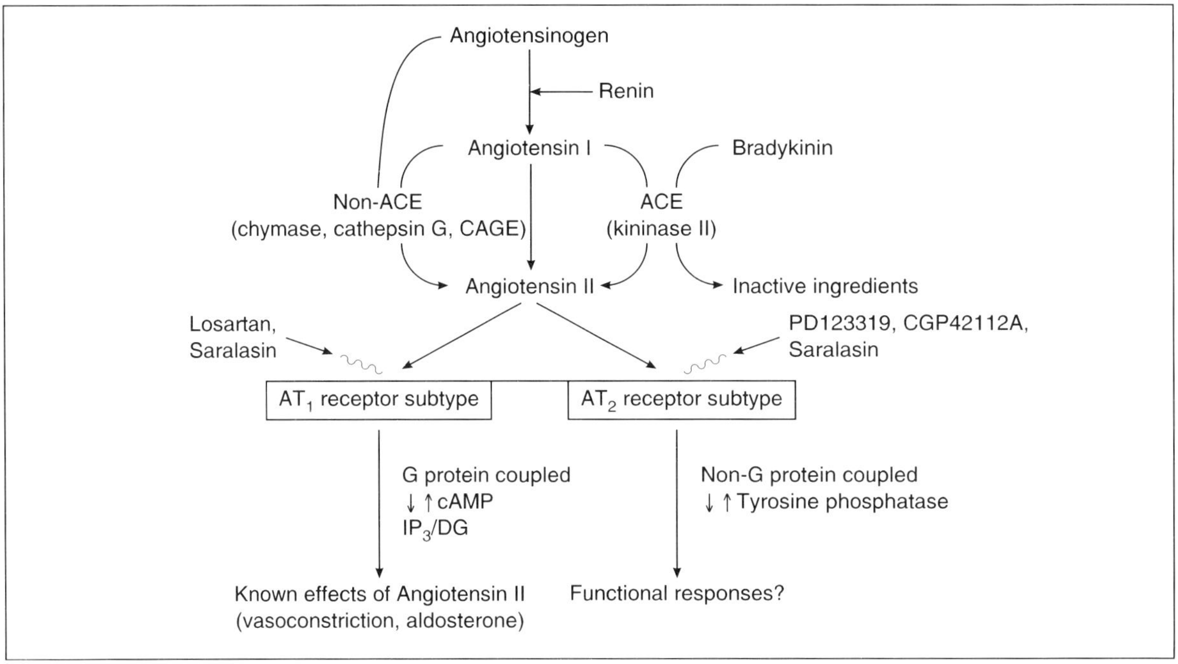

Fig. 18.1
The renin–angiotension–aldosterone system and angiotensin II receptor subtypes.

Short-term effects	Long-term effects
Increased platelet adhesion	Increased intimal lipid permeability
Secretion of PAI-1	Foam cell formation
Vasoconstriction	Vascular smooth muscle cell hypertrophy and hyperplasia
Sympathomimetic	Cardiac myocyte hypertrophy
Parasympatholytic	Myocardial fibrosis
Stimulates aldosterone	?Atherogenic
Stimulates vasopressin	
Salt and water retention	

Table 18.1
Actions of angiotensin II.

Short-term effects	Postulated long-term effects
Vasodilatation	Reduced vascular smooth muscle hyperplasia
Increased nitric oxide secretion	Reduced cardiac myocyte hypertrophy
Increased endothelial prostacyclin	Reduced myocardial fibrosis
Reduced platelet adhesion	?Anti-atherogenic

NB. The long-term effects of bradykinin remain uncertain owing to the lack of specific agonists and antagonists for long-term use.

Table 18.2
Actions of bradykinin.

inhibitors. Whether they are present in sufficient quantity to generate significant amounts of angiotensin II either systemically or at a local (tissue) level is uncertain. Studies suggest that mRNA for chymase is expressed at much lower levels than mRNA for ACE in human cardiac tissues,[1] although in rat experiments, Urata[2] has suggested that enough chymase exists to generate a considerable amount of angiotensin II.

Chymotrypsin angiotensin generating enzyme and cathepsin D are other pathways for angiotensin II production which are not blocked by ACE inhibitors (Fig. 18.2).[3]

Angiotensin II receptor subtypes

The principal classification of angiotensin II receptors is into AT_1 and AT_2 receptors, but the *c-mas* oncogene encodes a protein that binds angiotensin II,[4] and at least one other angiotensin II binding protein (APJ) has been described,[5] although these proteins have been discounted as a site of action for angiotensin II. The AT_1 receptor in rats (but not in humans) can be subdivided into AT_{1A} and AT_{1B} subtypes, and other 'atypical' subtypes have been found in mouse cell lines and amphibians. The human AT_1 receptor gene does show some sequence variation, leading to some structural heterogeneity, but the homology is strikingly high at over 95%.[6]

The AT_1 receptor appears to be responsible for the mediation of all the classical, acute effects of angiotensin II. In *in vitro* models of animal tissues, stimulation of the AT_1 receptor causes vasoconstriction and aldosterone release, and enhances salt and water absorption in the proximal renal tubule, inhibits collagenase, and stimulates prostaglandin release.[7] AT_2 receptor

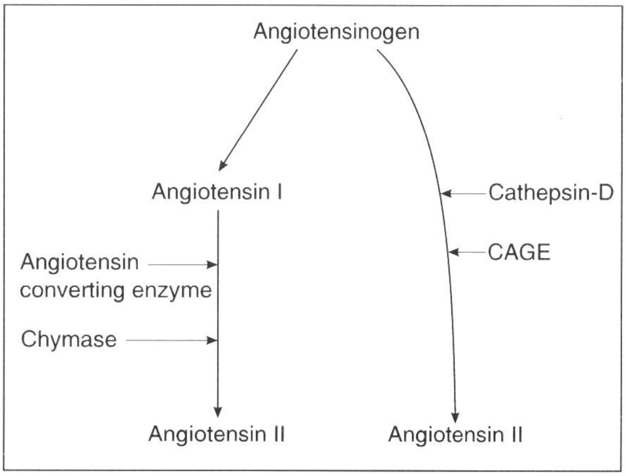

Fig. 18.2
Alternative pathways for the production of angiotensin II.

expression is enhanced relative to expression of AT_1 receptors in fetal life and during wound healing in animal experiments,[8,9] leading to the tentative suggestion that AT_2 receptors are involved in growth and development. Some have suggested that the AT_2 receptor[10] is a precursor of the AT_1 receptor,[11] although cloning studies now suggest that this is not the case.

Distribution of angiotensin II receptors in humans

Table 18.3 shows the distribution of different receptor sites as they are known to occur in humans. More is known about the tissue distribution in other animal species, in particular the rat, but species heterogeneity exists.

Angiotensin receptor antagonists: basic pharmacology

Currently, antagonists to the AT_1 and AT_2 receptors have been developed. Whereas the AT_1 receptor antagonists reduce vascular resistance and arterial pressure in humans, antagonists to the AT_2 receptor are without discernible effect in most animal models,[18] and have not yet been administered to humans.

At the time of writing, a substantial clinical experience exists only with losartan (MSD), although clinical studies with valsartan (Ciba–Geigy) and TCV-116 (Takeda) are well underway.

Losartan is 30 000 times more selective for AT_1 receptors than for AT_2 receptors[19] and appears devoid of antagonist actions for other vasoactive substances or affinity for other receptor systems. Losartan is moderately well absorbed by the oral route and is rapidly metabolized to a number of inactive compounds (Table 18.4).[20,21] However, about 14% is converted in the liver to an active metabolite, L-158 641, by oxidation.[7] L-158 641 (also known as EXP 3174) is also an effective AT_1 receptor antagonist and, despite the fact that only 14% of the parent compound is

Tissue	Predominantly AT_1 receptors	Mixed receptors	Predominantly AT_2 receptors	Other
Heart				
myocytes	12			
fibroblasts			12	
Arterioles	12			
Adrenal cortex		13		
Brain		14		5
Kidney				
glomeruli	15, 16			
afferent arterioles				
Platelets	12		12	
Adipocytes	12			
Uterus				
Placenta	17		13	

Table 18.3
Distribution of AT_1, AT_2, and other possible AT receptors in humans. (Numbers refer to references.)

Variable	Losartan	L-158 641
Absorption	20–35%*	NA
Excretion	Hepatic $\gg$ renal	Hepatic $\sim$ renal
Volume of distribution	34 litres	12 litres
Plasma half-life	2.1 hours	6.6 hours
Peak plasma concentration (oral dosing)	1 hour	4 hours
Protein binding	98.7%	99.8%

Table 18.4
Pharmacokinetics of losartan and its metabolite L-158 641 after oral dosing in humans. (– modest reduction after food, increased in hepatic disease.) (From references 20, 21.)*

metabolized by this route, owing to its longer half-life and smaller volume of distribution, plasma concentrations (area under the curve) of L-158 641 are four times higher than the parent compound.[7] About 1% of subjects studied so far produce little of this active metabolite, the implications of which are yet to be explored. Tissue concentrations of losartan and L-158 641 are generally lower than in plasma, apart from levels in liver and kidney.

The duration of the biological activity of losartan, valsartan and TCV-116 is much longer than the plasma half-life of the parent drugs would suggest,[20–25] indicating either that the drugs are tightly bound to the receptor and therefore inhibition persists despite elimination of free drug from the plasma or that the biologically active metabolites are important for the drug's duration of action. 80 mg of losartan or 40–80 mg of valsartan inhibit the pressor effects of exogenous angiotensin II for up to 24 hours.[20,22]

Hepatic disease increases oral bioavailability and increases the half-life of losartan but has little effect on L-158 641. Dose reduction is recommended. The relevance of these observations to patients with hepatic congestion due to heart failure has not been examined yet. Renal disease has little effect on the kinetics of losartan or its metabolite, even in patients requiring dialysis. Sex and age have only modest effects on pharmacokinetics, at least in patients without heart failure. No important interactions have been noted as yet with either warfarin or digoxin.

Valsartan, like losartan, has an active metabolite, and appears to be effective when given once daily. It too is mainly excreted by the liver.[22,25]

Similarities and differences between the actions of ACE inhibitors and AT_1 receptor antagonists

If the actions of ACE inhibitors are mediated entirely through angiotensin II and if the adverse effects of angiotensin II are mediated entirely through AT_1 receptors, then the effects of ACE inhibitors and angiotensin II receptor antagonists should be similar, though important pharmacodynamic differences may exist to favour the AT_1 receptor antagonists; the latter have a longer half-life of biological action which makes once-daily dosing theoretically more appropriate.

However, it is not certain that all the effects of ACE inhibition are mediated through the suppression of angiotensin II formation. For instance, enalapril and losartan exert similar effects on angiotensin-I-mediated vasoconstriction of the forearm but only enalapril enhances bradykinin-induced vasodilatation.[26] ACE inhibitors improve haemodynamics, symptoms, and prognosis in heart failure and the extent to which these clinical outcomes are interrelated is unclear. It is quite possible that different benefits of ACE inhibitors are mediated through different pathways. Thus, demonstration of equivalent haemodynamic action may suggest that the haemodynamic effects of ACE inhibitors are mediated through the AT_1 receptor, but this should not lead to the assumption that similar effects on symptoms and prognosis will be observed.

Effects of AT_1 receptor antagonists in experiments on animal tissues

In animal preparations at the tissue level, losartan inhibits the actions of angiotensin II, including smooth muscle cell growth, and vascular, non-vascular, and cardiac muscle contraction,[27] and cardiac myocyte necrosis.[28] Losartan inhibits adrenal medullary release of adrenaline in response to angiotensin II,[18] noradrenaline release from sympathetic nerve terminals,[29] and suppression of renal renin release by angiotensin II.[30] Losartan also blocks angiotensin II-mediated increases in proximal tubular salt and water retention.[7]

AT_1 receptor antagonists also have effects on cardiovascular structure. Losartan blocks angiotensin II-induced protein accumulation in cardiac myocytes,[31] collagen synthesis by myocardial fibroblasts,[32] and angiotensin II-induced increases in endothelin-1 mRNA from the endothelium.[33] Losartan reduces cardiac hypertrophy[34] although some studies have suggested that ACE inhibitors may be more effective.[35] Losartan also blocks angiotensin II-induced hypertrophy and hyperplasia of vascular smooth muscle cells[27] and it has favourable effects on the structure of resistance arteries.[36]

Effects of AT_1 receptor antagonists in animal models of heart failure

In experimental heart failure, losartan improves central haemodynamics,[37,38] reduces atrial natriuretic peptide,[38] increases renal blood flow,[39] and, in high-output models, increases urine volume.[40] Some reports suggest that AT_2 receptor antagonists may have effects on salt and water excretion.[41]

In a rat model of heart failure produced by coronary ligation, losartan and captopril produce similar haemodynamic effects[37] (although different effects on renal function[42]) but no difference in survival at 1 year. Using a similar model, another group failed to find a benefit on survival with losartan compared to captopril,[43] but this is difficult to interpret as a beneficial effect of ACE inhibitors on survival in the rat model of heart failure is inconsistent.[44,45] Antagonists of the AT_2 receptor more closely simulated the effects of an ACE inhibitor on post-infarction haemodynamics and myocardial collagen accumulation in one study, but this awaits confirmation in other studies.[46] However, Schieffer[47] noted a similar benefit from enalapril and losartan in terms of myocardial hypertrophy and interstitial fibrosis.

In a rat model of heart failure induced by aortocaval shunting, losartan reversed ventricular hypertrophy, reduced filling pressures and increased sodium excretion.[40,48,49] Similarly, in a murine model of myocarditis an AT_1

receptor antagonist helped preserve ventricular function.[50]

In sheep and dog models of heart failure induced by pacing, the haemodynamic effects of an AT_1 receptor antagonist and an ACE inhibitor were similar, and the AT_1 antagonist also induced diuresis.[38,51,52] In contrast in a dog model of heart failure induced by repeated DC shocks, ramipril delayed the onset of heart failure, but DuP 532, an AT_1 antagonist, did not.[53] AT_1 receptor antagonists do not appear to reduce infarct size – an inconsistant finding in animal studies of ACE inhibitors.[54]

Pharmacodynamic aspects of ACE inhibition and AT_1 receptor antagonists in humans

ACE inhibition

The pharmacokinetics of ACE inhibitors are complex and probably a poor guide to drug action.[3] Most ACE inhibitors are prodrugs and require hepatic de-esterification to their active moiety. The ACE inhibitor rapidly saturates the ACE and in general any unbound drug is excreted, mainly by the kidneys, fairly rapidly with a half-life of 1–12 hours, depending on the agent used. However, the actions of ACE inhibitors persist for longer than predicted from simple pharmacokinetic studies, because it is the fraction that is bound to the ACE that is important. ACE inhibitors such as quinapril, perindopril, and trandolapril are tightly bound to the ACE and therefore have a long terminal elimination half-life and a much longer duration of action than their plasma half-life would suggest.[55]

Surprisingly, after 15 years of research comparatively little is known about the most important aspects of the pharmacodynamic actions of ACE inhibitors. This is for at least two reasons:[55]

1. It is not known which fundamental aspects of ACE inhibition are critical for the beneficial effects of ACE inhibition. It is possible that the situation is even more complex – for instance, reduction of angiotensin II could be important for the effects of ACE inhibitors on symptoms and haemodynamics but increases in bradykinin may mediate the effects of ACE inhibitors on recurrent infarction and prognosis.
2. Pharmacodynamic studies have tended to be short-term and have studied mainly effects on ACE activity. It is known that over 80% of the ACE has to be inhibited, initially, for endogenous angiotensin II to fall or to inhibit the pressor actions of exogenous angiotensin I. It is also known that long-term ACE inhibition leads to an accumulation of angiotensin I and an induction of the ACE itself, so that much more than 80% inhibition may be required to prevent resumption of angiotensin II production during chronic ACE inhibition. Angiotensin II may also be produced by alternative pathways. There are few studies that have measured the effects on bradykinin.

There is little idea what the optimal dosage of any ACE inhibitor is, especially during long-term use. Several studies, including ATLAS, NETWORK, and ACHIEVE[55] are underway; these should give at least partial answers to the question of dosage. If these studies show a consistent treatment effect for one or other extreme of dosing, the optimal long-term dose will still be unknown. For instance, if the ATLAS study shows that 35 mg/day of lisinopril is more effective than 5 mg/day, it is possible that 100 mg/day of lisinopril would have been more effective still.

AT_1 receptor antagonists

If all the benefits of ACE inhibition are mediated by reducing angiotensin II-mediated AT_1 receptor stimulation, then an AT_1 receptor antagonist may be preferable to an ACE inhibitor for the treatment of heart failure for a variety of reasons:

- an AT_1 receptor antagonist will block the effects of angiotensin II, regardless of the pathway by which it is produced;
- the duration of action of AT_1 receptor antagonists may be longer; and
- if the side-effects of ACE inhibition, such as cough or angioneurotic oedema, are mediated through bradykinin, then AT_1 receptor antagonists may give rise to fewer side-effects.

Renin secretion is suppressed by angiotensin II, while AT_1 receptor antagonists increase renin by releasing it from this negative feedback loop. As renin rises, so does angiotensin I and, consequently, angiotensin II. Suggestions that reduced receptor sequestration of angiotensin II, a putative mechanism of catabolizing angiotensin II, may also contribute to a rise in angiotensin II have been refuted.[56] Just as the effects of ACE inhibition may be overcome by competition from rising concentrations of angiotensin I so AT_1 receptor inhibition may be overcome, at least in part, by rising concentrations of angiotensin II. The consequences of unopposed actions on the AT_2 receptor of rising concentrations of angiotensin II are unknown.

ACE inhibitors and AT_1 antagonists in combination

Rather than being alternatives, it is possible that AT_1 receptor antagonists and ACE inhibitors are complementary. The ACE inhibitor prevents excessive increases in plasma angiotensin II, reducing competition between AII and the antagonist for binding to the AT_1 receptor. The AT_1 receptor antagonist inhibits the effects of any residual angiotensin II at the receptor. Studies already show that the rise in angiotensin II induced by an AT_1 receptor antagonist can be attenuated by ACE inhibition, at least in the short term, while addition of an AT_1 receptor antagonist to an ACE inhibitor results in a further decline in aldosterone, indicating better renin–angiotensin system blockade.[57] Any adverse effect of angiotensin II on the AT_2 receptor will be ameliorated by ACE inhibition.

Clinical studies with AT_1 receptor antagonists

Actions of AT_1 receptor antagonists in heart failure

Little clinical information on angiotensin II antagonists in human heart failure yet exists. In hypertension, doses of losartan from 50–100 mg/day seem equally effective and as effective as enalapril 10–20 mg once daily.[58]

Haemodynamics studies with losartan

Two haemodynamic studies have been reported so far.[59,60] A single dose study[59] suggested that losartan 25 mg reduces systemic vascular resistance and arterial pressure; trends to an increase in cardiac output and reduction in pulmonary wedge pressure were not significant. The effects persisted for at least 24 hours. Worryingly, the haemodynamic effects of losartan 5 mg, 10 mg, 75 mg, and 150 mg were generally not significantly different from those of placebo (Fig. 18.3). A haemodynamic study before and after 3 months' dosing[60] with losartan at doses of 2.5 mg, 10 mg, 25 mg and 50 mg per day showed little improvement in haemodynamics

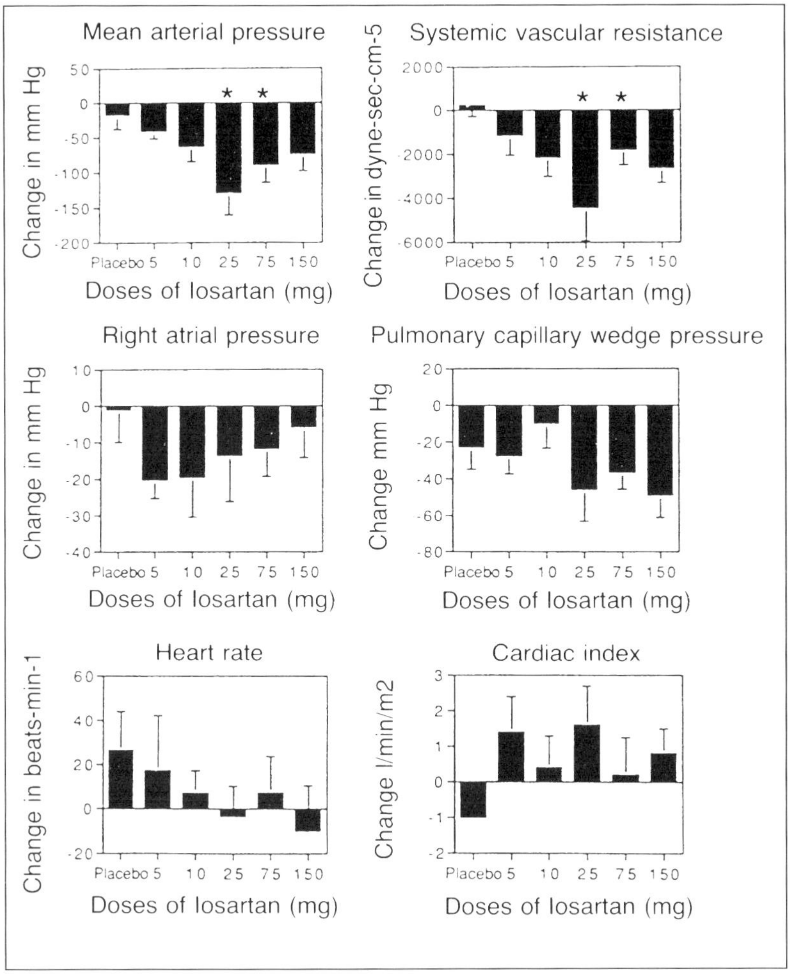

Fig. 18.3
Bar graphs of change in haemodynamic parameters by area-under-the-curve analysis after administration of placebo and five doses of losartan (5 mg, 10 mg, 25 mg, 75 mg, and 150 mg). Increasing vasodilator response was noted up to a dose of 25 mg. (– significance ($p < 0.05$) compared with placebo.) (From reference 62.)*

24 hours after the last dose, mean pulmonary capillary wedge pressure having fallen by no more than 3 mmHg with no significant effect on cardiac output or systemic vascular resistance. The 10 mg and 25 mg dose were associated with a reduction in heart rate. After 3 months' therapy and 6–12 hours after a further dose, 25 mg and 50 mg of losartan reduced systemic vascular resistance, pulmonary wedge pressures, and heart rate, and increased cardiac output (Fig. 18.4) compared to placebo. Effects of other dosages were inconsistent, although the 2.5 mg dose appeared to retain some effect in reducing wedge pressure. Only the 50 mg dose reduced cardiothoracic ratio significantly over 3 months. As with ACE inhibitors, the haemodynamic benefits were modest (Fig. 18.5).

Neuroendocrine effects

Neuroendocrine variables were measured in both of the above studies.[59,60] The single dose study[59] showed small increases in plasma renin activity and angiotensin II, as predicted, and a decline in aldosterone. As with ACE inhibitors, a fall in plasma noradrenaline was also noted

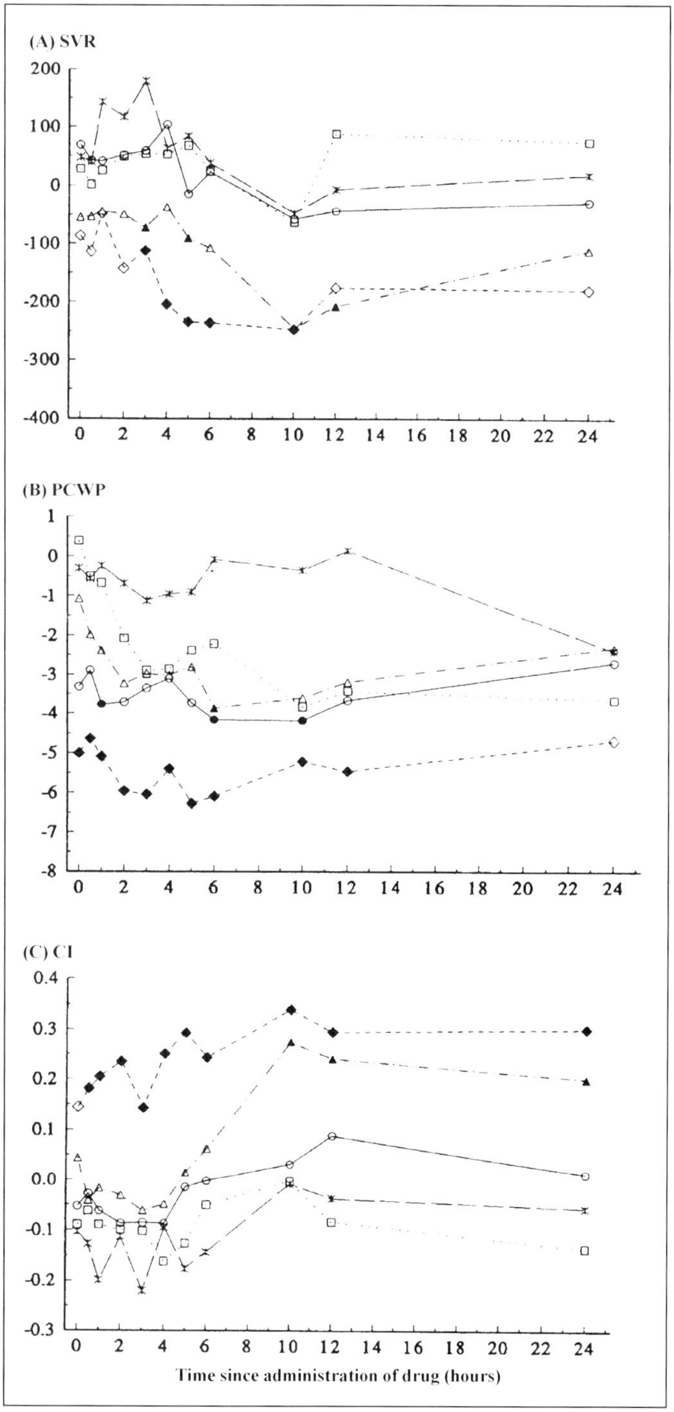

Fig. 18.4
Plots of mean change from pretreatment baseline levels after 12 weeks of therapy in (A) systemic vascular resistance (dyne · s^{-1} · cm^{-5}), (B) pulmonary capillary wedge pressure (mmHg), and (C) cardiac index (L · min^{-1} · m^{-2}). (placebo; ○ losartan 2.5 mg; □ losartan 10 mg; △ losartan 25 mg; ◇ losartan 50 mg.) Shaded symbols indicate a significant difference ($p \leq 0.05$) between losartan and placebo groups.*

Drug	CI	SVR	PVR	MAP	HR	PCWP	MRAP
Baseline	1.8	2200	400	85	85	28	12
Captopril	+0.3	−700	−75	−18	−6	−8	−4
Hydralazine	+0.9	−1000	ND	−15	+1	−5	−1
	*	*			*	*	*
Nitroprusside	+0.9	−1000	−150	−17	0	−8	−6
	*	*	*		*		*
ISDN	+0.5	−500	−150	−8	−2	−8	−6
	*		*	*	*		*
Prazosin	+0.7	−800	ND	−18	−5	−8	−5
	*	*					

Table 18.5
*Acute effects of different vasodilator agents in chronic heart failure. (CI – cardiac index (l/min/m^2); SVR – systemic vascular resistance (dyne/s/cm^{-5}); PVR – pulmonary vascular resistance (dyne/s/cm^{-5}); MAP – mean arterial pressure (mmHg); HR – heart rate (bpm); PCWP – pulmonary capillary wedge pressure (mmHg); MRAP – mean right atrial pressure (mmHg); * – significantly different from the response to captopril.) (From reference 3.)*

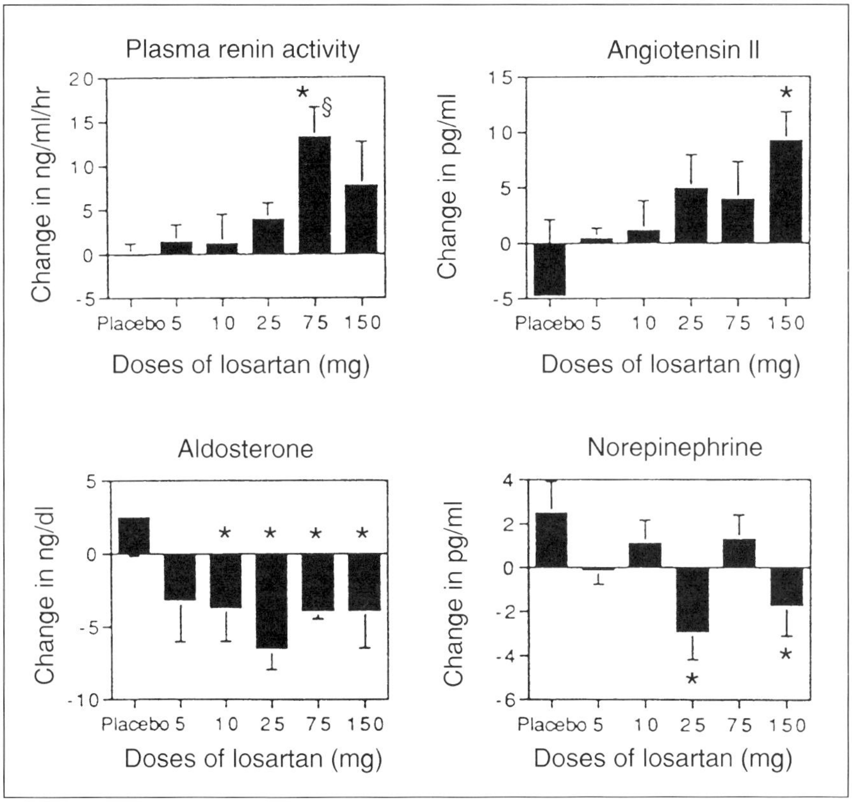

Fig. 18.5
Bar graphs of neurohormonal response by area-under-the-curve analysis after administration of placebo and five doses of losartan. Logarithmic values are displayed. Plasma renin activity and plasma angiotensin II concentrations increased with increasing doses of losartan. Aldosterone and noradrenaline concentrations decreased following losartan administration. (– significance ($p < 0.05$) compared with placebo; § – significance compared with 25 mg losartan.) (From reference 62.)*

with dosages of 25 mg and above. The fall in aldosterone 6 hours post-dosing was observed with doses as low as 10 mg. The long-term study[60] showed similar trends though only the 10 mg dosage reduced aldosterone significantly and only the 25 mg dosage reduced plasma noradrenaline significantly (Fig. 18.5).

These studies suggest that doses of losartan around 10 mg may be most effective in reducing aldosterone. This may reflect the ability of larger doses to cause a reflex increase in angiotensin II, which then competes with the antagonist at adrenal receptor sites. Alternatively, larger doses of losartan may conserve potassium more effectively, and small increases in potassium could stimulate aldosterone secretion.

Symptoms

As yet no study investigating the effects of losartan compared to placebo on symptoms or exercise performance in patients with heart failure exists. Data gleaned from the only moderately large, medium-term haemodynamic study in patients who have been treated for heart failure but who are not receiving an ACE inhibitor suggest that symptoms of heart failure are improved.[60] During 3 months of follow-up, 38% (11 of 29) on placebo reported worsening heart failure compared to 12% (7 of 61) of those on losartan 25–50 mg/day.

Two studies comparing the effects of losartan and enalapril on symptoms and exercise performance have been reported.[61,62] Both studies adopted a design whereby patients stabilized on enalapril were randomized to continue this treatment or to receive losartan 25–50 mg/day. Patients were followed for 12 weeks. Neither study showed a difference between losartan and enalapril. Although these data suggest that enalapril and losartan have similar benefits, some caution in interpretation is required. Several shorter-term studies have documented that exercise performance deteriorates within 6–8 weeks of withdrawing an ACE inhibitor;[63–65] deterioration may be slower after withdrawal from prolonged ACE inhibition, indicating that a prolonged 'carry-over' effect from ACE inhibition cannot be discounted.[66]

Morbidity and mortality data

In the haemodynamic studies described above,[59,60] five deaths occurred among 179 patients randomized to losartan, and none in 41 patients randomized to placebo. Death was the result of myocardial infarction or ventricular arrhythmia. However, only three of the five patients had received losartan around the time of death. All three died of ventricular fibrillation, after 10, 21 and 85 days of treatment. Two deaths occurred on the 2.5 mg dosage. As this dosage of losartan was associated with little evidence of a haemodynamic or neuroendocrine effect, it can be argued that the deaths that occurred are not relevant to patients on effective doses of losartan. The initial clinical trials do not give rise to concerns about the effects of losartan on other major morbid events. For the reasons outlined above, a mortality benefit from losartan, though possible, cannot be assumed.

Clinical studies: a comparison of the haemodynamic effects of ACE inhibitors and AT_1 receptor antagonists

Studies in patients with hypertension and in animal experimental models suggest that the effects of AT_1 receptor antagonists and ACE inhibitors are haemodynamically similar.[51,58] There are as yet no controlled studies comparing the haemodynamic effects of an AT_1 receptor antagonist and an ACE inhibitor in human heart failure. It is unwise to compare the haemodynamic effects from different studies, as the characteristics of the patients are likely to be different. Studies with ACE inhibitors were commonly conducted in patients with more severe heart failure, but the longer-term studies with AT_1 receptor antagonists recruited either patients with milder disease, in whom it was not deemed unethical at the time to withhold an ACE inhibitor for a few months, or patients who had had an adverse effect with an ACE inhibitor such as cough or angioneurotic oedema.

Adverse effect profile: are there advantages of AT_1 receptor antagonists over ACE inhibitors?

Cough

A persistent dry cough is undoubtedly a common side effect of ACE inhibitors, especially among women.[67] However, the amount of disability it causes is unclear. Cough is reported spontaneously as an adverse effect in large-scale studies of ACE inhibitors in only about 3% of cases, a rate that is little higher than with placebo.[68] Some patients have a severe cough caused by ACE inhibitors but surprisingly do not report it spontaneously, believing the side-effect to be part of their illness. Cough can be disabling, physically tiring the patient and disrupting sleep; undoubtedly some patients 'cough themselves to death'.

The mechanism underlying cough induced by ACE inhibitors is unclear. The most popular current theory is that ACE inhibitors increase pulmonary bradykinin and prostaglandins and that these in turn cause cough.[69] Non-steroidal anti-inflammatory drugs have enjoyed mixed success for the relief of cough but are of course strongly contraindicated in patients with heart failure because of their adverse renal effects. Changing to another ACE inhibitor occasionally helps but this may have more to do with the interruption of therapy than any real differences between ACE inhibitors. Anecdotally, ACE inhibitors may perpetuate cough initially caused by a respiratory tract infection; a drug-free interval may be all that is necessary to stop the cough, the patient then being able to resume the same treatment. A more recent approach is to use a mast cell stabilizer such as sodium cromoglycate.[70] Although angiotensin II has effects on mast cells, it is unclear how ACE inhibitors would induce cough by this mechanism; effects on mast cell stability or histaminase are possible.[71]

The author has personal experience of one patient with severe heart failure who did nearly 'cough himself to death' with an ACE inhibitor but who subsequently responded very well to losartan. Early reports in hypertension and heart failure support the contention that AT_1 receptor antagonists do not induce cough.

Angioneurotic oedema

Clinical trials of heart failure have suggested that this side-effect of ACE inhibitors is no commoner than in a placebo-treated population.[68] The mechanism underlying this reaction are also unclear, but an effect on histamine release by mast cells cannot be discounted. Patients on renal dialysis are at greater risk of angioneurotic-like reactions.[74] This appears to be related to the release of kinins particularly by polyacrylonitrile dialysis membranes.[73] Losartan has not been shown to precipitate angioneurotic-like reactions in this setting.

Hypotension

The incidence of first-dose hypotension with ACE inhibitors has declined dramatically from the 11% recorded in the first cohort of the

CONSENSUS study to around 2.2% in the SOLVD study (note that this was the combined incidence in the prevention and treatment arms; presumably the incidence would have been higher in the treatment arm as only these patients were receiving diuretics).[3] Unfortunately, the data provided in the studies do not help clinical practice very much as they fail to distinguish between syncope, haemodynamic crisis, and symptomless hypotension. Studies to resolve this problem are underway. Even if the incidence of first-dose syncope were 1% this would still be a major problem leading to thousands of life-threatening episodes worldwide each year.

First-dose syncope induced by ACE inhibitors appears temporally related to a rapid fall in angiotensin II and venous return.[74] Use of a longer-acting ACE inhibitor leads to a delay in the onset of action but the decline in angiotensin II due to inhibition of the final 10–20% of ACE appears no less abrupt.[75] Thus, longer-acting ACE inhibitors require a longer period of monitoring, and their use has not been shown to lead to a lower incidence of syncope.[75]

It is not clear at present whether AT_1 receptor antagonists are associated with a different incidence of first-dose syncope. However, it is possible that the occupation of AT_1 receptors occurs more slowly than the abrupt fall in angiotensin II that occurs with ACE inhibitors, and this may reduce the risk of syncope. The single dose haemodynamic study[59] discussed above noted a 3.7% (two patients out of 54) incidence of hypotension, though it is not clear if this led to disturbed consciousness. However, five of 125 (4%) patients discontinued losartan because of hypotension on the first or second day of treatment in the 12-week study, all of these episodes occurring with the 25 mg or 50 mg dosage. No episode resulted in permanent harm. It would appear that, as with ACE inhibitors, it is wise to initiate treatment with low doses, losartan 10 mg or less, and monitor the patient for 3–4 hours until wider experience is gained.

Renal dysfunction

Renal dysfunction is most likely to occur after ACE inhibition in elderly patients, patients with severe heart failure, and those with pre-existing renal disease.[3] Although this problem is not perceived to be a large one in the clinical studies with losartan so far, it is likely that patient selection has excluded many patients at risk of this side-effect. Renal dysfunction secondary to ACE inhibition is certainly perceived as a major problem by some renal physicians.[76]

ACE inhibitors reduce renal perfusion pressure and efferent arteriolar tone, which conspires to reduce glomerular filtration.[77] This is compensated for to some extent by a rise in renal blood flow. The increase in renal blood flow may be partly dependent on bradykinins and prostaglandins; non-steroidal anti-inflammatory drugs block vasodilator prostaglandin production and are particularly likely to cause renal failure in patients taking ACE inhibitors and diuretics.[3]

AT_1 receptor antagonists may not increase renal blood flow as much as ACE inhibitors, owing to the lack of effect on the bradykinin–prostaglandin pathway. Whether this has an adverse or beneficial effect on glomerular filtration will depend on whether the prostaglandin–bradykinin effect is predominantly an effect on the afferent or efferent arteriole. Efferent arteriolar dilatation will tend to cause a fall in filtration, whereas the opposite is true for afferent arteriolar dilatation. Prostaglandins probably exert more important effects on afferent tone and thus a greater fall in glomerular filtration might be predicted. However, during the initial haemodynamic studies in heart failure only one patient (receiving losartan 10 mg/day) developed a sufficient increase in creatinine to warrant withdrawal from the study. The cause of the problem was later identified as prostatic obstruction, probably (in this author's opinion) unrelated to the drug. Comparative studies suggest that treatment with losartan may be associated with a small fall in serum urea and creatinine as opposed to the small increase observed with enalapril.[24]

In non-diabetic hypertensive[78] patients, losartan, like the ACE inhibitors, appears to reduce proteinuria.

Gout

Losartan appears to increase uric acid secretion and to reduce serum uric acid.[79] Although this effect may be welcome, the risk of precipitating acute gout and renal calculi in the chronically hyperuricaemic patients must be borne in mind. The first medium-term study of losartan investigated 154 patients with heart failure, and it suggested a possible decrease in the incidence of gout.[79]

Conclusion

AT_1 antagonists undoubtedly appear to be a step forward in the treatment of heart failure. How big a step remains to be answererd. Ultimately, the most important use of an AT_1 antagonist may be in addition to rather than instead of an ACE inhibitor.

References

1 Morgan K, Wharton J, Webb JC, et al. Co-expression of renin–angiotensin system component genes in human atrial tissue. *J Hypertens Suppl* 1994;**12**:S11–S19.

2 Urata H, Healy B, Stewart RW, Bumpus FM, Husain A. Angiotensin II forming pathways in normal and failing human hearts. *Circ Res* 1990;**66**:883–890.

3 Morgan K. The mechanism of ACE inhibitor action. In: Cleland JGF, ed. *The Clinician's Guide to ACE Inhibition*. Churchill Livingstone, Edinburgh, 1993.

4 Jackson TR, Blair LAC, Marshall J, Goedert M, Hanley MR. The mas oncogene encodes an angiotensin receptor. *Nature* 1988;**335**:437–440.

5 O'Dowd BF, Heiber M, Chan A, et al. A human gene that shows identity with the gene encoding the angiotensin receptor is located on chromosome 11. Gene 1993;**136**:355–360.

6 Tiret L, Bonnardeux A, Poirier O, et al. Synergistic effects of ACE and angiotensin II type 1 receptor gene polymorphisms on risk of myocardial infarction. *Lancet* 1994; **344**:910–913.

7 Timmermans PBMWM, Benfield P, Chiu AT, Herblin WF, Wong PC, Smith RD. Angiotensin II receptors and functional correlates. *Am J Hypertens* 1992;**5**:2215–2355.

8 Kimura B, Sumners C, Phillips MI. Changes in angiotensin II (AII) receptors in skin during wound healing. *FASEB J* 1992;**6**:A1013.

9 Viswanathan M, Saavedra JM. Enhanced expression of angiotensin II AT_2 receptors in the skin of rats during experimental wound healing. *FASEB J* 1992;**6**:A1013.

10 Zemel S, Millan MA, Feuillan P, Aguilera G. Characterization and distribution of angiotensin II receptors in the primate fetus. *J Clin Endocrinol Metab* 1990;**71**:1003–1007.

11 Cook VI, Grove KL, McMenamin KL, Carter MR, Harding JW, Speth RC. The AT_2 angiotensin receptor subtype predominates in the 18 day gestation fetal rat brain. *Brain Res* 1991; **560**:334–336.

12 Smith RD, Timmermans PBMWM. Human angiotensin receptor subtypes. *Curr Opinion Nephrol Hypertens* 1994;**3**:112–122.

13 Whitebread S, Mele M, Kamber B, Degasparo M. Preliminary biochemical characterization of two angiotensin II receptor subtypes. *Biochem Biophys Res Commun* 1989;**163**:284–291.

14 Barnes JM, Barber PC, Barnes NM. Identification of angiotensin II receptor subtypes in human brain. *NeuroReport* 1991; **2**:605–608.

15 Grone HJ, Simon M, Fuchs E. Autoradiographic characterization of angiotensin receptor subtypes in fetal and adult human kidney. *Am J Physiol* 1992;**262**:326F–331F.

16 Chansel D, Czekalski S, Pham P, Ardaillou R. Characterization of angiotensin II receptor subtypes in human glomeruli and mesangial cells. *Am J Physiol* 1992;**262**:F432–F441.

17 Kalenga MK, Degasparo M, Dehertogh R, Whitebread S, Vankrieken L, Thomas K. Angiotensin II receptors in the human placenta are type AT_1. *Reprod Nutr Dev* 1991;**31**:257–267.

18 Wong PC, Hart SD, Zaspel A, Chiu AT, Smith RD, Timmermans PBMWM. Functional studies of nonpeptide angiotensin II receptor subtype-specific ligands: DuP 753 (AII-1) and PD123177 (AII-2). *J Pharmacol Exp Ther* 1990;**255**:584–592.

19 Chiu AT, McCall DE, Ardecky RJ, Duncia JV, Nguyen TT, Timmermans PBMWM. Angiotensin II receptor subtypes and their selective nonpeptide ligands. *Receptor* 1990; **1**:33–40.

20 Christen Y, Waeber B, Nussberger J, et al. Oral administration of DuP 753, a specific angiotensin II antagonist, to normal male volunteers: inhibition of pressor response to exogenous angiotensin I and II. *Circulation* 1991; **83**:1333–1342.

21 Munafo A, Christen Y, Nussberger J, Lee RJ, Timmermans PBMWM, Brunner HR. Dose–response relationship following oral administration of DuP 753 to normal humans. *Am J Hypertens* 1991;**4**:350S–353S.

22 Muller P, Cohen T, de Gasparo, Sioufi A, Racine-Poon A, Howald H. Angiotensin II receptor blockade with single doses of valsartan in healthy, normotensive subjects. *Eur J Clin Pharmacol* 1994;**47**:231–245.

23 Morimoto S, Ogihara T. TCV-116: a new angiotensin II type-1 receptor antagonist. *Cardiovasc Drug Rev* 1994;**12**:153–164.

24 Sweet CS, Rucinska EJ. Losartan in heart failure: preclinical experiences and initial clinical outcomes. *Eur Heart J* 1994;**15(suppl D)**:139–144.

25 Ogihara T, Higashimori K, Masuo K, Mikami H. Pilot study of a new angiotensin II receptor antagonist, TCV-116: effects of a single oral dose on blood pressure in patients with essential hypertension. *Clin Ther* 1994;**15**:684–691.

26 Cockcroft JR, Sciberras DG, Goldberg MR, Ritter JM. Comparison of angiotensin-converting enzyme inhibition with angiotensin II. *J Cardiovasc Pharmacol* 1993;**22**:579–584.

27 Chiu AT, Roscoe WA, McCall DE, Timmermans PBMWM. Angiotensin II-1 receptors mediate both vasoconstrictor and hypertrophic responses in rat aortic smooth muscle cells. *Receptor* 1991;**1**:133–140.

28 Kabour A, Hnenagr JR, Janicki JS. Angiotensin II induced myocyte necrosis: role of the AII receptor. *J Cardiovasc Pharmacol* 1994; **23**:547–553.

29 Schwieler JH, Kahan T, Nussberger J, Hjemdahl P. Converting enzyme inhibition modulates sympathetic neurotransmission in vivo via multiple mechanisms. *Am J Physiol Endocrinol Metab* 1993;**264**:E631–E637.

30 Koepke JP, Bovy PR, McMahon EG, et al. Central and peripheral actions of a nonpeptidic angiotensin II receptor antagonist. *Hypertension* 1991;**15(part 2)**:841–847.

31 Murphy DD, Shepard J, Smith SG III, Stephens GA. Effects of the AT_1 receptor antagonist losartan on angiotensin II induced hypertrophy of rat cardiomyocytes. *FASEB J* 1992; **6**:A1261.

32 Moscucci A, Moscucci M, Murphy MB, January CT. Angiotensin II receptor mediated effects on L-type CA current in canine ventricular myocytes: a study using DuP 753, a new, receptor specific, nonpeptide angiotensin II antagonist. *Biophys J* 1991;**59**:99a.

33 Chua CC, Chua BHL, Diglio CA, Siu BB. Induction of endothelin-1 transcripts by angiotensin II in rat heart endothelial cells. *FASEB J* 1992;**6**:A1636.

34 Morton JJ, Beattie EC, MacPherson F. Angiotensin II receptor antagonist losartan has persistent effects on blood pressure in the young spontaneously hypertensive rat: lack of relation to vascular structure. *J Vasc Research* 1992;**29**:264–269.

35 Linz W, Henning R, Scholkens BA, Becker RHA. ACE inhibition and angiotensin II receptor antagonism on development and regression of cardiac hypertrophy in rats. In: *Current Advances in ACE Inhibition* volume 2. Union of Physiological Sciences and American Physiological Societies, 1991:188–190.

36 Morton JJ, Beattie EC, MacPherson F. Treatment of young spontaneously hypertensive rats (SHR) with angiotensin receptor antagonist losartan reduces hypertension and vascular hypertrophy in adulthood. *J Hypertens* 1992;**10(suppl 4)**:S151.

37 Raya TE, Fonken SJ, Lee RW, et al. Hemodynamic effects of direct angiotensin II blockade compared to converting enzyme inhibition in rat model of heart failure. *Am J Hypertens* 1991;**4(part 2)**:334S–340S.

38 Fitzpatrick MA, Pademaker MT, Charles CJ, Yandle TG, Espiner EA, Ikram H. Angiotensin II receptor antagonism in ovine heart failure: acute hemodynamic, hormonal, and renal effects. *Am J Physiol* 1992; **263**:H250–H256.

39 Matsubara L, Brilla CG, Weber KT. Angiotensin II-mediated inhibition of collagenase activity in cultured cardiac fibroblasts. *FASEB J* 1992;**6**:A941.

40 Qing G, Garcia R. Chronic captopril and losartan (DuP 753) administration in rats with high output heart failure. *Am J Physiol* 1992; **263**:833H–840H.

41 Keiser JA, Biork FA, Hodges JC, Taylor DG Jr. Renal hemodynamic and excretory responses to

PD123319 and losartan, nonpeptide AT, and AT, subtype specific angiotensin II ligands. *J Pharmacol Exp Ther* 1992;**262**:1154–1160.
42 Deck CC, Gaballa MA, Raya TE. Renal function in rats with experimental heart failure: angiotensin II blockade versus ACE inhibition. *Circulation* 1993;**88(suppl)**:1–514.
43 Smits JFM, Vankrimpen C, Schoemaker RG, Cleutjens JPM, Daemen MJAP. Angiotensin II receptor blockade after myocardial infarction in rats: effects on hemodynamics, myocardial DNA synthesis, and interstitial collagen content. *J Cardiovasc Pharmacol* 1992; **20**:772–778.
44 Smits JFM, Schoemaker RG, Daemen MJAP, et al. Haemodynamic consequences of interference with the renin–angiotensin system following myocardial infarction in rats [abstract]. *Br J Pharmacol* 1991;**102(suppl)**:99P.
45 Linz W, Martorana PA, Wienre G, Grotsch H, Scholkens BA. The cardioprotective effects of the ACE inhibitor ramipril resemble those of bradykinin in ischaemic hearts. In: MacGregor GA, Sever PS, eds. *Current Advances in ACE Inhibition.* Churchill Livingstone, London, 1989;283–285.
46 Smits JFM, Passier PCJJ, Daemen MJAP. ACE inhibition and AT receptor inhibition following myocardial infarction: structural and functional consequences [abstract]. *Can J Cardiol* 1994; **10(suppl A)**:59A.
47 Schieffer B, Wirger A, Meybrunn M, et al. Comparative effects of chronic angiotensin converting enzyme inhibition and angiotensin II type 1 receptor blockade on cardiac remodelling after myocardial infarction in the rat. *Circulation* 1994;**89**:2273–2282.
48 Ruzicka M, Leenen FHH. Nonpeptide angiotensin II receptor blocker but not angiotensin converting enzyme inhibitor attenuates the hypertrophic response of the heart to cardiac volume overload in rats. *FASEB J* 1993;**7**:551.
49 Abassi ZA, Kelly G, Golomb E, et al. Losartan improves the natriuretic response to ANF in rats with high output heart failure. *J Pharmacol Exp Ther* 1994;**268**:224–230.
50 Tanaka A, Matsumori A, Wang W, Sasayama S. An angiotensin II receptor antagonist reduces myocardial damage in an animal model of myocarditis. *Circulation* 1994;**90**:2051–2055.
51 Murakami M, Suzuki H, Naitoh M, et al. Significance of action of angiotensin II in congestive heart failure in conscious dogs. *Circulation* 1991;**84(suppl II)**:107.
52 Matsumoto A, Suzuki H, Naitoh M, et al. Angiotensin II inhibition augments natriuretic effect of candoxatril in congestive heart failure with renal dysfunction [abstract]. *J Hypertens* 1994;**12(suppl 3)**:586.
53 McDonald KM, Francis GS, Carlyle PF, et al. Hemodynamic, left ventricular structural and hormonal changes after discrete myocardial damage in the dog. *J Am Coll Cardiol* 1992; **19**:460–467.
54 Richard V, Ghaleh B, Berdeaux A, et al. Comparison of the effects of EXP3174, an angiotensin II antagonist and enalaprilat on myocardial infarct size in anesthetised dogs. *Br J Pharmacol* 1993;**110**:969–974.
55 Cleland JGF, Poole-Wilson PA. ACE inhibitors for heart failure: a question of dose. *Br Heart J* 1994;**72**:106–110.
56 Vernace MA, Mento PF, Maita ME, Wilkes BM. Effects of angiotensin receptor subtype inhibitors on plasma angiotensin clearance. *Hypertension* 1994;**23**:853–856.
57 Menard J. Improving hypertension treatment: where should we put our efforts: new drugs, new concepts, or new management? *Am J Hypertens* 1992;**5(suppl II)**:252S–258S.
58 Burnier M, Waeber B, Brunner HR. The advantages of angiotensin II antagonism. *J Hypertens Suppl* 1994;**12**:S7–S15.
59 Gottlieb SS, Dickstein K, Fleck E, et al. Hemodynamic and neurohormonal effects of the angiotensin II antagonist losartan in patients with congestive heart failure. *Circulation* 1993;**88**:1602–1609.
60 Crozier I, Ikram H, Awan N, et al. Losartan in heart failure. Hemodynamic effects and tolerability. *Circulation* 1995;**91**:691–697.
61 Dickstein K, et al. Comparison of the effects of losartan and enalapril on clinical status and exercise performance in patients with moderate or severe chronic heart failure (In preparation).
62 Lang RM, Yellen LG, McKelvie RS, et al. Comparative effects of losartan and enalapril on exercise capacity and clinical status of patients with heart failure. *Circulation* 1994; **90(suppl)**:1–602.

63 Cleland JGF, Dargie HJ, Ball SG, et al. Effects of enalapril in heart failure: a double blind study of effects on exercise performance, renal function, hormones, and metabolic state. *Br Heart J* 1985;**54**:305–312.

64 Cleland JGF, Dargie HJ, Hodsman GP, et al. Captopril in heart failure. A double blind controlled trial. *Br Heart J* 1984;**52**:530–535.

65 Northridge DB, Rose E, Raftery ED, et al. A multicentre, double-blind, placebo-controlled trial of quinapril in mild, chronic heart failure. *Eur Heart J* 1993;**14**:403–409.

66 Pflugfelder PW, Baird MG, Tonkon MJ, DiBianco R, Pitt B. Clinical consequences of angiotensin-converting enzyme inhibitor withdrawal in chronic heart failure: a double-blind, placebo-controlled study of quinapril. *J Am Coll Cardiol* 1993;**22**:1557–1563.

67 Os I, Bratland B, Dahloff B, et al. Female sex as an important determinant of lisinopril-induced cough. *Lancet* 1992;**339**:372.

68 The SOLVD investigators. Effect of enalapril on survival in patients with reduced left ventricular ejection fractions and congestive heart failure. *N Engl J Med* 1991;**325**:303–310.

69 Israili ZH, Hall WD. Cough and angioneurotic edema associated with angiotensin-converting enzyme inhibitor therapy. A review of the literature and pathophysiology. *Ann Intern Med* 1992;**117**:234–242.

70 Hargreaves M. Sodium cromoglycate: a remedy for ACE inhibitor-induced cough. *Br J Clin Pract* 1993;**47**:319–320.

71 Cleland JGF. Lack of effect of nedocromil sodium in ACE inhibitor-induced cough. *Lancet* 1995;**345**:394.

72 Varma JR, Nixon GA. Angioedema and angiotensin-converting enzyme (ACE) inhibitors. *J Am Board Fam Pract* 1994;**7**:433–435.

73 Schulman G, Hakim R, Arias R, Silverberg M, Kaplan AP, Arbeit L. Bradykinin generation by dialysis membranes: possible role in anaphylactic reaction. *J Am Soc Nephrol* 1993;**3**:1563–1569.

74 Cleland J, Semple P, Hodsman P, et al. Angiotensin II levels, hemodynamics, and sympathoadrenal function after low-dose captopril in heart failure. *Am J Med* 1984;**77**:880–886.

75 Cleland JGF, Dargie HJ, McAlpine H, et al. Severe hypotension after first dose of enalapril in heart failure. *B M J* 1985;**291**:1309–1312.

76 Czapla K, Ahmed E, McMillan MA. Renal artery stenosis and congestive heart failure [letter]. *Lancet* 1993;**342**:302.

77 Cleland JGF, Dargie HJ, Gillen G, et al. Captopril in heart failure: a double-blind study of the effects on renal function. *J Cardiovasc Pharmacol* 1986;**8**:700–706.

78 Gansevoort RT, De Zeeuw D, De Jong PE. Is the antiproteinuric effect of ACE inhibition mediated by interference with the renin–angiotensin system? *Kidney Int* 1994;**45**:861–867.

79 Nakashima M, Uematsu T, Kosuge K, Kanamaru M. Pilot study of the uricosuric effect of DuP-753, a new angiotensin II receptor antagonist in healthy subjects. *Eur J Clin Pharmacol* 1992;**42**:333–335.

19

Where do we go from here with treatment? The ongoing trials and unanswered questions

Axel Sigurdsson, Karl Swedberg

Introduction

During the past decade considerable advances have been achieved in the treatment of chronic congestive heart failure. The angiotensin converting enzyme (ACE) inhibitors have been shown to improve survival among patients with mild, moderate and severe heart failure,[1–3] and heart transplantations are now being performed successfully at many centres throughout the world, although this method is still only available for a limited number of patients. In parallel with these therapeutic advances, our understanding of the epidemiology, natural history, and pathophysiology of chronic heart failure (CHF) has been expanding. Epidemiological studies have indicated that the prevalence of CHF is high and appears to be increasing.[4–6] These studies also clearly show that CHF becomes more frequent with age. When this fact is placed in the context of the current shift towards an ageing population and a 5-year mortality of 50% among patients with CHF,[7] the size of this important health care problem becomes obvious. Another recent epidemiological survey based on data from the Framingham Heart Study[8] has underscored the high age-adjusted mortality of chronic heart failure and indicated no significant therapeutic improvement during a 40-year period from 1948 to 1988.

The objectives of treatment for chronic heart failure may be considered to be threefold:

- prevention;
- relief of symptoms; and
- improvement of prognosis.

Preventative measures may be divided further into:

- measures that are capable of preventing the myocardial damage that is the underlying cause of the cardiac failure; and
- prevention of progression of heart failure that is already present.

Future research and treatment should focus primarily on these important main objectives. In order to improve therapy, increased knowledge of pathophysiological mechanisms involved in the development and progression of heart failure is essential. Basic research directed at myocardial as well as at peripheral mechanisms is therefore important, and the progress in molecular biology has added a new dimension to heart failure research.[9] At the same time, the importance of well-performed placebo-controlled clinical trials must be emphasized. These studies are essential to test the validity of therapeutic interventions, pathophysiological concepts and hypotheses. There are indeed several controlled studies on patients with myocardial dysfunction or heart failure which have shown increased mortality with active drug therapy compared to placebo.[10–12]

Furthermore, such studies may reveal a new potential therapeutic concept that may need further testing. An example is the prevention of coronary events achieved by treatment with ACE inhibitors in the SAVE (Survival and Ventricular Enlargement)[13] and SOLVD (Studies of Left Ventricular Dysfunction)[14] trials, which studied patients with left ventricular dysfunction after myocardial infarction on the one hand and patients with heart failure of mild or moderate severity on the other hand. As more knowledge is gained, a tailoring of preventive and therapeutic strategies for CHF may evolve. A tailored approach might be based on factors such as the degree of systolic dysfunction and possibly the degree of diastolic dysfunction, the cause of heart failure, the risk of sudden death from arrhythmias, the risk of further myocardial damage, the degree of neurohormonal activation, the architecture of the myocardium itself, and possibly on genetic factors.

Pathophysiological concepts and current treatment strategies

Apart from being disabling to the patient, heart failure is a progressive and lethal disorder. Most patients die because of progressive pump failure. However, death is often sudden, in which case it is most likely to be due to ventricular tachyarrhythmias or bradyarrhythmias.[15] Surprisingly little is known about the mechanism of the progression of heart failure. Moreover, it is not clear which patients will experience progression from ventricular dysfunction to overt heart failure, and, once heart failure has developed, which patients will follow a stepwise downhill course of progressive disease. Heart failure may progress because of repeated myocardial damage induced by the underlying cardiac disease (e.g. recurrent myocardial infarction, myocardial involvement of infectious origin) or because of continuous pressure or volume overload caused by a valvular disorder. Recent knowledge also indicates that heart failure may progress because of a complicated interaction between the heart and different peripheral counter-regulatory mechanisms that become maladaptive over time.[16] Endothelial dysfunction,[17–19] altered baroreceptor function,[20–22] and sustained activation of different neuroendocrine systems may all be important in this respect.[23-27]

From a pathophysiological viewpoint, CHF can be treated according to various concepts. The most important of these concepts can be divided into:

- preventive measures;
- relief of vascular congestion;
- inotropic support;
- haemodynamic unloading;
- correction of maladaptive responses such as excessive neurohormonal activation and endothelial and baroreceptor dysfunction;
- prevention of sudden death from arrhythmias; and
- other pathophysiological concepts that may lead to improved treatment.

Preventative measures

Primary prevention of heart failure should ideally be aimed at the underlying cause of the disease. Despite the diversity of aetiologies, the predominant cause of heart failure in industrialized nations is ischaemic heart disease. Therefore, measures capable of preventing atherosclerotic disease, plaque rupture, and thrombosis are of particular importance. If myocardial damage and left ventricular dysfunction have already occurred, preventative measures will have to aim at preventing the progression to symptomatic heart failure. The importance of measures with a potential capacity to prevent the development of symptomatic heart failure may be best illustrated by the fact that, in patients with left ventricular dysfunction, the prognosis is much worse among those with symptomatic failure than among those who are asymptomatic.[3,28]

Following an acute myocardial infarction, progressive left ventricular dilatation may occur.[29–33] During the first week, thinning and dilatation of the infarcted myocardium appears to predominate, whereas later on, remodelling of the non-infarcted contractile myocardium may be more important.[34] Increased left ventricular volume appears to be highly associated with adverse prognosis.[35] The exact mechanisms responsible for the dilatation of the left ventricle, often termed remodelling, are incompletely understood. Haemodynamic factors, which may lead to an increase in myocardial wall stress, might be important.[33] Furthermore, in the presence of myocardial dysfunction, a number of adaptive mechanisms are activated in order to maintain blood pressure and perfusion to vital organs. Among these compensatory responses are the activation of the sympathetic nervous system and the activation of the renin–angiotensin system.[23] This activation may initially increase myocardial contractility and raise heart rate and thus improve cardiac output. However, long-term activation of these neuroendocrine systems can be harmful to the myocardium and possibly increase the risk of development of symptomatic heart failure.[26] Thus, it appears that the transition from acute myocardial infarction to left ventricular dilatation is a highly complicated process, and one that probably also involves collagen synthesis and genetic mechanisms.[36,37] There is substantial evidence to indicate that therapy of patients with asymptomatic or symptomatic left ventricular dysfunction should aim at reducing the effects of neurohormonal activation by drugs such as ACE inhibitors.[38] A number of studies in patients with acute myocardial infarction have shown that left ventricular dilatation is capable of being modified and that progressive dilatation may be reduced by treatment with ACE inhibitors.[39–41]

Recently, the efficacy of ACE inhibitors following myocardial infarction has been studied in a number of large placebo-controlled trials.[13,42–45] These studies indicate that patients with symptomatic or asymptomatic left ventricular dysfunction after an acute myocardial infarction should receive long-term treatment with an ACE inhibitor, and that such treatment may improve survival, reduce the incidence of overt heart failure, and reduce the risk of reinfarction. In the early phase of myocardial infarction, efforts to reduce or limit infarct size are of prime importance and have been shown to improve both short-term and long-term outcomes.[46,47] Thrombolytic drugs and beta-adrenoceptor blockers have been shown to be particularly useful in this respect. In the ISIS-2 trial, early administration of aspirin was also shown to be highly beneficial.[47] Although studies with ACE inhibitors have expanded our understanding of pathophysiological mechanisms, the remodelling process and the importance of neurohormonal mechanisms, ACE inhibition may be only one of many possible treatments for the prevention of heart failure after myocardial infarction.

Relief of vascular congestion

For a long time, diuretics have remained a mainstay of heart failure treatment when fluid retention or pulmonary congestion is present. These agents are necessary for symptomatic relief, although their effects on the progression of heart failure or mortality is unknown.

Inotropic support

As the primary abnormality of heart failure is loss of functioning myocardium, enhancing the contractile performance of the remaining undamaged myocardium might appear as an attractive therapeutic concept. However, the results of long-term therapy with inotropic drugs, such as beta-adrenergic agonists and the phosphodiesterase inhibitors, has been disappointing, and placebo-controlled trials have indicated that these drugs may adversely affect survival.[11,12,48,49] The inotropic agent vesnarinone was recently shown to decrease mortality when used in low doses but to increase mortality when administered in doses that were twice as large.[50] This has led to the speculation that inotropic drugs might be beneficial when used in doses low enough not to increase the force of myocardial contraction at rest.[51] This may also underscore the growing opinion that a positive haemodynamic action of a drug should not be considered a prerequisite for the development of an effective drug for the treatment of CHF.[26]

Digitalis, the oldest drug with inotropic activity, has been in clinical use for more than 200 years.[52] Ironically, the first trial assessing the effects of digitalis on survival in patients with heart failure and sinus rhythm is only now in progress.[53] Digitalis is a relatively weak inotropic agent compared to catecholamines and phosphodiesterase inhibitors. However, digitalis may have other effects, which may be important for the treatment of patients with CHF. For example, it may inhibit excessive neurohormonal activity.[54–56] It also has an interesting influence on parasympathetic mechanisms, which may have positive therapeutic implications.[57] The RADIANCE (Randomized Assessment of [the effect of] Digoxin on Inhibitors of the Angiotensin Converting Enzyme)[58] and PROVED (Prospective Randomized Study of Ventricular Failure and the Efficacy of Digoxin)[59] trials studied the effects of withdrawal of digoxin from patients with CHF. In both these studies, patients were randomized in a double blind fashion to continue receiving digoxin or to be switched to placebo. Clinical deterioration and a worsening of exercise capacity were commoner among patients who were switched to placebo than among those who continued on digoxin.

Haemodynamic unloading

Another pathophysiological concept in the treatment of heart failure is the haemodynamic unloading of the heart by drugs with vasodilating activity. The haemodynamic alterations in CHF include elevated filling pressures and increased impedance to left ventricular ejection, the latter of which is primarily due to peripheral vasoconstriction. These alterations cause an increase in left ventricular wall stress, which may be an important underlying mechanism behind ventricular remodelling and dilatation.[60] These pathophysiological events provide the main rationale for the use of vasodilators in the treatment of CHF. Vasodilators reduce systemic vascular resistance by dilating the arteries and reduce filling pressures by dilating the veins. These effects should have a favourable influence on the mechanical performance of the heart, haemodynamical parameters, and myocardial metabolism. Vasodilators are usually classified according to their site of action. Thus, nitrates in low doses are primarily venodilators. Hydralazine and the first- and second-generation calcium channel blockers are mainly arterial dilators.

Examples of balanced vasodilators, which provide both venous and arterial dilation, are alpha-adrenergic blockers (such as prazosin, nitroprusside, and flosequinan) and nitrates when given in high doses. The effects of vasodilators on mortality and morbidity in patients with CHF have been tested in placebo-controlled trials. The combination of isosorbide dinitrate and hydralazine compared to placebo and prazosin was assessed in the V-HeFT I trial.[61] Treatment with the vasodilator combination produced an overall 28% reduction in mort-ality compared to placebo, but no beneficial effect was found with prazosin therapy. The effects of monotherapy with nitrates or hydralazine on mortality in CHF is unknown. Flosequinan, a vasodilator with some inhibiting activity on phosphodiesterase, was tested in the PROFILE (Prospective Randomized Flosequinan Longevity Evaluation) survival study. There was an adverse effect on survival and quality of life during long-term therapy with flosequinan 100 mg/day compared to placebo (M Packer, 1995, personal communication). The first-generation calcium channel blockers (verapamil, nifedipine and diltiazem) can produce short-term haemodynamic benefits which, however, are not necessarily sustained during long-term treatment.[62] In addition, many patients with severe heart failure exhibit haemodynamic and symptomatic deterioration when treated with these agents; some develop severe hypotension and cardiogenic shock.[63] Therefore, there is little evidence to support the use of these drugs in patients with CHF.

During recent years, second-generation calcium channel blockers have been developed. These drugs are less likely to depress left ventricular function, but they can cause coronary and systemic vasodilation similar to the effects of nifedipine and diltiazem and they have therefore often been characterized as being vasoselective. Examples of second-generation calcium channel blockers that have been developed are amlodipine, nicardipine, nisoldipine, nitrenipine, felodipine, and isradipine. Clinical trials testing the effects of these drugs on morbidity and mortality are currently ongoing or are being planned. Recently, the main results of the PRAISE trial (Prospective Randomized Amlodipine Survival Evaluation) were reported. 1153 patients were randomized and no overall effect was seen on survival. However, in a prespecified analysis, a significant reduction in mortality was found in patients classified as non-ischaemic. The reduction was 45% ($p<0.001$, M Packer, personal communication). The investigators concluded that amlodipine was safe in heart failure and that an effect in patients with non-ischaemic aetiology was likely.

Correction of maladaptive responses

A modern concept for the treatment of heart failure is targeted towards the correction of maladaptive responses that follow the myocardial injury. These maladaptive responses include sustained neurohormonal activation and endothelial and baroreceptor dysfunction. As indicated above, these responses appear to be related to the progressive nature of heart failure. Although the initial event in the development of left ventricular dysfunction is structural damage to the myocardium, heart failure is not only a disease of the heart. Patients with left ventricular dysfunction frequently have no symptoms of heart failure, probably because compensatory mechanisms enable maintenance of cardiac output and peripheral perfusion. These adaptive responses are the result of a complex interplay between myocardial, haemodynamic, and neurohormonal mechanisms, which are activated almost immediately following the myocardial injury.[64,65]

At some point of time, however, compensatory mechanisms tend to become exhausted and many patients ultimately develop symptoms of heart failure. At this stage, sustained activation of the sympathetic nervous system and the renin–angiotensin system appears to be maladaptive and may cause further harm to the myocardium, leading to progression of the disorder.[26,64–66]

Furthermore, baroreflex responses are not able to limit the magnitude of activation of the vasoconstrictor hormones, because baroreceptor function may be impaired.[20,67] During sympathetic activation, the beta-receptors are modified, both in numbers and function.[68] Thus, sustained neurohormonal activation is partly maintained by altered baroreceptor function, which may reduce inhibitory signals to the vasomotor centre and thereby diminish the inhibition to sympathetic outflow. It has repeatedly been shown that different neurohormonal systems are activated in patients with CHF.[69–74] Neurohormonal activation appears to be most pronounced among patients with severe symptoms, although the magnitude of activation varies widely.[75–77]

Factors other than the disease itself may influence neurohormonal mechanisms and it is well known that diuretic treatment may activate the renin–angiotensin system.[78,79] A strong association has been found between mortality and plasma concentrations of noradrenaline, atrial natriuretic peptide (ANP), angiotensin II, and plasma renin activity in both moderate and severe CHF.[66,80–82] Recently, using a multivariate model that included left ventricular ejection fraction, peak exercise oxygen consumption, and cardiothoracic ratio, plasma noradrenaline was found to be a significant predictor of mortality among patients with mild or moderate congestive heart failure.[82]

Although these data do not prove a causal relationship, a lot of available evidence indicates that activation of the sympathetic nervous system and the renin–angiotensin system is harmful to the myocardium and may be largely responsible for progress of the disorder.[26,83–85] The renin–angiotensin system is both a circulating and local tissue hormonal system. Plasma concentrations of the hormonal components and enzyme activities of this system have traditionally been used as indicators of activity. With an increased pathophysiological understanding, the importance of the tissue renin–angiotensin system has emerged during recent years.[86–90] Simultanously, understanding of local vasculatory mechanisms has expanded markedly and endothelial dysfunction has emerged as an important factor in this context. The regulatory function of nitric oxide[91] and the release of hormones such as endothelin[92] underscore the importance of the vascular endothelium in patients with heart failure.

A number of placebo-controlled clinical trials have shown that ACE inhibitors improve survival among patients with CHF,[1,3] and furthermore that these drugs appear to be superior to the combination of the direct-acting vasodilators isosorbide dinitrate and hydralazine in terms of reducing mortality.[2] At the same time, the vasodilator combination produced a more pronounced improvement in ejection fraction and peak exercise oxygen consumption than the ACE inhibitor enalapril, as shown in the V-HeFT II trial.[2] The modulation of neurohormonal activation and possibly improved baroreceptor reflex function induced by treatment with ACE inhibitors may be two important determinants of the effects of these drugs in chronic heart failure.[38,93] Moreover, treatment with ACE inhibitors may be related to an improvement in endothelial function (which increases the ability of the peripheral vessels to dilate, and treatment may indeed cause an improvement in peripheral oxygen utilization).[94]

Although treatment with beta-adrenergic blockers in patients with heart failure is still controversial, there has recently been growing interest concerning the use of these agents in the long-term therapy of patients with CHF. From a pathophysiologial viewpoint, modulation of excessive sympathetic activity by beta-adrenergic blockers might be beneficial. However, it may be difficult to determine exactly when sympathetic activity is maladaptive and when it is compensatory. Thus, treatment with beta-adrenergic blockers should be initiated carefully, beginning with low doses and then titrating the dose carefully upwards. The MDC (Metoprolol in Dilated Cardiomyopathy) trial[95] indicated positive results from metoprolol therapy among patients with heart failure caused by idiopathic dilated cardiomyopathy. The combined end point of death and the need for heart transplantation was significantly less common in patients on metoprolol than in patients on placebo. Earlier uncontrolled but smaller studies have indicated positive clinical and haemodynamic effects in a similar population of patients.[96–98] Furthermore, data from the Beta-blocker Heart Attack Trial (BHAT)[99] indicated improved survival with propranolol compared with placebo in patients with heart failure following myocardial infarction. The CIBIS (Cardiac Insufficiency Bisoprolol)[100] trial included 641 patients with chronic heart failure in NYHA class III–IV who were treated with diuretics and ACE inhibitors (90%), who had an ejection fraction < 40%. Overall, mortality was not reduced by the beta-blocker but prognosis was significantly improved in patients with idiopathic dilated cardiomyopathy. In the largest heart failure study with a beta-blocker so far, 1094 patients in the United States were randomized to carvedilol or placebo. Four trials were planned for 6–12 month follow-up. The study was terminated by the Safety Committee short of a complete recruitment because of beneficial effects on survival. Mortality was reduced from 8.2% to 2.9% (p=0.0001), a 67% reduction.[100a] An Australian/New Zealand trial of 415 patients previously reported six-month results where no effect on mortality or morbidity was observed.[100b] An update after 18 months showed a non-significant effect on mortality of 23%, with a positive significant effect on the combined end-point hospitalizations and mortality (N Sharpe, personal communication). A meta-analysis of beta-blocker trials in heart failure[101] has indicated beneficial effects that are strengthened by this additional data. Large clinical trials are in progress to confirm these promising results and to explore whether there is any difference in effect on survival between metoprolol and carvedilol.

Prevention of sudden death from arrythmias

Ventricular arrhythmias are common in patients with CHF. About 50% of the mortality is due to sudden death. The relative proportion of patients dying suddenly is higher among patients with milder forms of heart failure than among those with severe heart failure who more frequently die because of progressive disease.[15] Antiarrhythmic drug therapy for asymptomatic ventricular arrhythmias in the presence of heart failure has not been shown to positively influence survival or reduce the risk of sudden death. Instead, the CAST (Cardiac Arrhythmia Suppression Trial) studies[10,102] indicated an adverse effect on survival by treatment with the class I antiarrhythmic drugs flecainide, encainide and morizicine in patients after myocardial infarction. In patients with symptomatic ventricular arrhythmia there is a lack of well-designed trials assessing the possible value of antiarrhythmic drugs, and controversies exist about how to predict the efficacy of such therapy.[103] Currently, the class III antiarrhythmic agent amiodarone appears most promising.[104–106] Moreover, there are strong data indicating that beta-adrenergic blocking drugs may reduce the risk of sudden death among patients with heart failure following myocardial infarction.[99] The use

Name of trial	Patients planned (no).	Agent	Entry criteria	Duration of follow-up	Primary end points	Expected end date (month/ year)
ATLAS	3000	High- vs low-dose lisinopril	NYHA II–IV EF<30%	2 years	Mortality	12/96
ELITE	1000	Losartane vs captopril	NYHA II–IV EF<40%	1 year	Tolerability, efficacy, incidence of heart failure and death	1/96
DIG	7500	Digoxin vs placebo	CHF, sinus rhythm and stratified by EF $\leq$0.45/>0.45	2 years	Mortality	12/95
V-HeFT–III	800–900	Felodipine, digoxin, placebo (2×2 factorial design)	CT ratio$\geq$0.55, EF$\leq$30%	27 months	Exercise tolerance	1994
DEFIANT–II	400	Nisoldipine vs placebo	Post-MI:EF<50% No overt heart failure	6–12 months	Exercise tolerance	11/92
Proprionyl-L-carnitine	500	Carnitine vs placebo	NYHA II–III EF<40%	6 months	Exercise tolerance	9/96
RALES	50 (pilot) 3500 (main)	Spironolactone vs placebo	NYHA III–IV EF<35%	1 year (pilot) 3 years (main)	Safety (pilot) Mortality (main)	3/94
NETWORK	1500	Enalapril, comparison of different dosages	CHF requiring diuretics and an abnormal echocardiogram	6 months	Mortality, hospitalization, worsening CHF	5/95
WASH	3600	Aspirin vs warfarin vs no antithrombotic therapy	CHF and an impaired systolic function on echocardiography	3 years	Mortality	6/97

Table 19.2
Overview of ongoing, randomized, parallel, controlled trials in patients with CHF and left ventricular dysfunction with sample size of at least 300 patients.

(ATLAS – Assessment of Treatment With Lisinopril and Survival; ELITE – Evaluation of Losartane in the Elderly; DIG – Digitalis Investigators Group; V-HeFT III – third Vasodilator Heart Failure Trial; DEFIANT-II – Doppler Flow and Echocardiography and Functional Cardiac Insufficiency Assessment of Nisoldipine Therapy; RALES – Randomized Aldactone Evaluation Study; WASH – Warfarin/Aspirin Study in Heart Failure. EF – ejection fraction; CT ratio – cardio-thoracic index).

The unresolved questions – where do we go from here?

There are many questions about therapeutic interventions in patients with CHF that are still unresolved. Examples of such questions are:

- How can we improve preventative measures in order to reduce the incidence of chronic heart failure?
- How does diuretic therapy affect the natural history and mortality of patients with chronic heart failure?
- Is it possible that inotropic drugs may be helpful when used in doses that do not increase the force of myocardial contraction?
- How does digitalis affect mortality and morbidity in CHF?
- Can the addition of a vasodilator to treatment with diuretics and an ACE inhibitor further improve survival?
- Can morbidity and survival be influenced by further inhibition of sustained neurohormonal activation?
- How can the risk of sudden death be diminished?

How can we improve preventative measures in order to reduce the incidence of CHF?

In Western societies, prevention of atherosclerosis and coronary artery disease is an important goal in the primary prevention of CHF. In other parts of the world, prevention of myocardial failure of infectious origin may be more important. Among patients with established coronary artery disease, lipid lowering with simvastatin therapy appears to improve survival[112] and may affect coronary artery pathology.[113] The role of ACE inhibitors in preventing the development of heart failure has been established among patients with left ventricular dysfunction after myocardial infarction.[13] Whether further blockade of neurohormonal activation among patients with left ventricular dysfunction following myocardial infarction may additionally delay the transition to overt heart failure remains to be determined. Drugs such as angiotensin II receptor antagonists, neutral endopeptidase inhibitors, dopamine receptor agonists, and prostaglandin analogues may be particularly interesting in this respect, but controlled clinical trials are needed to resolve these questions. Studies with ACE inhibitors among patients with coronary artery disease in the absence of left ventricular dysfunction are also underway.[114,115]

How does diuretic therapy affect the natural history and mortality in CHF?

The ability of diuretic drugs to relieve fluid retention has made them a cornerstone in the treatment of chronic congestive heart failure and these drugs generally constitute first-line therapy of the disorder. It is completely unknown how long-term diuretic therapy affects the survival of patients with heart failure. Diuretics have a number of adverse effects that may indeed make them potentially hazardous. Hypokalaemia and hypomagnesaemia[116] are probably the commonest adverse effects. These electrolyte disturbances may predispose to the development of malignant ventricular arrhythmias. Although diuretic therapy has been shown to improve symptoms and quality of life among patients with congestive heart failure, many patients deteriorate clinically during long-term follow-up.[117] Diuretics are known to activate the renin–angiotensin system in patients with heart failure.[78,79] This activation may have adverse effects during long-term therapy.[26,38] However, the risk of clinical deterioration and the adverse metabolic effects of diuretic therapy can be reduced by simultaneous treatment with an ACE inhibitor.[118] The effect of diuretic therapy on survival of patients with CHF has never been tested in controlled clinical trials. Owing to the symptomatic relief provided by diuretic therapy, randomized placebo-controlled trials are almost impossible to perform. Atrial natriuretic peptide (ANP) has been administered intravenously to patients with heart failure and studies have demonstrated that exogenously administered ANP can improve cardiac function.[119] This endogenous polypeptide has both diuretic and vasodilating activity.[120,121] Increased intrarenal enzymatic degradation of ANP by neutral endopeptidase may explain the diminished diuretic and natriuretic effect of exogenously administered ANP in patients with heart failure. Attenuation of this enzyme activity by a synthetic endopeptidase inhibitor has been shown to increase significantly the renal effects of ANP, as evidenced by increased diuresis, natriuresis, and increased production of cyclic guanosine monophosphate.[122,123] Despite the diuretic effects of ANP and the endopeptidase inhibitors, these substances are not likely to replace the widespread use of traditionally used diuretic drugs for the treatment of CHF. However, more trials are needed to define the role of these recently discovered substances for the treatment of patients with heart failure.

Could inotropic drugs be helpful when used in doses that do not increase the force of myocardial contraction?

As previously pointed out, there are many theoretical reasons why agents with positive inotropic activity could be useful in patients with heart failure and reduced systolic function of the left ventricle. However, the depression of contractility in heart failure might also be considered as a compensatory mechanism intended to reduce the energy consumption of the 'starving' myocardium.[124] The results of a number of clinical trials have indicated adverse effects of long-term therapy with inotropic drugs with different mechanisms of action.[11,12,125,126] On the other hand, the PROFILE study (M Packer, personal communication) and the study with vesnarinone[50] both indicated that large doses of the drugs were associated with increased mortality, whereas this risk did not appear to be present with lower doses. Packer has indicated that dosage may be the critical determinant of the efficacy and safety of positive inotropic drugs in heart failure.[51] This hypothesis needs to be tested further in clinical trials. Low doses of drugs with inotropic activity may have actions on the heart and the circulation that are not associated with increased force of contraction. Examples of such effects are vasodilatation, modulation of neurohormonal activity, and possibly antiarrhythmic effects. However, a narrow therapeutic range could make it difficult to use these drugs in clinical practice.

How does digitalis affect mortality and morbidity in CHF?

Digitalis is a drug with a complicated mechanism of action. It has long since been used for the treatment of heart failure. There has been considerable debate concerning the clinical value of digitalis therapy for heart failure among patients in sinus rhythm. However, it is generally considered beyond dispute that digitalis is effective in the control of heart failure and ventricular rate when atrial fibrillation is present. Despite many available studies on the efficacy of digitalis in patients with CHF, including the previously mentioned withdrawal studies, we still have no clear answers on the effects of this drug on morbidity and mortality of the disorder. The results of the currently ongoing large DIG (Digitalis Investigators Group) trial are therefore eagerly awaited. The study plans to enroll 7500 patients, in a randomized placebo-controlled trial, to test the effect of digoxin on survival and major morbidity in patients with heart failure.[53]

Can the addition of a vasodilator to treatment with diuretics and an ACE inhibitor improve survival further?

Studies addressing this question are currently in progress. Results of trials such as the PRAISE, V-HeFT III and DEFIANT-II, using the 'second generation' calcium channel blockers felodipine, amlodipine and nisoldipine are eagerly awaited. On the other hand, results of the PROFILE study using flosequinan given orally and the FIRST (Flolan International Randomized Survival Trial) trial using epoprostenol (flolan) given by a continuous intravenous infusion were disappointing. The main results of the PRAISE trial have been mentioned previously.

Can morbidity and survival be influenced by further inhibition of sustained neurohormonal activation?

CHF results not only from an alteration in cardiac function, but also from a complicated interaction of haemodynamic and neurohormonal factors. A major characteristic feature of heart failure is the tendency to progression. No matter how stable the condition of an individual patient may appear initially, the underlying disease will ultimately progress. The neurohormonal hypothesis states that heart failure progresses because endogenous neurohormonal systems that are activated by the initial myocardial injury exert deleterious effects on the circulation and that these effects are independent of the haemodynamic actions of these systems.[26] ACE inhibitors are drugs that modulate neurohormonal activity, and they have been shown to have a positive influence on survival in CHF. The beneficial effects of the drugs have been shown to be most pronounced among patients with the highest plasma concentrations of hormones such as angiotensin II, noradrenaline, aldosterone, and ANP,[66] indicating that neurohormonal activation is an important determinant for the efficacy of ACE inhibitors in CHF. If this hypothesis is true, further modulation of neurohormonal activity in patients with heart failure might positively affect the progressive nature of the disorder and lead to a further reduction in mortality and morbidity. Of special interest in this respect is therapy with beta-adrenergic blockers, with or without alpha blocking activity, angiotensin II receptor antagonists, neutral endopeptidase inhibitors, and dopamine receptor agonists. It is to be hoped that the clinical efficacy of these drugs will be determined in clinical trials in the very near future.

Owing to a number of positive preliminary results and to the fact that beta-adrenergic blockers may inhibit some of the toxic effects of excessive sympathetic stimulation, the results of ongoing or planned placebo-controlled trials on the efficacy of these agents in CHF are awaited eagerly. Large studies are now underway with two beta-blockers with vasodilating activity: bucindolol and carvedilol.

Ibopamine has hitherto been the only dopaminergic drug to be investigated extensively in the treatment of CHF. Comprehensive reports are available discussing the pharmacological profile, clinical efficacy, and safety of this drug.[127] Ibopamine stimulates presynaptic dopamine receptors, thus inhibiting the release of noradrenaline from nerve terminals.[65] Furthermore, a reduction in plasma concentration of aldosterone,[128] plasma renin activity,[129] and noradrenaline has been reported.[130] In the DIMT trial (Double-blind placebo-controlled study of Ibopamine and digoxin in patients with mild to moderate heart failure: results of the Dutch Multicenter Trial)[131] the efficacy and safety of ibopamine were compared with those of digoxin and placebo in 161 patients. Ibopamine and digoxin were both found to inhibit neurohormonal activation in this population of patients with heart failure of mild to moderate severity. The authors concluded that the effects of the two drugs may be different though in both cases related to the degree of left ventricular dysfunction. The efficacy of dopamine receptor antagonists is still to be tested in controlled clinical trials.

Drugs that interfere with the activity of renin (renin inhibitors) or with the interaction of angiotensin II and its receptor (i.e. angiotensin II receptor antagonists), have been developed.[132,133] The efficacy of these drugs in CHF is unknown at the present time, but unlike ACE inhibitors, these new approaches do not lead to the accumulation of kinins and could therefore be less likely to produce some of the side-effects (e.g. cough and angioedema) associated with existing agents. The addition of the aldosterone antagonist spironolactone to conventional therapy with diuretics and an ACE inhibitor is also being evaluated.

How can the risk of sudden death be diminished?

Sudden death in patients with heart failure can result from a variety of potential mechanisms. The relative importance of these mechanisms may depend on the aetiology and the severity of the heart failure. Preventing deaths from primary arrrhythmias will extend survival of some patients but it is important to mention that sudden death may also be non-arrhythmic. At the present time it is not known whether an implantable cardiovertor–defibrillator, cardiac transplantation, or amiodarone therapy is the best option for any individual patient at the risk of sudden arrhythmic death.[134] Increased knowledge of the factors responsible for the arrhythmias is needed, and clinical trials comparing different treatment modalities are necessary.

Conclusion

Epidemiological studies have shown that CHF is a disorder that is being seen with increasing frequency. Although some promising new therapeutic concepts, such as treatment with ACE inhibitors, have been developed in recent years, CHF remains a disabling and lethal disorder. Despite the fact that the primary abnormality of the disorder is damage to the myocardium leading to myocardial dysfunction, therapy with inotropic drugs has been disappointing. On the other hand, long-term therapy with drugs with unloading effects on the heart appears more promising. In particular, drugs that are able to influence neurohormonal activity as well as improve baroreceptor and endothelial function will have to be tested in future clinical trials.

To date, most patients with clinical heart failure have been treated with diuretics and an ACE inhibitor. The efficacy of the addition of digitalis is currently being evaluated. Moreover, the addition of vasodilator therapy to treatment with an ACE inhibitor is currently under investigation. Apart from treatment with ACE inhibitors, other drugs that may modulate neurohormonal activity are being tested. The role of beta-adrenergic blockers in the therapy of CHF appears interesting in this respect and will be evaluated in future clinical trials.

The risk of sudden death remains a major problem among patients with heart failure, and this area is a field of major research. The recent increase in our knowledge of molecular biology may open the gate to new therapeutic concepts for the treatment of heart failure. The results of heart transplantations performed during the last decade appear promising, but the limited availability of donor organs is a major problem. In the future, tailoring of therapeutic strategies for the treatment of CHF may evolve. A tailored approach may be based on factors such as the degree of left ventricular dysfunction, the underlying cause of heart failure, the estimated risk of sudden death, the risk of further myocardial damage, the degree of neurohormonal activation, and possibly on genetic mechanisms.

References

1 CONSENSUS Trial Study Group. Effects of enalapril on mortality in severe congestive heart failure: results of the Cooperative North Scandinavian Enalapril Survival study (CONSENSUS). *N Engl J Med* 1987;**316**: 1429–1435.

2 Cohn JN, Johnson G, Ziesche S, et al. A comparison of enalapril with hydralazine–isosorbide dinitrate in the treatment of congestive heart failure. *N Engl J Med* 1991; **325**:303–310.

3 The SOLVD Investigators. Effect of enalapril on survival in patients with reduced left ventricular ejection fractions and congestive heart failure. *N Engl J Med* 1991;**325**:293–302.

4 Eriksson H, Svärdsudd K, Larsson B, et al. Risk factors for heart failure in the general population. The study of men born in 1913. *Eur Heart J* 1989;**10**:647–656.

5 Kannel WB, Belanger AJ. Epidemiology of heart failure. *Am Heart J* 1991;**121**:951–957.

6 Remes J, Reunanen A, Aromaa A, et al. Incidence of heart failure in eastern Finland: a population based surveillance study. *Eur Heart J* 1992;**13**:588–593.

7 Schocken DD, Arrieta ML, Leaverton PE. Prevalence and mortality rate of congestive heart failure in the United States. *J Am Coll Cardiol* 1992;**20**:301–306.

8 Ho KKL, Anderson KM, Kannel WB, Grossman W, Levy D. Survival after the onset of congestive heart failure in Framingham Heart Study Subjects. *Circulation* 1993; **88**:107–115.

9 Schwartz K, Chassagne C, Boheler KR. The molecular biology of heart failure. *J Am Coll Cardiol* 1993;**22(suppl A)**:30A–33A.

10 The Cardiac Arhythmia Suppression Trial (CAST) Investigators. Effect of encainide and flecainide on mortality in a randomized trial of arrhythmia suppression after myocardial infarction. *N Engl J Med* 1989;**321**:406–412.

11 The Xamoterol in Severe Heart Failure Study Group. Xamoterol in severe heart failure. *Lancet* 1990;**336**:1–6.

12 Packer M, Carver J, Rodeheffer R, et al. Effects of oral milrinone on mortality in severe chronic heart failure. *N Engl J Med* 1991;**325**:1468–1475.

13 Pfeffer MA, Braunwald E, Moyé L, et al. Effect of captopril on mortality and morbidity in patients with left ventricular dysfunction after myocardial infarction. *N Engl J Med* 1992;**327**:669–677.

14 Yusuf S, Pepine C, Pouleur H, et al. Effect of enalapril on myocardial infarction and unstable angina in patients with low ejection fractions. *Lancet* 1992;**340**:1173–1178.

15 Kjekshus J. Arrhythmias and mortality in congestive heart failure. *Am J Cardiol* 1990;**65**:42–48.

16 Cohn JN. Has the problem of heart failure been solved? *Am J Cardiol* 1994;**73**:40C–43C.

17 Kubo SH, Rector TS, Bank AJ, Williams RE, Heifetz SM. Endothelium-dependent vasodilation is attenuated in patients with heart failure. *Circulation* 1991;**84**:1589–1596.

18 Katz SD, Biasucci L, Sabba C, et al. Impaired endothelium-mediated vasodilation in the peripheral vasculature of patients with congestive heart failure. *J Am Coll Cardiol* 1992;**19**:918–925.

19 Treasure CB, Alexander RW. The dysfunctional endothelium in heart failure. *J Am Coll Cardiol* 1993;**22(suppl A)**:129A–134A.

20 Hirsch AT, Dzau VJ, Creager MA. Baroreceptor function in congestive heart failure: effect on neurohormonal activation and regional vascular resistance. Circulation 1987;**75(suppl IV)**:36–48.

21 Zucker I, Wang W, Chen J-S. Baroreceptor and cardiac receptor abnormalities in experimental heart failure. *Heart Failure* 1990;17–32.

22 Wrobleski H, Kastrup J, Mortensen SA, Haunsö S. Abnormal baroreceptor-mediated

vasodilation of the peripheral circulation in congestive heart failure secondary to idiopathic dilated cardiomyopathy. *Circulation* 1993; **87**:849–856.

23 Francis GS, Goldsmith SR, Levine TB, Olivari MT, Cohn JN. The neurohormonal axis in congestive heart failure. *Ann Intern Med* 1984; **101**:370–377.

24 Packer M, Lee WH, Kessler PD, Gottlieb SS, Bernstein JL, Kukin ML. Role of neurohormonal mechanisms in determining survival in patients with severe chronic heart failure. *Circulation* 1987;**75(suppl IV)**:80–92.

25 Packer M. Neurohormonal interactions and adaptions in congestive heart failure. *Circulation* 1988;**77**:721–730.

26 Packer M. The neurohormonal hypothesis: a theory to explain the mechanism of disease progression in heart failure. *J Am Coll Cardiol* 1992;**20**:248–254.

27 Sigurdsson A. Neurohormonal activation in acute myocardial infarction or chronic congestive heart failure, with special reference to treatment with ACE inhibitors. *Blood Pres* 1995;(**suppl**):1–45.

28 The SOLVD Investigators. Effect of enalapril on mortality and the development of heart failure in asymptomatic patients with reduced left ventricular ejection fractions. *N Engl J Med* 1992;**327**:685–691.

29 Eaton LW, Weiss JL, Bulkley BH, Garrison JB, Weisfeldt ML. Regional cardiac dilatation after acute myocardial infarction. *N Engl J Med* 1979;**300**:57–62.

30 Erlebacher JE, Weiss JL, Eaton LW, Kallman C, Weisfeldt ML, Bulkley BH. Late effects of acute infarct dilatation on heart size: a two dimensional echocardiographic study. *Am J Cardiol* 1982;**49**:1120–1126.

31 McKay RG, Pfeffer MA, Pasternak RC, et al. Left ventricular remodeling after myocardial infarction: a corollary to infarct expansion. *Circulation* 1986;**74**:693–702.

32 Pfeffer M, Pfeffer J. Ventricular enlargement following a myocardial infarction. *J Cardiovasc Pharmacol* 1987;**9(suppl 2)**:S18–S20.

33 Sharpe N. Ventricular remodeling following myocardial infarction. *Am J Cardiol* 1992; **70**:20C–25C.

34 Sigurdsson A, Swedberg K. Left ventricular remodelling, neurohormonal activation and early treatment with enalapril (CONSENSUS II) following myocardial infarction. *Eur Heart J* 1994;**15(suppl B)**:14–19.

35 White HD, Norris RM, Brown MA, Brandt PWT, Whitlock RML, Wild CJ. Left ventricular end-systolic volume as the major determinant of survival after recovery from myocardial infarction. *Circulation* 1987;**76**:44–51.

36 Francis GS, McDonald KM, Cohn JN. Neurohormonal activation in preclinical heart failure. Remodeling and the potential for intervention. *Circulation* 1993;**87(suppl IV)**: 90–96.

37 Sigurdsson A, Swedberg K. ACE inhibitors in patients with minimally or asymptomatic left ventricular dysfunction. *Coron Artery Dis* 1995;**6**:288–294.

38 Sigurdsson A, Swedberg K. Is neurohormonal activation a major determinant of the response to ACE inhibition in left ventricular dysfunction and heart failure. *Br Heart J* 1994; **72(suppl)**:75–80.

39 Sharpe N, Murphy J, Smith H, Hannan S. Treatment of patients with symptomless left ventricular dysfunction after myocardial infarction. *Lancet* 1988;**i**:255–259.

40 Pfeffer MA, Gervasio LA, Vaughan DA, Parisi AF, Braunwald E. Effect of captopril on progressive ventricular dilatation after anterior myocardial infarction. *N Engl J Med* 1988; **319**:80–86.

41 Sharpe N, Smith H, Murphy J, Greaves S, Hart H, Gamble G. Early prevention of left ventricular dysfunction after myocardial infarction with angiotensin-converting-enzyme inhibition. *Lancet* 1991;**337**:872–876.

42 AIRE Study Investigators. Effect of ramipril on mortality and morbidity of survivors of acute myocardial infarction with clinical evidence of heart failure. *Lancet* 1993;**342**:821–828.

43 Gruppo per Italiano per lo Studio della Sopravivenza nell'Infarto Miocardico. GISSI-3: effects of lisinopril and transdermal glyceryl trinitrate singly and together on 6-week mortality and ventricular function after acute myocardial infarction. *Lancet* 1994;**343**:1115–1122.

44 ISIS-4 (Fourth International Study of Infarct Survival) Collaborative Group. ISIS-4: a randomized factorial trial assessing early captopril, oral mononitrate, and intravenous magnesium sulphate in 58 050 patients with suspected acute myocardial infarction. *Lancet* 1995;**345**:669–685.
45 Swedberg K, Held P, Kjekshus J, et al. Effects of early administration of enalapril on mortality in patients with acute myocardial infarction. *N Engl J Med* 1992;**327**:678–684.
46 Fibrinolytic Therapy Trialists (FTT) Collaborative Group. Indications for fibrinolytic therapy in suspected acute myocardial infarction: collaborative overview of early mortality and major morbidity results from all randomised trials of more than 1000 patients. *Lancet* 1994;**343**:311–322.
47 ISIS-2 Collaborative Group. Randomised trial of intravenous streptokinase, oral aspirin, both or neither among 17 187 cases of suspected acute myocardial infarction: ISIS–2. *Lancet* 1988;**ii**:349–360.
48 Dies F, Krell MJ, Whitlow P, et al. Intermittent dobutamine in ambulatory outpatients wuth chronic cardiac failure. *Circulation* 1986; **74(suppl II)**:38.
49 Krell MJ, Kline EM, Bates ER, et al. Intermittent ambulatory dobutamine infusions in patents with severe congestive heart failure. *Am Heart J* 1986;**112**:787–791.
50 Feldman AM, Bristow MR, Parmley WW, et al. Effects of vesnarinone on morbidity and mortality in patients with heart failure. *N Engl J Med* 1993;**329**:149–155.
51 Packer M. The development of positive inotropic agents for chronic heart failure: how have we gone astray? *J Am Coll Cardiol* 1993; **22(suppl A)**:119A–126A.
52 Withering W. *An Account of the Foxglove, and Some of its Medical Uses: With Practical Remarks on Dropsy and Other Diseases*. M Swinney, Birmingham, 1785.
53 Yusuf S, Garg R, Held P, Gorlin R. Need for a large randomized trial to evaluate the effects of digitalis on morbidity and mortality in congestive heart failure. *Am J Cardiol* 1992;**69**:64G–70G.
54 Ribner HSA, Plucinski DA, Hsieh AM, et al. Acute effects of digoxin on total systemic vascular resistance in congestive heart failure due to dilated cardiomyopathy: a hemodynamic–hormonal study. *Am J Cardiol* 1985;**56**:896–904.
55 Ferguson DW, Berg WJ, Sanders JS, Roach PJ, Kempf JS, Kienzle MG. Sympathoinihibitory responses to digitalis glycosides in heart failure patients: direct evidence from sympathetic neural recordings. *Circulation* 1989;**80**:65–77.
56 Gheorghiade M, Ferguson D. Digoxin, a neurohormonal modulator in patients with heart failure. *Circulation* 1991;**84**:2181–2186.
57 Ferguson DW. Digitalis and neurohormonal abnormalities in heart failure and implications for therapy. *Am J Cardiol* 1992;**69**:24G–32G.
58 Packer M, Gheorghiade M, Young J, et al. Withdrawl of digoxin from patients with chronic heart failure treated with angiotensin-converting-enzyme-inhibitors. *N Engl J Med* 1993;**329**:1–7.
59 Uretsky BF, Young JB, Shahidi FE, et al. Randomized study assessing the effect of digoxin withdrawl in patients with mild to moderate chronic congestive heart failure: results of the PROVED Trial. *J Am Coll Cardiol* 1993;**22**:955–962.
60 Sharpe N. Myocardial infarction and heart failure. The common ground. *Circulation* 1993; **87**:1037–1039.
61 Cohn JN, Archibald DG, Ziesche S, et al. Effect of vasodilator therapy on mortality in chronic congestive heart failure. Results of a Veterans' Administration Cooperative Study (V-HeFT). *N Engl J Med* 1986;**314**:1547–1552.
62 Packer M. Second generation calcium channel blockers in the treatment of chronic heart failure: are they better than their predecessors? *J Am Coll Cardiol* 1989;**14**:1339–1342.
63 Packer M, Lee W, Medina N, Yushak M, Bernstein JL, Kessler PD. Prognostic importance of the immediate hemodynamic response to nifedipine in patients with severe left ventricular dysfunction. *J Am Coll Cardiol* 1987; **10**:1303–1311.
64 Sigurdsson A, Held P, Swedberg K. Short and long term neurohormonal activation following acute myocardial infarction. *Am Heart J* 1993; **126**:1068–1076.

65 Francis G. Neurohumoral mechanisms involved in congestive heart failure. *Am J Cardiol* 1985; **55**:15A–21A.

66 Swedberg K, Kjekshus J. Cardiovascular hormones in relation to mortality in severe heart failure. *J Am Coll Cardiol* 1989;**13**:246A.

67 Ferguson DW. Baroreflex-mediated circulatory control in human heart failure. *Heart Failure* 1990;3–11.

68 Bristow MR, Ginsburg R, Minobe W, et al. Decreased catecholamine sensitivity and β-adrenergic-receptor density in failing human hearts. *N Engl J Med* 1982;**307**:205–211.

69 Curtiss C, Cohn JN, Vrobel T, Franciosa JA. Role of the renin–angiotensin system in the systemic vasoconstriction of chronic congestive heart failure. *Circulation* 1978;**58**:763–770.

70 Thomas JA, Marks BH. Plasma norepinephrine in congestive heart failure. *Am J Cardiol* 1978; **41**:233–243.

71 Levine TB, Francis GS, Goldsmith SR, Simon AB, Cohn JN. Activity of the sympathetic nervous system and renin–angiotensin system assessed by plasma hormone levels and their relation to hemodynamic abnormalities in congestive heart failure. *Am J Cardiol* 1982; **49**:1659–1666.

72 Remes J, Tikkanen I, Fyhrquist F, Pyörälä K. Neuroendocrine activity in untreated heart failure. *Br Heart J* 1991;**65**:249–255.

73 Goldsmith SR, Fracis GS, Cowley A, Levine TB, Cohn JN. Increased plasma arginine vasopressin levels in patients with congestive heart failure. *J Am Coll Cardiol* 1983;**1**:1385–1390.

74 Anand IS, Ferrari R, Kalra GS, Wahi PL, Poole-Wilson PA, Harris PC. Edema of cardiac origin. Studies of body water and sodium, renal function, hemodynamic indexes, and plasma hormones in untreated congestive cardiac failure. *Circulation* 1989;**80**:299–305.

75 Brown JJ, Davies JL, Johnson VW, Lever F. Renin relationships in congestive heart failure, treated and untreated. *Am Heart J* 1970;**80**: 329–342.

76 Swedberg K, Eneroth P, Kjekshus J, et al. Hormones regulating cardiovascular function in patients with severe congestive heart failure and their relation to mortality. *Circulation* 1990;**82**:1730–1736.

77 Sigurdsson A, Amtorp O, Gundersen T, Nilsson B, Remes J, Swedberg K. Neurohormonal activation in patients with mild or moderately severe congestive heart failure and effects of ramipril. *Br Heart J* 1994;**72**:422–427.

78 Bayliss J, Norell M, Canepa-Anson R, Sutton G, Poole-Wilson P. Untreated heart failure: clinical and neuroendocrine effects of introducing diuretics. *Br Heart J* 1987;**57**:17–22.

79 Broqvist M, Dahlström U, Karlberg BE, Karlsson E, Marklund T. Neuroendocrine response in acute heart failure and the influence of treatment. *Eur Heart J* 1989;**10**:1075–1083.

80 Cohn JN, Levine TB, Olivari MT, et al. Plasma norepinephrine as a guide to prognosis in patients with chronic congestive heart failure. *N Engl J Med* 1984;**311**:819–823.

81 Gottlieb SS, Kukin ML, Ahern D, Packer M. Prognostic importance of atrial natriuretic peptide in patients with chronic heart failure. *J Am Coll Cardiol* 1989;**13**:1534–1539.

82 Francis GS, Cohn JN, Johnson G, et al. Plasma norepinephrine, plasma renin activity and congestive heart failure. Relations to survival and the effects of therapy in V-HeFT II. *Circulation* 1993;**87(suppl VI)**:40–48.

83 Gavras H, Kremer D, Brown JJ, et al. Angiotensin- and norepinephrine-induced myocardial lesions: experimental and clinical studies in rabbits and man. *Am Heart J* 1975;**89**:321–332.

84 Kabour A, Henegar JR, Janicki JS. Angiotensin II (A-II)-induced myocyte necrosis: role of the A-II receptor. *J Cardiovasc Pharmacol* 1994; **23**:547–553.

85 Packer M. Pathophysiology of chronic heart failure. *Lancet* 1992;**340**:88–92.

86 Dzau V. Circulating versus local renin–angiotensin system in cardiovascular homesostasis. *Circulation* 1988;**77(suppl I)**: C–13C.

87 Dzau VJ. Autocrine and paracrine mechanisms in the pathophysiology of heart failure. *Am J Cardiol* 1992;**70**:4C–11C.

88 Hirsch AT, Pinto YM, Schunkert H, Dzau VJ. Potential role of the tissue renin–angiotensin system in the pathophysiology of congestive heart failure. *Am J Cardiol* 1990;**66**:22D–32D.

89 Hirsch AT, Talsness CE, Schunkert H, Paul M, Dzau VJ. Tissue-specific activation of cardiac angiotensin converting enzyme in experimental heart failure. *Circ Res* 1991;**69**:475–482.
90 Schunkert H, Igelfinger JR, Hirsch AT, et al. Evidence for tissue-specific activation of renal angiotensinogen mRNA expression in chronic stable experimental heart failure. *J Clin Invest* 1992;**90**:1523–1529.
91 Knowles RG, Moncada S. Nitric oxide as a signal in blood vessels. *Trends Biochem Sci* 1992;**17**:399–402.
92 Underwood RD, Chan DP, Burnett JC Jr. Endothelin: an endothelium-derived vasoconstrictor peptide and its role in congestive heart failure. *Heart Failure* 1991:50–58.
93 Cody RJ, Franklin KW, Kluger J, Laragh JH. Mechanisms governing the postural response and baroreceptor abnormalities in chronic congestive heart failure: effects of acute an long term converting enzyme inhibition. *Circulation* 1982;**66**:135–142.
94 Drexler H, Hayoz D, Münzel T, Just H, Zelis R, Brunner HR. Endothelial function in congestive heart failure. *Am Heart J* 1993;**126**: 761–764.
95 Waagstein F, Bristow M, Swedberg K, et al for the Metoprolol in Dilated Cardiomyopathy (MDC) trial study group. Beneficial effects of metoprolol in idiopathic dilated cardiomyopathy. *Lancet* 1993;**342**:1441–1446.
96 Swedberg K, Hjalmarson Å, Waagstein F, Wallentin I. Adverse effects of beta-blockade withdrawal in patients with congestive cardiomyopathy. *Br Heart J* 1980;**44**:134–142.
97 Swedberg K, Hjalmarson Å, Waagstein F, Wallentin I. Beneficial effects of long-term beta-blockade in congestive cardiomyopathy. *Br Heart J* 1980;**44**:117–133.
98 Waagstein F, Caidahl K, Wallentin I, Bergh C-H, Hjalmarson Å. Long-term β-blockade in dilated cardiomyopathy. *Circulation* 1989; **80**:551–563.
99 Chadda K, Goldstein S, Byington R, Curb JD. Effect of propranolol after acute myocardial infarction in patients with congestive heart failure. *Circulation* 1986;**73**:503–510.
100 CIBIS Investigators and Committees. A randomized trial of β-blockade in heart failure. The cardiac insufficiency bisoprolol study (CIBIS). *Circulation* 1994;**90**:1765–1773.
100a Packer M, Bristow MR, Cohn JN, et al. Effect of carvedilol on the survival of patients wich chronic heart failure. *Circulation* 1995;**92**:1–142.
100b Australia – New Zealand Heart Failure Research Collaborative Group. Effects of carvedilol, a vasodilator – β-blocker, in patients with congestive heart failure due to ischemic heart disease. *Circulation* 1995;**92**:212–218.
101 Doughty RN, MacMahon S, Sharpe N. Beta-blockers in heart failure, promising or proved? *J Am Coll Cardiol* 1994;**23**:1814–1821.
102 The Cardiac Arrhythmia Suppression Trial II Investigators. Effect of the antiarrhythmic agent moricizine on survival after myocardial infarction. *N Engl J Med* 1992;**327**:227–233.
103 The ESVEM Investigators. The ESVEM trial. Electrophysiologic study versus electrocardiographic monitoring for selection of antiarrhythmic therapy of ventricular arrhythmias. *Circulation* 1989;**79**:1354–1360.
104 Hamer AWF, Arkles LB, Johns JA. Beneficial effects of low dose amiodarone in patients with congestive cardiac failure a placebo controlled trial. *J Am Coll Cardiol* 1989;**14**: 1768–1774.
105 Gottlieb S, Riggio DW, Lauria S, et al. High dose oral amiodarone loading exerts important hemodynamic actions in patients with congestive heart failure. *J Am Coll Cardiol* 1994; **23**:560–564.
106 Doval HC, Nul D R, Grancelli HO, et al. Randomized trial of low dose amiodarone in severe congestive heart failure. *Lancet* 1994; **344**:493–498.
107 Anderson JL, Karagounis LA, Roskelly M, Osborn JS, Handrahan D. Effect of prophylactic antiarrhythmic therapy on time to implantantable cardiovertor – defibrillator discharge in patients with ventricular tachyarrhythmias. *Am J Cardiol* 1994;**733**:683–687.
108 Katz A. Changing strategies in the management of heart failure. *J Am Coll Cardiol* 1989; **13**:513–523.
109 Katz AM. Heart failure in 2001: a prophecy. *Am J Cardiol* 1992; **70**:126C–131C.

110 Katz A. Cardiomyopathy of overload. A major determinant of prognosis in congestive heart failure. *N Engl J Med* 1990;**322**:100–110.

111 Garg R, Yusuf S. Current and ongoing randomized trials in heart failure and left ventricular dysfunction. *J Am Coll Cardiol 1993*;**22(suppl A)**:194A–197A.

112 The Scandinavian Simvastatin Survival Study Group. Randomised trial of cholesterol lowering in 4444 patients with coronary heart disease: the Scandinavian Simvastatin Survival Study (45). *Lancet* 1994;**344**:1383–1389.

113 MAAS Investigtors. Effect of simvasttin on coronary atheroma. The Multicentre Anti-Atheroma Study (MAAS). *Lancet* 1994; **344**:633–638.

114 Texter M, Lees RS, Pitt B, Dinsmore RE, Uprichard ACG. The Quinapril Ischemic Event Trial (QUIET). Design and methods: evaluation of chronic ACE inhibitor therapy after coronary artery intervention. *Cardiovasc Drugs Ther* 1993;**7**:273–282.

115 Lonn EM, Yusuf S, Prabhat J, et al. The emerging role of angiotensin converting enzyme inhibitors in cardiac and vascular protection. *Circulation* 1994;**90**:2056–2069.

116 Dyckner T, Webster PO. Potassium/magnesium depletion in patients with cardiovascular disease. *Am J Med* 1987;**82(suppl 3A)**:11–17.

117 Captopril–Digoxin Multicenter Research Group. Comparative effects of therapy with captopril and digoxin in patients with mild to moderate heart failure. *JAMA* 1988;**259**:539–544.

118 Packer M. Treatment of chronic heart failure. *Lancet* 1992;**340**:92–95.

119 Cody RJ, Atlas SA, Laragh JH, et al. Atrial natriuretic factor in normal subjects and heart failure patients. Plasma levels and renal, hormonal and hemodynamic responses to peptide infusion. *J Clin Invest* 1986;**78**:1362–1374.

120 Martin DR, Pevahouse JB, Trigg DJ, Vesely DL, Buerkert JE. Three peptides from the ANF prohormone NH_2 terminus are natriuretic and/or kaliuretic. *Am J Physiol* 1990; **258**:F1401–F1408.

121 Weidman P, Gnädinger M, Ziswiler H, et al. Cardiovascular, endocrine and renal effects of atrial natriuretic peptide in essential hypertension. *J Hypertens* 1986;**4(suppl 2)**:S71–S83.

122 Granger JP. Inhibitors of ANF metabolism. *Circulation* 1990;**82**:313–315.

123 Cavero PG, Margulies KB, Winaver J, Seymour M, Delaney NG, Burnett JCJ. Cardiorenal effects of neutral endopeptidase inhibition in experimental congestive heart failure. *Circulation* 1990;**82**:196–201.

124 Katz AM. Biochemical 'defect' in the hypertrophied and filing heart: deleterious or compensatory? *Circulation* 1973;**47**:1076–1079.

125 Massie B, Bourassa M, DiBianco R, et al. Long-term oral administration of amrinone for congestive heart failure: lack of efficacy in a multicenter controlled trial. *Circulation* 1985; **71**:963–971.

126 Uretsky BF, Jessup M, Konstam MA, et al. Multicenter trial of oral enoximone in patients with moderate to moderately severe congestive heart failure. *Circulation* 1990;**82**:774–780.

127 Godfraind T, Spano PF, Carruba MO, et al. Inodilators: a new strategy in the therapy of heart failure. *J Cardiovasc Pharmacol* 1990; **14(suppl 8)**:S1–S132.

128 Rolandi E, Marchetti G, Franceschinis R, et al. Inhibition of prolactin and aldosterone secrection by the dopamine derivative, ibopamine. *Eur J Clin Pharmacol* 1986;**29**:629–630.

129 Caponnetto S, Terrachini V, Canale C, et al. Long-term treatment of congestive heart failure with oral ibopamine. Effects on rhythm disorders and neurohumoral alterations. *Cardiology* 1990;**77(suppl 5)**:43–48.

130 Rafjer SI, Rossen JD, Douglas FL, Goldberg LI, Karrison T. Effects of long-term therapy with oral ibopamine on resting hemodynamics and exercise capacity in patients with heart failure: relationship to the generation of N-methyl-dopamine and to plasma norepinephrine levels. *Circulation* 1986;**73**:740–748.

131 van Veldhuisen DJ, Veld MI, Dunselman PHJM, et al. Double-blind placebo-controlled study of ibopamine and digoxin in patients with mild to moderate heart failure: results of the Dutch Ibopamine Multicenter Trial (DIMT). *J Am Coll Cardiol* 1993;**22**:1564–1573.

132 Eberhardt RT, Kevak RM, Kang PM, Frishman WH. Angiotensin II receptor block-

ade: an innovative approach to cardiovascular therapy. *J Clin Pharmacol* 1993;**33**:1023–1038.

133 Kang PM, Landau AJ, Eberhardt RT, Frishaman WH. Angiotensin II receptor antagonist, a new approach to blockade of the renin–angiotensin system. *Am Heart J* 1994; **127**:1368–1401.

134 Stevenson WG, Stevenson LW, Middlekauff HR, Saxon LA. Sudden death prevention in patients with advanced ventricular dysfunction. *Circulation* 1993;**88**:2953–2961.

Index